Textbook of Pharmacology and Toxicology

Textbook of Pharmacology and Toxicology

Edited by **Abby Calvin**

SYRAWOOD
PUBLISHING HOUSE

New York

Published by Syrawood Publishing House,
750 Third Avenue, 9th Floor,
New York, NY 10017, USA
www.syrawoodpublishinghouse.com

Textbook of Pharmacology and Toxicology
Edited by Abby Calvin

© 2016 Syrawood Publishing House

International Standard Book Number: 978-1-68286-191-2 (Hardback)

Printed in the United States of America.

Contents

Permissions

List of Contributors

Preface

The world is advancing at a fast pace like never before. Therefore, the need is to keep up with the latest developments. This book was an idea that came to fruition when the specialists in the area realized the need to coordinate together and document essential themes in the subject. That's when I was requested to be the editor. Editing this book has been an honour as it brings together diverse authors researching on different streams of the field. The book collates essential materials contributed by veterans in the area which can be utilized by students and researchers alike.

Toxicology forms an integral part of pharmacology. It plays a crucial role in drug development as well. This book integrates the applications of toxicology and pharmacology through researches collected from across the globe. Some of the areas covered in this book are drug safety, drug interactions, drug reaction and monitoring, evaluation of drugs, ecotoxicology, etc. This text will prove to be a beneficial resource material for students, scholars, pharmacologists, researchers and anyone else who wants to delve deeper into the advancements in pharmacology and toxicology.

Each chapter is a sole-standing publication that reflects each author's interpretation. Thus, the book displays a multi-facetted picture of our current understanding of applications and diverse aspects of the field. I would like to thank the contributors of this book and my family for their endless support.

Editor

Drug safety of rosiglitazone and pioglitazone in France: a study using the French PharmacoVigilance database

Stephanie Berthet[1], Pascale Olivier[1,2], Jean-Louis Montastruc[1,2] and Maryse Lapeyre-Mestre[1,2]*

Abstract

Background: Thiazolidinediones (TZDs), rosiglitazone (RGZ) and pioglitazone (PGZ) are widely used as hypoglycemic drugs in patients with type 2 diabetes mellitus. The aim of our study was to investigate the profile of adverse drug reactions (ADRs) related to TZDs and to investigate potential risk factors of these ADRs.

Methods: Type 2 diabetic patients were identified from the French Database of PharmacoVigilance (FPVD) between 2002 and 2006. We investigated ADR related to TZD, focusing on 4 ADR: edema, heart failure, myocardial infarction and hepatitis corresponding to specific WHO-ART terms.

Results: Among a total of 99,284 adult patients in the FPVD, 2295 reports concerned type 2 diabetic patients (2.3% of the whole database), with 161 (7%) exposed to TZDs. The frequency of edema and cardiac failure was significantly higher with TZDs than in other patients (18% and 7.4% versus 0.8% and 0.1% respectively, $p < 0.001$) whereas the frequency of hepatitis was similar (5.9% versus 4%, NS). A multiple logistic regression model taking into account potential confounding factors (age, gender, drug exposure and co-morbidities) found that TZD exposure remained associated with heart failure and edema, but not with hepatitis or myocardial infarction.

Conclusions: Thiazolidinediones exposure is associated with an increased risk of edema and heart failure in patients with type 2 diabetes even when recommendations for use are respected. In contrast, the risk of hepatic reactions and myocardial infarction with this class of drugs seems to be similar to other hypoglycemic agents.

Background

Thiazolidinediones (TZDs) are peroxisome proliferator-activated receptor (PPAR) agonists which regulate transcription of genes encoding proteins involved in glucose and lipid metabolism. Troglitazone, the first agent of this class, caused serious liver toxicity leading to its withdrawal in 2000, less than 3 years after its marketing [1]. The use of the 2 other TZDs, rosiglitazone (RGZ) and pioglitazone (PGZ), has sharply increased during the last few years. These 2 drugs seem to present a lower risk of hepatotoxicity than troglitazone [2].

TZDs could also induce adverse drug reactions (ADRs) related to the cardiovascular system including edema and heart failure [3,4]. Edema is more frequent when the TZD is used in combination therapy and its incidence is higher in association with insulin. [4]. Because of the risk of congestive heart failure [5], the use of RGZ and PGZ was initially contraindicated in France in patients with a cardiac insufficiency corresponding to classes I to IV of the NYHA classification. The European Medicines Agency recommended the suspension of marketing authorizations for rosiglitazone-containing anti-diabetes medicines in Europe in September 2010 [6]. This decision followed the publication of 2 studies finding an increased cardiovascular risk of rosiglitazone [7,8]. In view of the restrictions already in place on the use of rosiglitazone in Europe, no additional measures have been identified that could reduce this cardiovascular risk.

The aim of our study was to investigate the profile of adverse drug reactions (ADRs) related to TZDs as reported to the French PharmacoVigilance System in type 2 diabetic patients, with a special focus on congestive

---

* Correspondence: lapeyre@cict.fr
[1]Unité INSERM 1027, Equipe de Pharmacoépidémiologie, Université de Toulouse (Université Paul Sabatier), Toulouse, France
Full list of author information is available at the end of the article

heart failure and myocardial infarction, and to investigate factors associated with these ADRs.

Methods

We used the data from the French national system of PharmacoVigilance, which has been described before [9,10]. All suspected ADRs are evaluated using a French standardized scale of causality assessment and registered in the French PharmacoVigilance Database (FPVD) [11]. For each report, information on patient's data (age, gender, medical history) and drug exposure (suspected and concomitantly used drugs) is recorded along with a brief clinical description. ADRs are coded according to ADR Terminology of the World Health Organization (WHO-ART) [12].

RGZ was the first TZD marketed at the end of 2001 in France. Therefore we performed searches in the French PharmacoVigilance Database for ADRs reported from January 2002 to December 2006. Among all cases of ADRs reported in the database, patients exposed to drugs approved in the treatment of diabetes in France were short-listed, and we selected only patients with type 2 diabetes. The following data were collected: age, gender, medical history (coded ICD 10th), and all drugs (coded according to the ATC classification) used, whether or not they were related to the present ADR. Several co morbidities were identified from medical history and use of drugs. The ADR were described according to the WHO-ART classification and presented as SOC terms. Several WHO-ART codes were retained to specifically describe edema (SOC term cardiovascular disorders and metabolic and nutritional disorders: edema, peripheral edema, low limbs edema), heart failure (SOC term cardiovascular disorders: cardiac failure, congestive cardiac failure, pulmonary edema), myocardial infarction (SOC term cardiovascular disorders and myocardia : myocardial infarction, cardiac death), and hepatitis (SOC term Liver and biliary system disorders: abnormal hepatic functions, abnormal ASAT-ALAT values, hepatitis).

The demographic and clinical characteristics of diabetic patients exposed and non-exposed to TZDs were compared using the $\chi2$ test or Fisher's exact test for qualitative variables and using the Student's t-test for quantitative variables. In a further step, association between use of TZDs and occurrence of edema, hepatitis, cardiac failure or myocardial infarction was examined in a bivariate analysis. In order to take into account potential confounding factors (age, gender, cardiovascular co-morbidities and other drugs), a multivariate analysis was performed using a backward logistic regression model. The Hosmer and Lemeshow procedure [13] was used to check the good fitting of the models. All analyses were done with the SAS® software version 9.1.

Results

Out of 99,284 adult patients registered in the FPVD between January 2002 and December 2006, 2295 were patients with type 2 diabetes (2.3% of the database). Table 1 presents the demographic and clinical characteristics of this population: half of the patients were men; the mean age was 67 (± 13) years, they presented a high frequency of comorbidities, with 27.0% suffering from other metabolic disorders than diabetes, 25.9% with previous heart attack, and 10.8% with cardiac insufficiency. Half of the population was exposed to sulfamides, 40% to metformin and 5% was also treated with insulin. One hundred and sixty-one patients (7%) were exposed to TZDs: 46.6% used pioglitazone, 44.7% used rosiglitazone, and 11.2% used roziglitazone + metformin (4 patients were exposed successively to rosiglitazone alone then to roziglitazone + metformin). These patients were younger, less frequently exposed to sulfamides and glinides, to statins and to NSAIDs than other diabetic patients. They presented less frequently cardiac insufficiency, but they were more frequently obese.

The number of reports containing ADRs related to TZDs increased from 2002 to the end of 2006, with 4 reports in 2002, 25 in 2003, 29 in 2004, 45 in 2005 and 58 in 2006 (Figure 1). Table 2 presents the most reported ADR which concerned "Body as a whole - general disorders", followed by "Metabolic and nutritional disorders", "Cardiovascular disorders" and "Skin and appendages disorders". Among the 5 ADRs related to sense disorders, 4 were macular edema, and there was no report of fractures. The degree of seriousness of reactions was similar whatever the groups, with 2.53% of ADR leading to death, 6.93% life-threatening, 0.61% leading to sequellae or disability, except for ADRs leading to hospitalization which were less frequent in TZD exposed patients (40.37% versus 53.51%, p < 0.0001) and non-serious ADRs which were more frequent in TZD exposed patients (53.42% versus 36.13%, p < 0.0001).

When considering specific ADR, heart failure was significantly more frequent in TZD patients (5 exposed to RGZ and 7 exposed to PGZ, 7.45% versus 0.14% in non-exposed patients; p < 0.001), as well as edema (9 exposed to RGZ and 20 to PGZ, 18.01% versus 0.84% in non-exposed patients; p < 0.0001). We did not find any difference for hepatitis (4 patients exposed to RGZ and 4 to PGZ 4.97% versus 5.39% in non-exposed patients) and for myocardial infarction (only 1 case exposed to PGZ 0.62% versus 1.18% in non-exposed patients).

Table 3 presents the results of the multivariate analysis concerning the association between TZD exposure and 4 ADRs: heart failure, myocardial infarction, edema and hepatitis. Only edema and heart failure were significantly and independently associated with TZD respectively with

Table 1 Demographic and clinical characteristics of patients identified in the French PharmacoVigilance Database with type 2 diabetes

	Total population N = 2295 (%)	TZD exposed N = 161 (%)	TZD not exposed N = 2134 (%)
Age (years)	67.2 (13.4) [19-97]	63.3 (14.2) **** [32-87]	67.5 (13.8) [19-97]
Gender (men)	1155 (49.7)	92 (57.1)	1063 (49.8)
Cardiovascular comorbidities			
Cardiac arrhythmia	128 (5.58)	8 (5)	120 (5.6)
Cardiac insufficiency	248 (10.81)	9 (5.6)*	239 (11.2)
Hypertension	596 (25.97)	33 (20.5)	563 (26.4)
Metabolic disorders	621 (27.06)	30 (18.7)*	591 (27.7)
Angina pectoris	154 (6.71)	6 (3.7)	148 (6.9)
Atherosclerosis	6 (0.26)	0 (0)	6 (0.28)
Obesity	76 (3.31)	10 (6.2)*	66 (3.1)
Heart valve disorders	7 (0.31)	1 (0.6)	6 (0.28)
Renal disorders	62 (2.7)	2 (1.2)	60 (2.8)
Drugs used for type 2 diabetes			
Sulfamides	1227 (53.46)	44 (27.33) ****	1183 (55.43)
Alpha glucosidase inhibitor	207 (9.02)	4 (2.48)**	203 (9.5)
Glinides	192 (8.37)	6 (3.7)*	186 (8.7)
Metformin	900 (39.22)	58 (36)	842 (39.5)
Benfluorex	227 (9.89)	4 (2.5)**	223 (10.45)
Insulin	115 (5.01)	4 (2.94)	111 (5.20)
Cardiovascular drugs			
Diuretics	627 (27.32)	34 (21.1)	593 (27.7)
ACE inhibitors	456 (19.87)	20 (12.4)*	436 (20.4)
Angiotensin II inhibitors	339 (14.77)	23 (14.3)	316 (14.8)
Digitalics	105 (4.58)	3 (1.9)	102 (4.8)
Betablockers	300 (13.07)	9 (5.6)**	291 (13.6)
Calcium inhibitors	321 (13.99)	16 (9.94)	305 (14.3)
Trinitrin	48 (2.09)	3 (1.9)	45 (2.1)
Amiodarone	103 (4.49)	2 (1.24)*	101 (4.73)
Central antihypertensive drugs	73 (3.18)	5 (3.1)	68 (3.2)
Antiarrythmia drugs	25 (1.09)	1 (0.6)	24 (1.12)
Other drugs			
Steroidal and Non Steroidal Anti-Inflammatory Drugs	232 (10.1)	8 (4.96)*	224 (10.5)
Statins	403 (17.56)	17 (10.6)*	386 (16.8)
Fibrates	142 (6.19)	7 (4.35)	135 (6.3)

* p < 0.05.

** p < 0.01.

*** p <0.001.

**** p < 0.0001.

Quantitative variables are presented as mean (SD), [min-max] and qualitative variables as number (%).

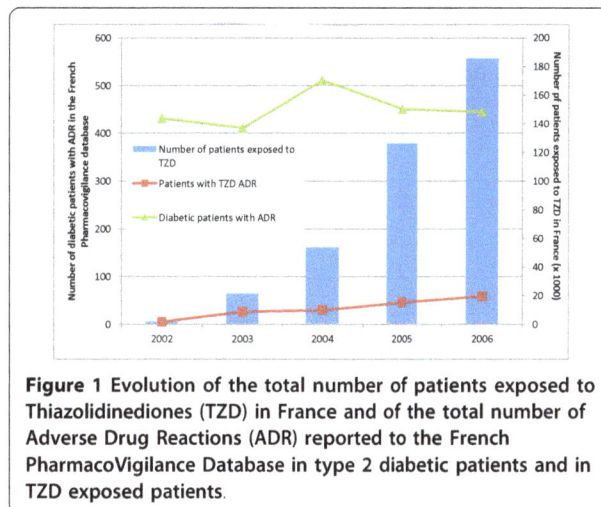

Figure 1 Evolution of the total number of patients exposed to Thiazolidinediones (TZD) in France and of the total number of Adverse Drug Reactions (ADR) reported to the French PharmacoVigilance Database in type 2 diabetic patients and in TZD exposed patients.

an OR of 25.09 and 65.39. Age and obesity were also associated with heart failure, and obesity with edema. Patients treated with biguanides were less exposed to risk of edema. We did not find any association between TZD and myocardial infarction (only heart

Table 2 Number and percentage of adverse drug reactions reported in the 161 patients exposed to thiazolidinediones in the French PharmacoVigilance database from 2002 to 2006

System Organ Classification terms	Number of patients (%)
Body as a whole - general disorders 1810	69 (42.8)
Metabolic and nutritional disorders 0800	64 (39.7)
Cardiovascular disorders, general 1010; Myo-, endo-, pericardial & valve disorders 1020; Heart rate and rhythm disorders 1030	42 (26.1)
Skin and appendages disorders 0100	35 (21.7)
Central & peripheral nervous system disorders 0410	33 (20.5)
Red blood cell disorders 1210; White cell and reticulo-endotelial system disorders 1220; Platelet, bleeding & clotting disorders 1230	26 (16.1)
Gastro-intestinal system disorders 0600	21 (13.0)
Liver and biliary system disorders 0700	15 (9.3)
Psychiatric disorders 0500	13 (8.1)
Respiratory system disorders 1100	11 (6.8)
Urinary system disorders 1300	7 (4.3)
Vascular (extra-cardiac) disorders 1040	6 (3.7)
Vision disorders 0431; Hearing and vestibular disorders 0432; Special senses other, disorders 0433	5 (3.1)
Endocrine disorders 0900	4 (2.5)
Immune system	3 (1.9)
Muscular-skeletal system disorders 0200	2 (1.2)
Fetal disorders 1500	2 (1.2)
Total number of adverse drug reactions	358

Table 3 Results of the multiple logistic regression models concerning the association between TZD exposure and 4 ADRs: Heart Failure, Myocardial Infarction, Edema and Hepatitis

Heart failure	Odds ratio	(95% CI)	P
Age	1.04	(0.99 - 1.09)	0.0705
Obesity	**5.69**	**(1.34 - 24.20)**	**0.0185**
Thiazolidinediones	**65.39**	**(17.678 - 241.93)**	**<0.0001**
Hosmer and Lemeshow procedure			*0.32*
Myocardial infarction			
Age	0.97	(0.95 - 1.00)	0.1076
Gender	1.73	(0.78 - 3.84)	0.1727
Thiazolidinediones	0.42	(0.05 - 3.17)	0.4039
Heart valve disorders	**25.95**	**(2.63 - 255.47)**	**0.0053**
Hypertension	0.34	(0.09 - 1.19)	0.0929
Hosmer and Lemeshow procedure			*0.8254*
Edema			
Obesity	1.89	(0.58 - 6.17)	0.2863
Thiazolidinediones	**25.09**	**(13.50 - 46.63)**	**<0.0001**
Biguanides	0.42	(0.20 - 0.87)	0.02
Hosmer and Lemeshow procedure			*0.8043*
Hepatitis			
Age	0.99	(0.97 - 1.00)	0.1167
Angina pectoris	0.43	(0.13 - 1.39)	0.1620
Cardiac arrhythmia	0.36	(0.08 - 1.52)	0.1686
Cardiac insufficiency	0.58	(0.25 - 1.37)	0.2217
Thiazolidinediones	0.84	(0.40 - 1.78)	0.6645
Non Steroidal Anti-Inflammatory Drugs	**1.85**	**(1.13 - 3.01)**	**0.0134**
Diuretics	0.58	(0.32 - 1.06)	0.0796
Calcium inhibitors	0.63	(0.32 -1.23)	0.1798
Angiotensin II inhibitors	0.68	(0.35 - 1.32)	0.2804
Hosmer and Lemeshow procedure			*0.4397*

Potential confounding factors retained in the final model are indicated in the first column.

valve disorders were significantly associated) or hepatitis (as expected, there was a significant association between hepatitis and NSAID).

Discussion

Among this population of diabetic patients registered in the French Pharmacovigilance database due to the occurrence of an adverse drug reaction, seven percent was exposed to TZDs. In these patients, the reactions were less frequently serious than in patients exposed to other antidiabetic agents. TZD exposure is associated with edema and heart failure in patients with type 2 diabetes, but the risk of hepatic reactions or myocardial infarction with this class of drugs is the same with other hypoglycemic agents.

TZDs can potentially lead to the development of congestive heart failure [1]. In clinical trials, the incidence of edema ranged from 2 to 5% in TZD monotherapy, 6 to 8% with metformin or sulfonylurea and 15% in combination with insulin. In our study, edema represented 18% of ADR related to TZD, and concerned mainly patients exposed to PGZ. Fluid retention can occur even at the lowest TZD dose, and diuretics and ACE inhibitors have variable effects on edema caused by TZDs [1,3].

We found only one case of myocardial infarction in a patient exposed to PGZ, and this event should not be related to this drug. It concerned a 46-year-old man, treated by lamivudine-zidovudine-nevirapine for a HIV infection, and presenting high serum levels of triglycerides 4,57 mmol/l (N< 1,74 mmol/l), cholesterol 8,80 mmol/l (N< 6,56 mmol/l), with a normal value for HDL-cholesterol. He was also treated by glicazide and benfluorex. After one year of treatment with TGZ, he presented a myocardial infarction successfully treated by angioplasty and a drug-eluting stent. The treatment with PGZ was maintained with a favorable evolution. We did not found any other cases with RGZ or PGZ, whereas 26 myocardial infarctions potentially related to drugs were reported in the population of diabetic patients in this study. Two meta-analyses have suggested that RGZ increases the risk of myocardial infarction but did not reach statistical significance for cardiovascular death [14,15], but the reviews published in 2010 led to the rosiglitazone withdrawal from the European market in September 2010. The final results of the RECORD trial, which compared cardiovascular outcomes in patients with type 2 diabetes treated with RGZ and metformin or sulfonylurea, confirm the increasing risk of heart failure with RGZ, but do not identify any statistically significant differences in the overall risk of cardiovascular morbidity or mortality [16]. Lincoff's meta-analysis on the effect of PGZ on ischemic cardiovascular events found that PGZ is associated with a significantly lower risk of death, myocardial infarction, or stroke [17]. In their review of the literature in order to estimate the association between hypoglycemic agents and morbidity and mortality in patients with heart failure and diabetes, Eurich et al [18] concluded that metformin is the only hypoglycemic agent not associated with harm in patients with heart failure. A nested case-control study in older patients found that both PGZ and RGZ were associated with an increased risk of congestive heart failure, acute myocardial infarction, and mortality when compared to other combinations of oral hypoglycemic agents [19].

Cases of hepatotoxicity with second generation TZDs have been few in number and less severe when compared to troglitazone [2,20]. Troglitazone, unlike PGZ and RGZ, induces the cytochrome P450 isoform 3A4, which is partly responsible for its metabolism, and may be prone to drug interactions. Floyd et al examined reports of liver failure reported to the FDA during

10 years and estimated that the rate of acute liver failure observed with RGZ or PGZ was about 17 times higher than the background rate for idiopathic acute liver failure in the general population [21]. By contrast, in our study, we did not find any association between hepatitis and TZD in comparison with other drugs used for diabetes. Even if no reliable estimates of the background rate of liver failure in diabetic patients are available in the literature, some have postulated that liver disease may be more frequent in this population with obesity and insulin resistance, due to non-alcoholic steato-hepatitis [2]. Moreover, this population may be exposed to other drugs, some of which are suspected to increase the risk of hepatic injuries [22], as observed in our data with NSAID.

Some limitations of our study should be discussed. First, limitations are due to the spontaneous reporting system itself, although the reporting rate in France is one of the highest among the European countries [23,24]. Given the small number of patients treated by TZDs in France, the number of ADR reports with TZD is relatively low, in comparison with the results obtained through the Health Canada's spontaneous adverse event reporting system (195 ADR with pioglitazone and 830 with rosiglitazone up to September 2006) [25]. Underreporting can affect validity of results since it can be related either to the drug or to the degree of seriousness of reactions. We did not find any case of myocardial infarction or fracture related to TZD in the database. This is not surprising, since in any spontaneous reporting system, clinicians are unlikely to report this kind of event related to TZD, and instead attribute them to the baseline risk of type 2 diabetes. The absence of fractures reported to the French pharmacovigilance system does not mean that this risk is not real. As demonstrated in the meta-analysis of 10 randomized controlled trials and 2 observational studies, long-term use of TZD doubles the risk of fractures among women with type 2 diabetes, without a significant increase in the risk of fractures in diabetic men [26]. In our study, reported ADRs in the exposed population has increased year by year since the marketing authorization of TZDs in France. This increase can be explained by the increased use of TZDs but also biased by reports related to the notoriety of TZD ADRs. This last point is limited as reports with TZD seem to be less frequently serious than for other diabetic patients.

Populations of patients with specific disease identified through the FPVD are very similar to that obtained through population-based studies in France [27,28]. This population of type 2 diabetic patients with ADR related to their medications presents characteristics comparable to those observed in other studies about French type 2 diabetes [29-31]: for example, we found that 11% of the

patients suffered from cardiac insufficiency, which is very similar to the 12% observed in the ENTRED national survey [30]. Moreover, the patterns of exposure to drugs in this population are in agreement with the guidelines for TZD use at the time of the study (in particular, TZDs are contraindicated with insulin and for patients with NYHA class I to IV). In our study, patients exposed to TZDs were less likely to present risk factors of heart failure and cardiovascular comorbidities, 5.6% had a cardiac insufficiency, and less than 3% were treated concomitantly with insulin.

Conclusions

In the French Pharmacovigilance database, adverse drug reactions reported in diabetic patients exposed to thiazolidinediones (rosiglitazone and pioglitazone) present a degree of seriousness similar to that observed with other anti diabetic drugs. Thiazolidinediones exposure is associated with an increased risk of edema and heart failure in patients with type 2 diabetes even when recommendations for use are respected, and this risk concerns much rosiglitazone as pioglitazone. In contrast, the risk of hepatic reactions and myocardial infarction, which has been discussed with this class of drugs, is not higher than with other hypoglycemic agents.

Acknowledgements
The authors acknowledge the assistance of all 31 regional centres of the French Pharmacovigilance System through the "Association Française des Centres Régionaux de Pharmacovigilance" (AFCRPV).
The authors acknowledge Ms. Pascale Morandi for editing the manuscript.

Author details
[1]Unité INSERM 1027, Equipe de Pharmacoépidémiologie, Université de Toulouse (Université Paul Sabatier), Toulouse, France. [2]Centre Régional de Pharmacovigilance, de Pharmacoépidémiologie et d'Information sur le Médicament, Service de Pharmacologie Clinique, Hôpitaux de Toulouse, Toulouse, France.

Authors' contributions
PO and MLM planed the study, SB managed the data, performed the statistical analysis and wrote the main results, JLM and MLM wrote the final manuscript. JLM is the head of the regional pharmacovigilance center and gave his support to access the French pharmacovigilance database. All authors read and approved the final manuscript.

Competing interests
None of the authors have any relevant conflict of interest.
SB received a grant from the "Fondation de France" to perform this study during her Master Research training in Clinical Epidemiology (University of Toulouse).

References
1. CV Rizos, MS Elisaf, DP Mikhailidis, EN Liberopoulos, How safe is the use of thiazolidinediones in clinical practice. Expert Opin Drug Saf. 8, 15–32 (2009).

2. AJ Scheen, Hepatotoxicity with thiazolidinediones: is it a class effect? Drug Saf. 24, 873–88 (2001).

3.   NV Niemeyer, LM Janney, Thiazolidinedione-induced edema. Pharmacotherapy. **22**, 924–9 (2002).

4.   TE Delea, JS Edelsberg, M Hagiwara, G Oster, LS Phillips, Use of thiazolidinediones and risk of heart failure in people with type 2 diabetes: a retrospective cohort study. Diabetes Care. **26**, 2983–9 (2003).

5.   P Raskin, M Rendell, MC Riddle, JF Dole, MI Freed, J Rosenstock, A randomized trial of rosiglitazone therapy in patients with inadequaly controlled insulin-treated type2 diabetes. Diabetes Care. **24**, :1226–32 (2001).

6.   European Medicines Agency, European Medicines Agency recommends suspension of Avandia, Avandamet and Avaglim. Anti-diabetes medication to be taken off the market. http://www.ema.europa.eu/docs/en_GB/document_library/Press_release/2010/09/WC500096996.pdf (2010). EMA/585784/2010 (accessed on May 17, 2011)

7.   DJ Graham, R Ouellet-Hellstrom, TE MaCurdy, F Ali, C Sholley, C Worrall, JA Kelman, Risk of acute myocardial infarction, stroke, heart failure, and death in elderly Medicare patients treated with rosiglitazone or pioglitazone. JAMA. **304**, 411–8 (2010).

8.   SE Nissen, K Wolski, Rosiglitazone revisited. An updated meta analysis of risk for myocardial infarction and cardiovascular mortality. Arch Intern Med. **170**, 1191–1201 (2010).

9.   F Thiessard, E Roux, G Miremont-Salame, A Fourrier-Reglat, F Haramburu, P Tubert-Bitter, B Begaud, Trends in spontaneous adverse drug reaction reports to the French PharmacoVigilance system (1986-2001). Drug Saf. **28**, 731–740 (2005).

10. IR Edwards, JK Aronson, Adverse drug reactions: definitions, diagnosis, and management. Lancet. **356**, 1255–1259 (2000).

11. B Begaud, JC Evreux, J Jouglard, G Lagier, Imputation of the unexpected or toxic effects of drugs. Actualization of the method used in France. Therapie. **40**, 111–118 (1985)

12. WHO collaborating Center for International Drug monitoring, WHO International monitoring of adverse reactions to drugs: adverse reaction terminology Uppsala. (2011)

13. S Lemeshow, DW Hosmer, A review of goodness of fit statistics for use in the development of logistic regression models. Am J Epidemiol. **115**, 92–106 (1982)

14. SE Nissen, K Wolski, Effect of rosiglitazone on the risk of myocardial infarction and death from cardiovascular causes. N Engl J Med. **356**, 2457–71 (2007).

15. S Singh, YK Loke, CD Furberg, Long-term risk of cardiovascular events with rosiglitazone: a meta-analysis. JAMA. **298**, 1189–95 (2007).

16. PD Home, SJ Pocock, H Beck-Nielsen, PS Curtis, R Gomis, M Hanefeld, NP Jones, M Komadja, JJV McMurray, for the RECORD Study Group, Rosiglitazone evaluated for cardiovascular outcomes in oral combination therapy for type 2 diabetes (RECORD): a multicentre, randomized, open-label trial. Lancet. **373**, 2125–35 (2009).

17. AM Lincoff, K Wolski, SJ Nicholls, SE Nissen, Pioglitazone and risk of cardiovascular events in patients with type 2 diabetes mellitus: a meta-analysis of randomized trials. JAMA. **298**, 1180–8 (2007).

18. DT Eurich, FA McAlister, DF Blackburn, SR Majumdar, RT Tsuyuki, J Varney, JA Johnson, Benefits and harms of antidiabetic agents in patients with diabetes and heart failure: systematic review. BMJ. **335**, 497 (2007).

19. LL Lipscombe, T Gomes, LE Lévesque, JE Hux, DN Juurlink, DA Alter, Thiazolidinediones and cardiovascular outcomes in older patients with diabetes. JAMA. **298**, 2634–43 (2007).

20. R Rajagopalan, S Iyer, A Perez, Comparison of pioglitazone with other antidiabetic drugs for associated incidence of liver failure: no evidence of increased risk of liver failure with pioglitazone. Diabetes Obes Metab. **7**, 161–9 (2005).

21. JS Floyd, E Barbehenn, P Lurie, SM Wolfe, Case series of liver failure associated with rosiglitazone and pioglitazone. Pharmacoepidemiol Drug Saf. **18**, 1238–43 (2009).

22. M Lapeyre-Mestre, AM de Castro, MP Bareille, JG Del Pozo, AA Requejo, LM Arias, JL Montastruc, A Carvajal, Non-steroidal anti-inflammatory drug-related hepatic damage in France and Spain: analysis from national

spontaneous reporting systems. Fundam Clin Pharmacol. **20**, 391–5 (2006).

23. B Bégaud, K Martin, F Haramburu, N Moore, Rates of spontaneous reporting of adverse drug reactions in France. JAMA. **288**, 1588 (2002).

24. KJ Belton, Attitude survey of adverse drug-reaction reporting by health care professionals across the European Union. Eur J Clin Pharmacol. **52**, 423–427 (1997).

25. S Singh, YK Loke, CD Furberg, Thiazolidinediones and heart failure. A teleo-analysis. Diabetes Care. **30**, 2148–2153 (2007).

26. YK Loke, S Singh, CD Furberg, Long-term use of thiazolidinediones and fractures in type 2 diabetes: a meta-analysis. CMAJ. **180**, 32–9 (2009)

27. M Gony, M Lapeyre-Mestre, JL Montastruc, Risk of serious extrapyramidal symptoms in patients with Parkinson's disease receiving antidepressant drugs : a pharmacoepidemiologic study comparing serotonin reuptake inhibitors and other antidepressant drugs. Clin Neuropharmacol. **26**, 142–5 (2003).

28. S Berthet, S Grolleau, C Brefel-Courbon, JL Montastruc, M Lapeyre-Mestre, Prevalence of Diabetes in France and Drug Use: Study Based on the French PharmacoVigilance Database. Therapie. **62**, 483–488 (2007).

29. C Marant, I Romon, S Fosse, A Weill, D Simon, E Eschwège, M Varroud-Vial, A Fagot-Campagna, French medical practice in type 2 diabetes: the need for better control of cardiovascular risk factors. Diabetes Metab. **34**, 38–45 (2008)

30. Institut de Veille Sanitaire, Le diabète. Echantillon national témoin représentatif des personnes diabétiques (Entred) 2007-2010.

31. http://www.invs.sante.fr/surveillance/diabete/entred_2007_2010/index.html. (accessed on May 17, 2011)

32. Agence Nationale d'Accréditation et d'Evaluation en Santé, Principes de dépistage du diabète de type 2. Paris : ANAES. (2003)

2

Validation of a transparent decision model to rate drug interactions

Elmira Far[1†], Ivanka Curkovic[1†], Kelly Byrne[1], Malgorzata Roos[2], Isabelle Egloff[1], Michael Dietrich[3], Wilhelm Kirch[4], Gerd-A Kullak-Ublick[1] and Marco Egbring[1*]

Abstract

Background: Multiple databases provide ratings of drug-drug interactions. The ratings are often based on different criteria and lack background information on the decision making process. User acceptance of rating systems could be improved by providing a transparent decision path for each category.

Methods: We rated 200 randomly selected potential drug-drug interactions by a transparent decision model developed by our team. The cases were generated from ward round observations and physicians' queries from an outpatient setting. We compared our ratings to those assigned by a senior clinical pharmacologist and by a standard interaction database, and thus validated the model.

Results: The decision model rated consistently with the standard database and the pharmacologist in 94 and 156 cases, respectively. In two cases the model decision required correction. Following removal of systematic model construction differences, the DM was fully consistent with other rating systems.

Conclusion: The decision model reproducibly rates interactions and elucidates systematic differences. We propose to supply validated decision paths alongside the interaction rating to improve comprehensibility and to enable physicians to interpret the ratings in a clinical context.

Keywords: Algorithm, Severity, Validation, Drug, Interaction, Decision, Model, Mmx, Epha.ch

Background

The management of adverse drug events (ADEs) is an important issue in healthcare [1]. While some ADEs are unpredictable (e.g. anaphylaxis), ADEs caused by drug-drug interactions (DDI) are likely to be preventable [2]. Nevertheless, DDIs continue to present a major problem in medical treatment. One Swiss study estimated that 17% of all ADEs occurring in hospitalized patients are provoked by DDIs [3], while a Dutch study found that 28% of patients admitted to the hospital experienced at least one DDI [4]. Clinical decision support software (CDSS) has been used as a supportive measure to improve medication safety [5,6]. The information provided by CDSS focuses on management advice rather than alerts, since more prevalent alerts may dominate less common but equally dangerous ones [4].

In the past, DDIs were classified according to their potential severity e.g. minor, moderate, or major. In 2001 a new management-oriented approach to DDI classification was advanced by Hansten and Horn [7]. More than 75% of majorly severe interactions are considered manageable [8]; therefore this approach seems reasonable. Recently, a separate group in our department developed ZHIAS (Zurich Interaction System), an extension of the clinical management approach, which is based on Operational Classification of Drug Interactions (ORCA) [9,10]. Another management-oriented classification system is based on types of adverse drug reactions [8]. Even with multiple classifications being available, the assessment of DDIs depends on both the experience and the interpretation of the assessor as well as the sources of information used in the assessment [11]. The discrepancies between different DDI ratings are well-documented [7,12-14]. No two DDI databases use the same set of criteria to assign severity ratings [15]. For example, the assigned interaction severity between alprazolam and

* Correspondence: marco.egbring@usz.ch
†Equal contributors
[1]Department of Clinical Pharmacology and Toxicology, University Hospital Zurich, Rämistrasse 100, 8091 Zurich, Switzerland
Full list of author information is available at the end of the article

digoxin ranges from "no interaction" to "major interaction", depending on database [16-19]. It remains unclear whether these rating discrepancies arise from inconsistent study results or from the use of different DDI classification algorithms. One case report and one study showed that plasma digoxin concentrations significantly increase in the presence of alprazolam [20]. A separate study involving healthy volunteers reported no clinically relevant change in digoxin plasma concentrations [21]. In the past 30 years, more than 15,000 papers on DDIs have been published [7]. The problem we face today is not the lack of information on DDIs or the type of classification, but the incompatibility of DDI rating systems. Alerts are often disregarded by physicians, if background information on the decision layer and practical management recommendations are lacking [22,23]. In order to increase user acceptance, the DDI rating must be consistent and comprehensible, and the decision model must be transparent [24].

To improve rating comprehensibility, we developed a transparent decision model (DM) to rate drug interactions. The model is based on previous research by van Roon and colleagues [25]. The aim of our current research is to validate the transparent decision model in terms of reproducibility and identification of systematic differences between DDI ratings.

Methods
Design of decision model
In designing the DM, we developed a list of binary questions which we considered would impact on the interaction rating. Similar questions were constructed iteratively, and six sets of clinically relevant questions were ultimately retained. The questions were evaluated regarding their relevance to a robust and comprehensible DDI rating system. The sequential order of the six binary questions (see Figure 1) was permuted by a review team consisting of one pharmacist, two clinical pharmacologists and one physician, until consensus regarding the rating outcome of the DM was achieved.

The six question sets are outlined as follows:

1. Apparent interaction (AIA) comprised two sub-questions:
   Only one "yes" answer is required to progress down the decision path to the next question.

   a) *Has this interaction been described in the scientific literature (e.g. credible clinical studies and credible case reports)?*

   b) *Can one postulate a plausible, hypothetical mechanism of pathogenic interaction?*

2. Serious adverse event (SAE) inquires into the clinical severity of the interaction: *Is there an increased risk for the occurrence of an SAE within the normal patient population?*
3. Action (ACT) determines whether medical intervention is necessary: *Does the interaction outcome necessitate medical intervention, other than simple precautionary measures?*
4. Surveillance (SUR) ascertains whether the consequences of the interaction can be easily monitored: *Is the interaction risk difficult to assess in an out-patient setting and within a short time-frame?*
5. Alternative (ATE) questions whether a safer alternative to either one of the drugs exists. It comprises two sub-questions.
   Both questions must be answered "yes" in order to proceed to the final step of the decision model.

   a) *Does a suitable alternative exist (within the same ATC category), which carries a lower potential for interaction?*
   b) *Are credible dose adjustment guidelines unavailable?*

6. Risk-benefit ratio (RBR): *Does the risk outweigh the potential benefit?*

The DM presents 13 possible decision paths leading to 5 possible interaction ratings: DM: A (no action required), DM: B (precautionary measures), DM: C (clinical monitoring), DM: D (avoid) and DM: E (contraindicated). For statistical analysis numbers 1 up to 5 were assigned to the ratings. The ratings are defined to avoid ambiguity and are based on clinical management. A rating of DM: A indicates that co-administration is safe, based on currently available scientific data. When an interaction is rated DM: B, precautionary monitoring for unusual side effects is sufficient. DM: C signifies that, although no alternative therapies are available, the likely effect of the interaction is easily monitored. Necessary medical action will be guided by the relevant published medical guidelines. DM: D indicates that co-administration should be avoided and only undertaken when deemed imperative. DM: E states clearly that the drugs must not be co-administered in any clinical situation. The interaction ratings were standardized to ensure consistency in rating outcomes by different physicians/pharmacists. The DDI rating was designed for integration into a network of additional decision support systems, such as patient-specific risk factors (e.g. old age, obesity, or renal insufficiency) or drug-disease state contraindications, whereas the DM refers to the low-risk normal population. A serious adverse event is defined as a life-threatening or debilitating

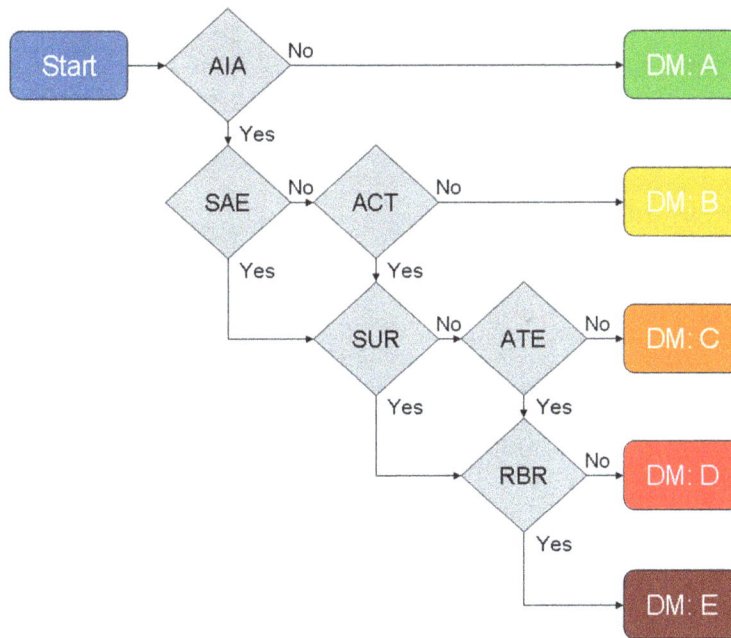

Figure 1 Visualisation of proposed action-oriented decision model to rate drug-drug interactions. The six question sets relate to: AIA (apparent interaction), SAE (serious adverse event), ACT (action), SUR (surveillance), ATE (alternative), RBR (risk-benefit ratio). Five possible ratings are DM: **A** (no action required), DM: **B** (precautionary measures), DM: **C** (clinical monitoring), DM: **D** (avoid) and DM: **E** (contraindicated).

event, resulting in death, inpatient hospitalization or prolongation of existing hospitalization, or persistent or significant disability/incapacity. Risk/benefit defines the balance between the effectiveness of a medicine and the risk of harm as specified by the World Health Organization Uppsala Monitoring Centre (WHO-UMC) in Sweden.

Other ratings

One of our assessors, a clinical pharmacologist, classified DDIs into five categories, namely: "no interaction", "minor", "moderate", "major" and "contraindicated", based on her personal clinical experience and interpretation of the available literature relating to drug interactions. The Micromedex DrugDex (MMX) database classifies DDIs as "unknown", "minor", "moderate", "major" or "contraindicated". MMX also estimates the quality of DDI documentation, rating it as either "excellent", "good", "fair" or "unknown".

Validation of decision model

In our study we randomly selected 200 potential drug interactions and compared the individual rating outcomes generated by three different rating methods. Clinical relevance of the drug interactions was assessed from queries received at the Department of Clinical Pharmacology and Toxicology at the University Hospital in Zurich, raised by pharmacists and physicians in primary and secondary care and from ward rounds at the University

Hospital. In the first rating method, one pharmacist applied our DM to manually rate the 200 interactions. The ratings were then reviewed and revised for plausibility by a team comprising two clinical pharmacologists and one physician. The second rating was performed by an independent senior clinical pharmacologist who was blinded with respect to the DM and who assigned each interaction rating based on her clinical experience and knowledge. The clinical pharmacologist was not permitted use of an interaction database, but was allowed access to available scientific sources such as PubMed database, Excerpta Medica database (Embase), European Public Assessment Reports (EPARs) and summary of product characteristics. The same information sources were accessible to the pharmacist. In the third rating method, a physician rated the 200 interactions using the commercially available MMX database [16].

Statistical methods

The concordance between all three ratings was determined using cross-tables, together with ordinary and weighted Cohen's Kappa coefficients. Cohen's Kappa measures the extent to which any two rating systems agree by chance alone. It ranges from zero (agreement no better than chance) to one (perfect agreement). In the tables, values adjacent to the diagonal (ratings differing by a single category) are considered less serious than deviations of two or more categories. Cohen's Kappa evaluates inter-rater agreement as follows: 0.01–0.2

slight agreement; 0.21–0.40 fair agreement; 0.41–0.60 moderate agreement; 0.61–0.80 substantial agreement and 0.81–1 perfect agreement [26]. To identify systematic differences between the rating systems, Bland–Altman plots, which illustrate agreement limits, were constructed. Identified systematic differences were reviewed individually by the aforementioned review team and were excluded from further analysis. The relative frequencies and confidence intervals of the remaining disagreements were determined by the Wilson method [27].

Results

The pharmacist, physician and the clinical pharmacologist independently assessed all cases of potential drug interactions (n = 200). 62 of the interactions yielded no information from MMX regarding possible DDIs. The ratings evaluated by the pharmacist and the clinical pharmacologist ranged from DM: B (precautionary measures) to DM: E (contraindicated).

Concordance

Agreement between the DM and the clinical pharmacologist was high, with a ordinary Kappa coefficient of 0.692 (95% CI [0.611, 0.744]) and weighted Kappa of 0.805 (95% CI [0.747, 0.863]). Agreement between the DM and MMX was fair with a ordinary Kappa coefficient of 0.315 (95% CI [0.233, 0.397]) and weighted Kappa of 0.363 (95% CI [0.276, 0.449]). The DM was concordant with the clinical pharmacologist and with MMX in 156 (78% (95% CI [72, 83])) and 94 cases (47% (95% CI [40, 54])), respectively. Likewise the clinical pharmacologist and MMX agreed in 89 (45% (95% CI [38, 51])) of the 200 interaction cases. Tables 1 and 2 show the DDI cross-ratings between DM and clinical pharmacologist and DM and MMX, respectively.

Divergence

We corrected the rating of the pharmacist in two cases, where the DM was applied incorrectly. The application error rate occurred in 1% of all 20 cases (95% CI [0, 3]). The first error, in the assessment of roxithromycin and simvastatin co-administration, was caused by incorrect interpretation of the DM question. The pharmacist applied the serious adverse events (SAEs) question to the "at-risk" population instead of to the "normal patient" population. Therefore the rating of DM: D (avoid) assigned to this interaction by the pharmacist, required correction to DM: B (precautionary measures). No further information about this rating was extracted from MMX, so a third rating was unavailable for comparison. The second error regarded the combination of atenolol and bupropion. The pharmacist did not use all available information to rate the interaction and in particular did not consider that co-administration can induce blood pressure changes, and thus may alter the effect of atenolol. Therefore the rating of DM: A (no action required) assigned to this interaction by the pharmacist, required correction to DM: B (precautionary measures).

Systematic difference

Systematic differences between the ratings of DM and MMX are displayed as a Bland–Altman plot in Figure 2. The mean difference is 0.9 and perfect agreement (zero) lies outside the confidence interval. The rankings differed by up to three classification categories. The limits of agreement were [−1.6, 3.4], indicating that the DM tends to rate a higher severity. Not shown are the systematic differences for clinical pharmacologist versus MMX (mean difference: 0.8, limits of agreement [−1.5, 3.1]), and DM versus clinical pharmacologist (mean difference: 0.13, limits of agreement [−0.8, 1.05]).

Systematic-difference based disagreements in DM versus MMX and DM versus clinical pharmacologist

Table 1 Cross correlation of drug-drug interaction ratings for clinically identified cases (n = 200) between the proposed decision model (DM) and a clinical pharmacologist

		Clinical Pharmacologist					
		A	B	C	D	E	Total
DM	A	18	3	0	0	0	21
	B	2	10	0	0	0	12
	C	0	0	49	5	0	54
	D	0	1	**30**	60	2	93
	E	0	0	0	1	19	20
	Total	20	14	79	66	21	**200**

Ratings are A (no action required), B (precautionary measures), C (clinical monitoring), D (avoid) and E (contraindicated). Systematic differences between ratings are highlighted.

Table 2 Cross correlation of drug-drug interaction ratings for clinically identified cases (n = 200) between the proposed decision model (DM) and Micromedex (MMX)

		MMX					
		A	B	C	D	E	Total
DM	A	21	0	0	0	0	21
	B	**8**	0	4	0	0	12
	C	**18**	4	26	6	0	54
	D	**32**	1	**25**	34	1	93
	E	**4**	0	0	3	13	20
	Total	83	5	55	43	14	**200**

Ratings are A (no action required), B (precautionary measures), C (clinical monitoring), D (avoid) and E (contraindicated). The rating X from MMX has been labeled E. Missing ratings from MMX have been labeled A. Systematic differences between ratings are highlighted.

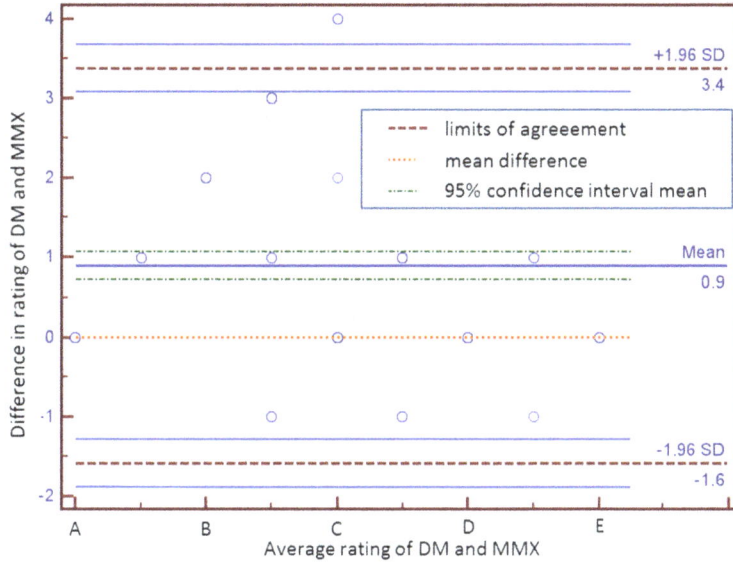

Figure 2 Bland-Altman plot of differences in ratings assigned to clinically identified drug-drug interactions (n = 200) by the proposed decision model (DM) and Micromedex (MMX). Data includes those interactions for which MMX had no rating (n = 62) as highlighted in cells (A,B),(A,C),(A,D) and (A,E) from Table 2.

assessments were excluded from further analysis. The corresponding cells are highlighted in Tables 1 and 2. Figure 3 shows the Bland–Altman plot of the remaining data set for DM and MMX. The mean difference decreased to –0.02, statistically the same as perfect agreement, while limits of agreement narrowed down to [–0.89, 0.85]. The rankings differed by at most one rating.

The remaining 14 (of the 200 ratings) disagreed between the DM and clinical pharmacologist for reasons not explained by systematic differences (these non-systematic discrepancies account for 7% (95% CI [4,11]) of all ratings). The remaining 19 non-systematic disagreements between DM and MMX constitute 9.5% (95%CI: [6,14]).

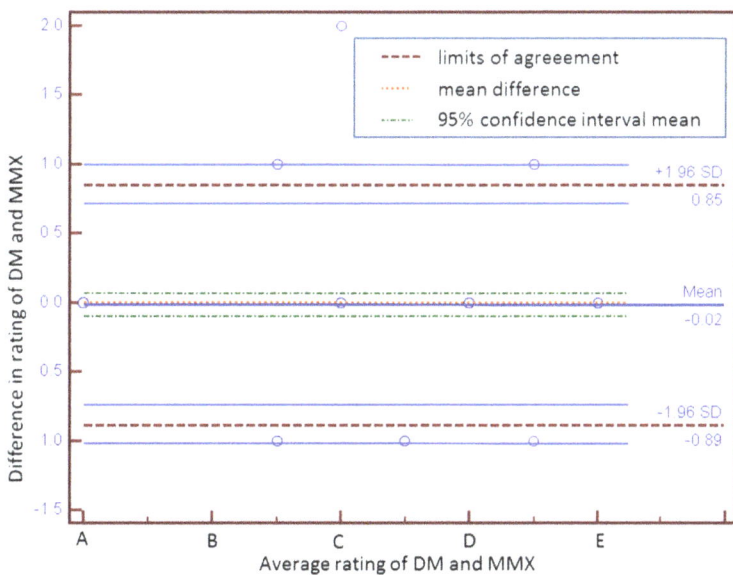

Figure 3 Bland-Altman plot of differences in ratings assigned to clinically identified drug-drug interactions (n = 113) by the proposed decision model (DM) and Micromedex (MMX). Data is based on 200 drug-drug interactions, but excludes those interactions for which MMX had no rating (n = 62) and those ratings with systematic differences (n = 25) (highlighted cells in Table 2).

Discussion

We evaluated a transparent decision model that reproducibly rates drug interactions and identifies systematic rating discrepancies. Altman [26] suggests that kappa is the appropriate means of judging agreement or reproducibility between classification categories obtained by two different rating methods and is supported by the higher weighted Kappa values, which strengthened the approach in the present study. No systematic differences showed up on the Bland–Altman plot of DM versus MMX, following removal of the systematic differences. Divergence in decision making remains an issue and review of certain cases is unavoidable. The review time, however, decreases as a result of the standardization. When comparing two ratings, our visualization of the decision path enables rapid comprehension of one side of the differences [28], thus clarifying (at least partially) the rating discrepancies. Such transparency improves the clinical value of the interpretation of the rating [29,30]. To our knowledge, we publish the first visualized decision model that is comparable with other ratings. Previously published ratings, though based on expert group decisions, are not guided by specified rules of an algorithm. The output of the decision model, corrected for systematic differences between rating systems, closely resembles that of other ratings. To illustrate the systematic nature of these differences, we summarize the most important ones (highlighted in the cross tables) below.

Systematic differences

If more than simple precautionary measures are required in first line therapy, or if complex monitoring of a likely side-effect is required, we assume that a suitable drug alternative precludes co-administration, because the latter disproportionately raises patient risk or health care costs. This explains why DM rated 30 cases of higher severity than the clinical pharmacologist (Table 1) and 25 cases of higher severity than MMX (Table 2).

Interactions requiring complex monitoring were rated of higher severity by DM than either the clinical pharmacologist (DM rated 18 of 30 cases more severely) or MMX (DM rated 21 of 25 cases more severely). (i) The clinical pharmacologist assigned a rating of C ("moderate") to the combination of citalopram and tramadol, whereas both DM and MMX recommended avoiding this combination (ratings: DM: D and "major", respectively), since co-administration increases the risk of serotonin toxicity. Monitoring for SAEs such as hyperreflexia, CNS symptoms, myoclonus, sweating and hyperthermia is imperative and is complex in an outpatient setting. (ii) Risk of amiodarone and phenytoin co-administration was rated C ("moderate") by MMX and C ("precautionary measures") by the clinical pharmacologist. The DM assigned a rating of D

("avoid"), since amiodarone concentrations in plasma may be reduced to as low as 30% in the presence of phenytoin. This effect can occur several weeks into phenytoin therapy, therefore amiodarone concentrations must be monitored for several weeks to enable dose adjustment. Furthermore, phenytoin toxicity can occur and surveillance requires considerable effort. (iii) Co-administration of duloxetine and amitriptyline increases the risk of anticholinergic or serotonin syndrome and may lead to elevated amitriptyline plasma concentrations. Because of the complex clinical surveillance required, this interaction was rated D by the DM, whereas MMX assigned a C rating.

The inclusion of suitable treatment alternatives in the decision process caused DM to rate an interaction more severely than the clinical pharmacologist in 12 of 30 cases, and more severely than MMX in 4 of 25 cases. (i) Co-administration of digoxin and alprazolam was rated C by the clinical pharmacologist, since alprazolam interferes with digoxin levels and therefore requires drug concentration monitoring at the initiation and discontinuation of alprazolam therapy. The DM rated this interaction as D, because a suitable alternative (lorazepam) exists. (ii) MMX rated the combination of midazolam and phenytoin as "moderate". Although the co-presence of phenytoin depresses midazolam levels, alternative benzodiazepines are available which carry a lower potential for interaction.

In one case, a rating discrepancy of two categories was found (the drug combination was rated B by MMX and D by DM). The drugs in question were fluconazole and fluvastatin, for which co-administration increases the risk of severe myopathy while an alternative to fluvastatin exists.

Study limitations

This study focused solely on the decision making process, and the positive contribution of the rating output to medical therapy was not evaluated. Although every attempt has been made to ensure that the categories are objective (i.e. they represent a consensus between four clinical specialists in three different fields), they are nonetheless subject to user interpretation and should not be regarded as a "gold standard", but as an approach to standardize ratings with defined rules. We hope that publication of this decision model will stimulate other groups to test the models' reproducibility. The feasibility of the decision model to illustrate system differences has been tested with a single database, MMX. In future, the DM may elucidate systematic differences between other rating discrepancies reported in the literature [11,13,14]. Concordance between the DM and expert assessment has been validated by only one pharmacist from our group.

The agreement between DM and MMX was evaluated as "fair", which can be explained partly by systematic differences in 25 cases, but which must also consider the missing information from MMX in 62 cases. The omission of information in MMX regarding a specific drug combination cannot be considered as the absence of a DDI. Therefore our database distinguishes between missing information and a safe combination (DM: A). No information was yielded by MMX for the following complications of drug co-administration. (i) The combination of phenobarbital and acetaminophen increases the risk of hepatotoxicity. (ii) The concurrent use of phenobarbital and mirtazepine may inhibit mirtazepine efficacy and therefore requires clinical monitoring. (iii) Duloxetine increases the area under the plasma concentration time curve (AUC) of metoprolol 1.8-fold. As a result, blood pressure and heart rate monitoring are required, particularly at the start and cessation of duloxetine therapy. Drugs that are used in Europe but not in the U.S. explain a portion of the missing data.

Conclusions

The decision model reproducibly rates interactions and identifies systematic differences. Ratings are based on critical indicators of clinical significance, namely; the risk of an SAE, the extent of medical intervention required, the clinical surveillance required, the existence of a safer alternative and the risk-benefit ratio. The decision model is consistent with other rating systems, following removal of systematic differences between methods. We propose to supply the decision path alongside the interaction rating, to facilitate rating comprehensibility and to assess mortality and morbidity rates in a clinical setting. If factors such as length of hospital stay or risk of complications are improved by using the model, then the model represents a significant advance over existing models.

Abbreviations

ADE: Adverse drug event; DDI: Drug-drug interaction; DM: Decision model; MMX: Micromedex DrugDex.

Competing interests

Gerd Kullak-Ublick, Michael Dietrich and Marco Egbring are shareholders of the spin-off EPha.ch, which develops prescribing services. The cases in this publication have been included in the interaction database, which is published under a Creative Commons Attribution-Share Alike 3.0 Unported License. The other authors declare that they have no competing interests.

Authors' contributions

EF and IC performed the study, analyzed the data, discussed the results and drafted the manuscript. EF and IC contributed equally. KB helped to analyze the data and revised the manuscript. MR analyzed the statistical data and revised the appropriate paragraphs. IE participated in the design of the study and collected data. MD drafted the concept and revised the manuscript. WK provided valuable external expertise regarding the development. GK participated in the design and coordination of the study and revised the manuscript. ME designed the concept, analyzed data statistically and participated in the draft and revision of the manuscript. All authors read and gave final approval of the submitted version of the manuscript.

Acknowledgements

All authors are funded by their listed institutions and did not receive any additional funding.

Author details

[1]Department of Clinical Pharmacology and Toxicology, University Hospital Zurich, Rämistrasse 100, 8091 Zurich, Switzerland. [2]Division of Biostatistics, ISPM, University Zurich, Hirschengraben 8, 8001 Zurich, Switzerland. [3]Department of Orthopaedic, Balgrist University Hospital, Forchstrasse 340, 8008 Zurich, Switzerland. [4]Institute of Clinical Pharmacology, Medical Faculty Technical University of Dresden, Fiedlerstrasse 27, D - 01307 Dresden, Germany.

References

1. Bates DW, Spell N, Cullen DJ, Burdick E, Laird N, Petersen LA, Small SD, Sweitzer BJ, Leape LL: The costs of adverse drug events in hospitalized patients. Adverse Drug Events Prevention Study Group. *JAMA* 1997, **277**(4):307–311.
2. Juurlink D, Mamdani M, Iazzetta J, Etchells E: Avoiding drug interactions in hospitalized patients. *Healthc Q* 2004, **7**(2):27–28.
3. Krahenbuhl-Melcher A, Schlienger R, Lampert M, Haschke M, Drewe J, Krahenbuhl S: Drug-related problems in hospitals: a review of the recent literature. *Drug safety: an international journal of medical toxicology and drug experience* 2007, **30**(5):379–407.
4. Zwart-van Rijkom JE, Uijtendaal EV, ten Berg MJ, van Solinge WW, Egberts AC: Frequency and nature of drug-drug interactions in a Dutch university hospital. *Br J Clin Pharmacol* 2009, **68**(2):187–193.
5. Bates DW, Leape LL, Cullen DJ, Laird N, Petersen LA, Teich JM, Burdick E, Hickey M, Kleefield S, Shea B, *et al*: Effect of computerized physician order entry and a team intervention on prevention of serious medication errors. *JAMA* 1998, **280**(15):1311–1316.
6. Garg AX, Adhikari NK, McDonald H, Rosas-Arellano MP, Devereaux PJ, Beyene J, Sam J, Haynes RB: Effects of computerized clinical decision support systems on practitioner performance and patient outcomes: a systematic review. *JAMA* 2005, **293**(10):1223–1238.
7. Hansten PD, Horn JR, Hazlet TK: ORCA: Operational Classification of drug interactions. *J Am Pharm Assoc (Wash)* 2001, **41**(2):161–165.
8. Bergk V, Gasse C, Rothenbacher D, Loew M, Brenner H, Haefeli WE: Drug interactions in primary care: impact of a new algorithm on risk determination. *Clin Pharmacol Ther* 2004, **76**(1):85–96.
9. Guzek MZO, Semmler A, Gonzenbach R, Huber M, Kullak-Ublick GA, Weller M, Russmann S: Evaluation of Drug Interactions and Dosing in 484 Neurological Inpatients Using Clinical Decision Support Software and an Extended Operational Interactions Classification System (ZHIAS). *Pharmacoepidemiol Drug Saf* 2011, in press.
10. Frolich T, Zorina O, Fontana AO, Kullak-Ublick GA, Vollenweider A, Russmann S: Evaluation of medication safety in the discharge medication of 509 surgical inpatients using electronic prescription support software and an extended operational interaction classification. *Eur J Clin Pharmacol* 2011, **67**(12):1273–1282.
11. Vitry AI: Comparative assessment of four drug interaction compendia. *Br J Clin Pharmacol* 2007, **63**(6):709–714.
12. Chan A, Tan SH, Wong CM, Yap KY, Ko Y: Clinically significant drug-drug interactions between oral anticancer agents and nonanticancer agents: a Delphi survey of oncology pharmacists. *Clin Ther* 2009, **31**(Pt 2):2379–2386.
13. Olvey EL, Clauschee S, Malone DC: Comparison of critical drug-drug interaction listings: the Department of Veterans Affairs medical system and standard reference compendia. *Clin Pharmacol Ther* 2010, **87**(1):48–51.
14. Fulda TR: Disagreement among drug compendia on inclusion and ratings of drug-drug interactions. *Curr Ther Res* 2000, **61**(8):540–548.
15. Horn JR: *Reducing Drug Interactions Alerts: Not So Easy*.; Available at http://www.hanstenandhorn.com/hh-article06-07.pdf.
16. Drug-Reax System: *Micromedex Healthcare Series (database on CD-ROM) Version 5.1*. Greenwood Village, Colorado: Thomson Reuters (Healthcare) Inc; 2007.

17. Pharmavista Interactions:; 2010. Available at: http://www.pharmavista.ch.
18. Hansten PD, Horn JR (Eds): *Drug Interactions Analysis and Management*. St. Louis, MO: Facts & Comparisons; 2011.
19. Baxter K (Ed): *Stockley's drug interactions*. 8th edition. London: Pharmaceutical Press; 2009.
20. Tollefson G, Lesar T, Grothe D, Garvey M: **Alprazolam-related digoxin toxicity.** *Am J Psychiatry* 1984, 141(12):1612–1613.
21. Ochs HR, Greenblatt DJ, Verburg-Ochs B: **Effect of alprazolam on digoxin kinetics and creatinine clearance.** *Clin Pharmacol Ther* 1985, 38(5):595–598.
22. Hansten PD: **Drug interaction management.** *Pharm World Sci* 2003, 25(3):94–97.
23. Isaac T, Weissman JS, Davis RB, Massagli M, Cyrulik A, Sands DZ, Weingart SN: **Overrides of medication alerts in ambulatory care.** *Arch Intern Med* 2009, 169(3):305–311.
24. Smithburger PL, Buckley MS, Bejian S, Burenheide K, Kane-Gill SL: **A critical evaluation of clinical decision support for the detection of drug-drug interactions.** *Expert Opin Drug Saf* 2011, 10(6):871–882.
25. van Roon EN, Flikweert S, le Comte M, Langendijk PN, Kwee-Zuiderwijk WJ, Smits P, Brouwers JR: **Clinical relevance of drug-drug interactions: a structured assessment procedure.** *Drug safety: an international journal of medical toxicology and drug experience* 2005, 28(12):1131–1139.
26. Altman D: *Practical statistics for medical research*. London: Chapman & Hall; 1991.
27. Wilson EB: **Probable inference, the law of succession, and statistical inference.** *JASA* 1927, 22:209–212.
28. Larkin JH, Simon HA: **Why a Diagram is (Sometimes) Worth Ten Thousand Words.** *Cogn Sci* 1987, 11(1):65–100.
29. Weingart SN, Seger AC, Feola N, Heffernan J, Schiff G, Isaac T: **Electronic drug interaction alerts in ambulatory care: the value and acceptance of high-value alerts in US medical practices as assessed by an expert clinical panel.** *Drug safety: an international journal of medical toxicology and drug experience* 2011, 34(7):587–593.
30. Seidling HM, Phansalkar S, Seger DL, Paterno MD, Shaykevich S, Haefeli WE, Bates DW: **Factors influencing alert acceptance: a novel approach for predicting the success of clinical decision support.** *Journal of the American Medical Informatics Association: JAMIA* 2011, 18(4):479–484.

3

The future of pharmaceutical care in France: a survey of final-year pharmacy students' opinions

Clémence Perraudin[1,2,3,4*], Françoise Brion[5,6], Olivier Bourdon[5,6] and Nathalie Pelletier-Fleury[2,3,4]

Abstract

Background: In the last decades, the provision of pharmaceutical care by community pharmacists has developed in OECD countries. These developments involved significant changes in professional practices and organization of primary care. In France, they have recently been encouraged by a new legal framework and favored by an increasing demand for health care (increase in the number of patients with chronic diseases) and reductions in services being offered (reduction in the number of general practitioners and huge regional disparities). Objectives: This study aimed to investigate final-year pharmacy students' opinions on 1/expanding the scope of pharmacists' practices and 2/the potential barriers for the implementation of pharmaceutical care. We discussed these in the light of the experiences of pharmacists in Quebec, and other countries in Europe (United Kingdom and the Netherlands).

Methods: All final-year students in pharmaceutical studies, preparing to become community pharmacists, at the University Paris-Descartes in Paris during 2010 (n = 146) were recruited. All of them were interviewed by means of a questionnaire describing nine "professional" practices by pharmacists, arranged in four dimensions: (1) screening and chronic disease management, (2) medication surveillance, (3) pharmacy-prescribed medication and (4) participation in health care networks. Respondents were asked (1) how positively they view the extension of their current practices, using a 5 point Likert scale and (2) their perception of potential professional, technical, organizational and/or financial obstacles to developing these practices.

Results: 143 (97.9%) students completed the questionnaire. Most of practices studied received a greater than 80% approval rating, although only a third of respondents were in favor of the sales of over-the-counter (OTC) drugs. The most significant perceived barriers were working time, remuneration and organizational problems, specifically the need to create a physical location for consultations to respect patients' privacy within a pharmacy.

Conclusions: Despite remaining barriers to cross, this study showed that future French pharmacists were keen to develop their role in patient care, beyond the traditional role of dispensing. However, the willingness of doctors and patients to consent should be investigated and also rigorous studies to support or refute the positive impact of pharmaceutical care on the quality of care should be carried out.

Background

Faced with increasing demand for health care and reductions in services being offered, particularly by general practitioners (GPs), questions are increasingly being raised in various regions of France about the health care principles of proximity, availability and access. To alleviate these problems, a health-care reform law was adopted in 2009 (known as the *"Hôpital, Patients, Santé, Territoires"* or "HPST" law). Primary care is at the forefront of this reform, and for the first time, a legislative framework is broadening the role of pharmacists in providing these services. After being merely a dispenser of medications (article R4235-48 of the Public Health law), the pharmacist is now being assigned responsibilities in front-line health care, health-care coordination, screening and therapeutic education (article 38 of the HPST law).

In 2009, there were 22,386 pharmacies in metropolitan France and 53,460 practicing pharmacists, with an average of one pharmacy for every 2,849 inhabitants [1]. The geographical distribution of pharmacies in France is

* Correspondence: clemence.perraudin@gmail.com
[1]Faculté de Médecine Paris-Sud Paris XI, Le Kremlin-Bicêtre, France
Full list of author information is available at the end of the article

relatively homogeneous because the licensing of pharmacies is regulated by demographic criteria, with one pharmacy per 2,500 or 3,000 inhabitants according to the size of the locality (law of September 11, 1941). With these figures, France has one of the highest pharmacy densities in Europe. The over-the-counter (OTC) market in France is different from neighboring European countries. Drugs provided without prescription account for only 17% of the volume of items sold in pharmacies [2].

The challenge today is to understand the conditions and consequences of a number of technical, organizational and social innovations. No scientific study has examined this issue with respect to the pharmacists' professional practices in France. One could hypothesize that the pharmacist model, in the meaning used by Hepler and Strand [3] as a dispenser of pharmaceutical care, may become the practice in France as well. In any case, the current discrepancies between the demand for and supply of health care provide a context that is conducive to this model, and the legal framework encourages this trend. However, the opposite hypothesis may also be valid; the redefinition of the pharmacist's profession [4] and professional, economic and/or organizational boundaries together with normal resistance to change may become obstacles to the implementation of this reform [5].

The objective of the present study was to analyze the opinions of final-year pharmacy students on expanding the scope of pharmacists' practices in France and thereby assess the potential barriers to adopting new practices.

Methods

Survey population

The survey population consisted of all final-year students in pharmaceutical studies who were preparing to become community pharmacists at the University of Paris-Descartes in Paris during 2010 (n = 146). All of these students were questioned at the end of their 6-month, final-year practical experience of working in a community pharmacy. We took advantage of the fact that these students were required to return to the university between June 21 and 28 for an oral examination to validate their practical experience. During this week, after we obtained their oral consent, we administered a printed questionnaire to all the students. These questionnaires were collected at the end of the examination.

Questionnaire

In France, the pharmacist's mission already extends beyond merely the sale of medications. They also provide advice to patients and sell OTC drugs without medical prescriptions. However, their mission is far from providing patient-centered services [6]. Drawing on the HSPT law and experience in other countries [7-9], we developed a questionnaire describing nine practices of pharmacists. These are summarized in Table 1 and are arranged in four dimensions: (1) screening and chronic disease management, (2) medication surveillance, (3) pharmacy-prescribed medication and (4) participation in health-care networks.

The respondents were asked two questions: (1) how positively they view the extension of their current practices (using a 5-point Likert scale from "strongly favorable" to "strongly unfavorable") and (2) their perception of potential professional, technical, organizational and/ or financial obstacles to developing these practices. For this latter variable, several response categories were provided. Upon completion of the questionnaire, we collected data on the respondents' characteristics, such as age, gender, motivation for selecting the community-pharmacy option in their studies (four alternatives) and the degree to which their practical experience working in a community pharmacy reflected their expectations (using a Likert scale with five choices from "completely" to "not at all").

Results

The questionnaire was completed by 143 of the 146 the students (97.9%) enlisted. The three remaining students left before the examination was completed and did not complete the questionnaire.

Sample characteristics

The majority of the respondents were women (73.9%), and the average age was 25.1 ± 1.6 years. These students chose the community-pharmacy option in their studies because of their desire for patient contact (46.1%), their wish to create an enterprise (11.2%) or a combination of these reasons (28.7%). Only 8.4% chose the community-pharmacy option by default, and 5.6% did not know how to answer this question. For the majority (79.2%), their experience working in a community pharmacy met their expectations "completely" or "almost completely," but 17.1% indicated "averagely" and 3.5% answered "little" or "not at all."

Opinions on expanding the scope of pharmacists' practices

Figure 1 shows the respondents' opinions on expanding the scope of the pharmacist's practices. Eight of the 9 practices studied received a greater than 80.0% approval rating ("favorable" or "strongly favorable"). However, only 34.3% had "favorable" or "strongly favorable" opinions about expanding the sales of OTC drugs. We should note that 14.7% felt "Strongly unfavorable" about this practice.

Table 1 Description of the nine pharmacists' practices

Dimension 1: Screening and chronic disease management

The pharmaceutical consultation	Individual interview in a confidential area to inform and counsel the patient by explaining the treatment, its side effects, and drug interactions, and any follow-up to be adopted.
Therapeutic education	Practical tools for the patient to acquire skills to manage their disease and its care and supervision in partnership with health-care providers.
The pharmacist as a coordinator of care	A protocol allowing the community pharmacist, chosen by the patient, to periodically renew chronic treatments, adjust dosage (if necessary), and make medication-use reviews (side effects, observance, follow-up) at a doctor's request or with his consent.
Screening	Offering screening procedures for certain ailments to patients using easily administered tests such as blood pressure, expiratory flow rate, and blood-sugar levels.

Dimension 2: Medication surveillance

The electronic pharmaceutical record (e-pr)	Making an electronic file for each patient containing all drugs dispensed to the patient during the last four months for his or her own personal consumption, with or without medical prescription, in any pharmacy that is equipped for such recording.
The pharmaceutical opinion	A professional opinion, under the pharmacist's authority, on the pharmaceutical appropriateness of one or a series of treatments to be dispensed by the pharmacist. This is to be communicated on a standardized form to the prescriber of the medication and/or to the patient when the pharmacist recommends a revision or to justify his refusal to dispense a medication as prescribed.

Dimension 3: Pharmacy-prescribed medication

Prescription for minor ailments	Dispensing certain medications without a medical prescription or advising patients to consult a doctor, following appropriate questioning of the patient to determine the gravity of the symptoms of his or her ailment.
Sales of over-the-counter drugs	Direct public access to medications referred to as "pharmaceutical products" in specific, clearly identified locations in very close proximity to where medications are dispensed, and providing the public with information from respected health-care authorities relative to the appropriate use of these products.

Dimension 4: Participation in health-care networks

Pharmacotherapeutic consultation groups	Group discussions with GPs and/or other specialists to discuss the clinical situation of patients for whom they jointly provide care, such as in the framework of health-care networks.

Obstacles to developing new practices

Figure 2 summarizes the potential obstacles to developing new pharmacists' practices. Lack of time and appropriate remuneration constitute the major barriers to developing the four practices under the "screening and chronic disease management" heading. These items were respectively checked by 77.0% and 61.2% of respondents with respect to "pharmaceutical consultation" and by 75.2% and 51.8% for developing "therapeutic education."

Also, organizational obstacles, specifically the need to create a physical location for consultations to respect patients' privacy within a pharmacy, were seen by most respondents (56.8%) as a brake on "pharmaceutical consultation" and by more than a third (36.4%) as limiting the development of "screening." Finally, lack of training and competition with doctors were considered to be significant impediments to developing "pharmacists as coordinators of care," with 30.0% of the respondents

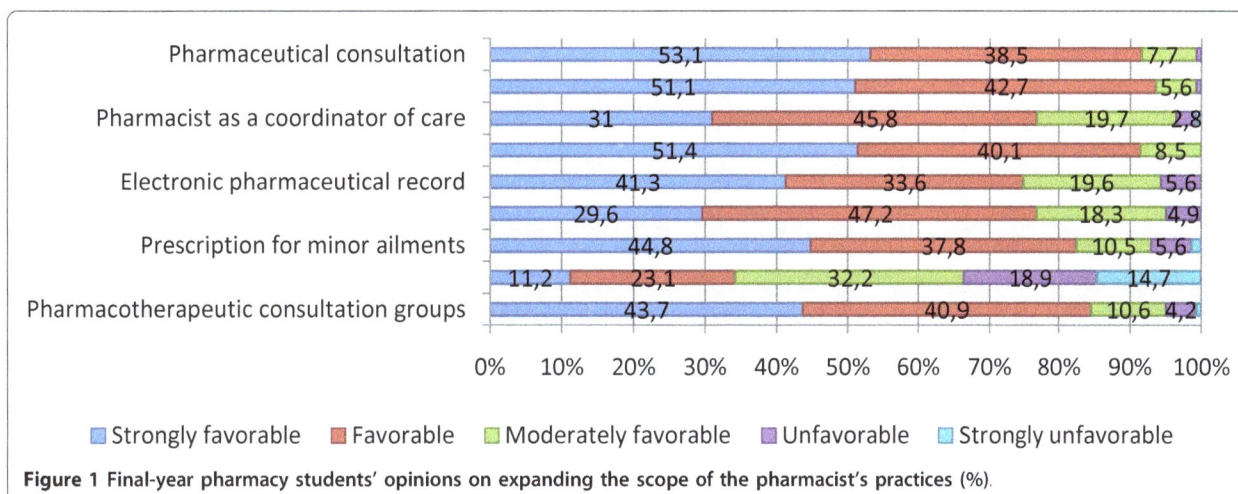

Figure 1 Final-year pharmacy students' opinions on expanding the scope of the pharmacist's practices (%).

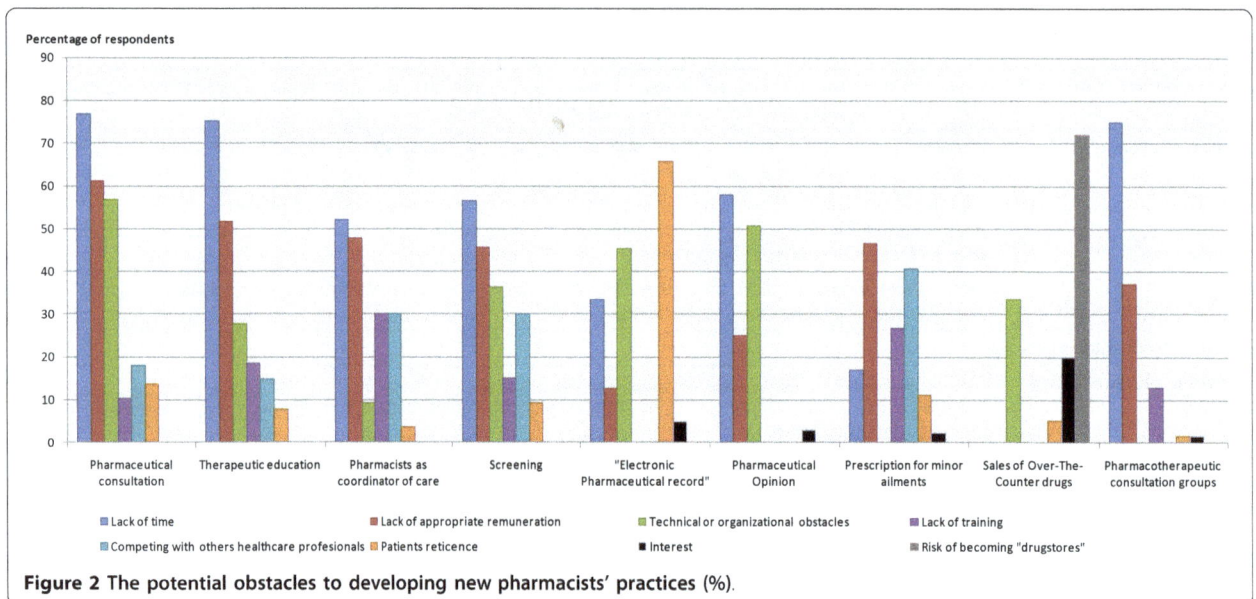

Figure 2 The potential obstacles to developing new pharmacists' practices (%).

checking these two items. Competition with doctors was cited by 30.0% as an obstacle for "screening."

With respect to the "medication surveillance" dimension, half of the respondents checked technical obstacles, specifically those involving computer hardware and the problem of sharing information between health-care professionals. These were cited by 45.5% as factors limiting "electronic pharmaceutical record" (e-pr) development and by 50.7% as factors limiting "pharmaceutical opinion." Time was also mentioned as a factor constraining e-pr development by a third of the respondents (33.6%), and by more than 50.0% (57.9%) as limiting "pharmaceutical opinion," whereas remuneration was infrequently selected as a limiting factor. It is particularly striking that nearly two-thirds of the respondents (65.7%) considered patient reticence as a potential obstacle to e-pr development.

As for the "pharmacy-prescribed medication" dimension for minor ailments, in addition to the lack of remuneration, which was considered by nearly half (46.5%) of the respondents as a barrier, we also found problems with competing with doctors (40.8%) and, to a lesser extent, lack of training (26.8%). Less than one-fifth of the respondents (16.9%) mentioned lack of time for this dimension. For "selling OTC medications," the notable finding was the high percentage (72.1%) who perceived the risk of pharmacies becoming "drugstores" as an obstacle to its development. Added to this were organizational problems, specifically the space available for these items in pharmacies (33.6% of respondents). Finally, for "participation in health-care networks," time and (to a lesser degree) remuneration were seen as the principal obstacles (75.0% and 37.1%, respectively).

Discussion

Pharmaceutical care

The concept of pharmaceutical care originated in an article by Hepler and Strand [3]. Although there are several definitions of this concept, most agree that a pharmacist's commitment to the patient is to attain the patient's health objectives. This concept has become widely used in North America, particularly in Quebec, but it has received less recognition in Europe [10], with the exception of the United Kingdom and the Netherlands [8]. The pharmacists' practices considered in the present study are integrated into the concept of pharmaceutical care that is defined by the *Ordre des Pharmaciens du Québec* (The College of Pharmacists in Quebec) as: "all the acts and services that the pharmacist is required to provide to patients, in order to improve the quality of their lives by attaining the pharmacotherapeutic objectives of prevention, cure or the provision of palliative care." [11]

Screening and chronic disease management

In Quebec, community pharmacists can, during a private pharmaceutical consultation with a patient, provide the following: develop a pharmaceutical care plan and the objectives to be attained; write a pharmaceutical opinion with suggestions to the patient's doctor to revise the patient's treatment; conduct simple tests in follow-up treatment, such as blood pressure; take the time to explain the treatment and the ailments; and listen to what the patient has to say [12,13]. The pharmacist can also participate in therapeutic education projects by showing patients how to modify their lifestyle to reduce their symptoms and improve their short-, medium- and long-term health status [14]. New approaches that give pharmacists the right to write out prescriptions are emerging elsewhere, such as in the United States and the United Kingdom, through establishing a protocol between the doctor, the pharmacist and the patient, defining the procedures and responsibilities of each person and developing the health-care project to be adopted. Collaborative drug-therapy management is practiced throughout the United States and is officially recognized in 25 states and by the federal government (Armed Forces and Veterans Affairs) [15]. In the United Kingdom, following a public consultation and under advice from the Committee on Safety of Medicines and the Medicines Commission, Ministers in 2003 agreed to the implementation of supplementary prescribing [9]. The procedures can be followed to different degrees, such as ranging from the initiation of treatment through to modifying and/or renewing the medication therapy.

In France, the pharmacist's involvement in providing care for patients with chronic ailments is one of the pillars of this recently adopted legislation. Due to health-care professionals' initiatives (pharmacists, doctors and nurses), co-operation agreements (defined since July 21, 2009 by Article 4011-1 of the Public Health law) may be signed, which follow the consultation with the *Haute Autorité de Santé* (French National Authority for Health) and authorization by the *Agence Régionale de Santé (Regional Health Agency)*. The objective is to transfer activities and/or care and to reorganize intervention procedures with patients between the different health-care professionals according to their respective knowledge and experience levels. In our study, the great majority of young pharmacists look favorably on implementing these measures. Nonetheless, according to our respondents, lack of time and remuneration constitute barriers for developing these new practices. In France today, pharmacists are essentially remunerated through profit margins on the medications they sell; therefore, the present remuneration system would have to be modified, and several alternatives can be envisaged. In Quebec, pharmacists are moving towards a system of being paid per pharmaceutical act [16]. In 2009, pharmacist representatives in France proposed (in the Rapport Rioli [17]) a mixed system of remuneration, which would make distinctions between the profit margins on medications sold, the fees for pharmaceutical acts and reimbursements for services provided. This proposal was inspired by the 2005 agreement signed between the National Health Service (NHS) and pharmacists [18] in the United Kingdom. This agreement identifies three levels of intervention, which differ according to the services offered, the source of funding and the agreements signed with the government. The *Rapport Rioli* also considered the roles that the compulsory health insurance system and complementary health plans should play in providing these services. This agreement was signed by eight pharmacist associations and was approved by the Ministry of Health. There are already a few initiatives wherein pharmacists are remunerated independently of medication sales. The insurance company GMF-Allianz has developed a model contract that remunerates pharmacists for their pharmaceutical consultations [19]. *La Mutuelle de la Région Lyonnaise* (complementary health plan of the Region of Lyon) is proposing a personalized prevention assessment for pharmacists. This assessment is made when a new contract is signed, it is renewed every two years, and each act is reimbursed up to a maximum of 22€ per beneficiary. Thus, a debate regarding a new system of remuneration for pharmacists is taking place in France.

In our study, the lack of appropriate training was perceived to represent a significant obstacle to developing chronic disease management, particularly in the context of increasing the coordinating role of pharmacists. In 2006, the World Health Organization and the International Pharmaceutical Federation (FIP) called for a new paradigm in pharmaceutical care that would require pharmacists to go beyond their training as experts in chemistry and their knowledge of pharmaceutical products. This paradigm called on pharmacists to understand and apply the principles involved in managing medical therapies, such as the clinical and social roles of pharmacies, communication, health promotion and ethics [20,21]. The FIP also recommended increasing vocational training for pharmacists [22]. In the United Kingdom, for example, pharmacists can only provide supplementary prescriptions after they train at a higher education institution and complete a "period of learning in practice" in accordance with the Royal Pharmaceutical Society of Great Britain curriculum. Currently, the practice of clinical pharmacy is poorly developed in France, in both hospitals and in the community. Starting in the fall of 2010, a common first year may be established for all students in medicine, pharmacy, dentistry and midwifery, and this may become an opportunity to create a common basis for these future health-care professionals and encourage tomorrow's collaborative practices.

Pharmacies are providing more screening practices in France, which are resulting from the combined initiatives of pharmacies collaborating with each other [23] or during awareness campaigns such as "Diabetes Day." In light of what has been happening in Germany, pharmacies could offer their patients the possibility of monitoring their blood pressure, blood-sugar levels, lipid values, body mass index or waistline [24]. In addition to the problems of remuneration and available working-time, the principal obstacles mentioned by our respondents concerning these practices were pharmacy layout, lack of space for meeting patients confidentially and competition with GPs, which is discussed below (see Pharmacy-prescribed medication). Designated spaces in pharmacies for respecting privacy or separate rooms for these consultations have to be created to develop this screening activity and to provide care for chronic ailments. The *Ordre des Pharmaciens* (The College of Pharmacists in France) mentioned this need in July 2006 [25]. Rapport et al. (2009) [26] were concerned with the impact of the community pharmacy setting on professional practice and sense of self. They emphasized the importance of separate enclosed consultation rooms in pharmacies in the United Kingdom. Providing such space would increase the degree of confidentiality during consultations and heighten the professional's sense of being a valuable consultant and diagnostician. However, typically, these spaces are not clearly reserved for consultations, and they are often used for stocking products due to the lack of space in small pharmacies. Rapport *et al.* concluded that, unlike in the case of GPs, a consultation room in a pharmacy tends to be a place where the patient is encouraged to buy, be served and move on instead of a place where the patient can expect to spend time with a health-care professional.

Medication surveillance

For many years, strategies for using electronic health records (e-hr) have been very different from one country to another. One of the first uses of e-hr was for medical prescriptions [27]. In France, an initial e-hr project *Dossier Médical Personnalisé* was adopted into law on August 13, 2004. It was abandoned due to problems with its application, such as deadlines not being respected and divergent interpretations of the limits and uses of the e-hr. The purpose was to create an e-hr for each person in France, which would include all of his or her past and present medical information. The e-pr developed independently of the e-hr. The e-pr is a pharmacist's professional tool designed to ensure the safe dispensing of medications. It records all medications delivered to a patient during the last four months from every pharmacy, which are linked into the system. By consulting the e-pr, the pharmacist can identify medicinal interactions and treatment redundancies. The National Consultative Committee of the *Ordre des Pharmaciens*, which initiated the e-pr, has been mandated by law (n° 2007-127 of January 30, 2007) to use this system. In the future, this will facilitate the implementation of the e-hr program. In our study, the great majority of the young pharmacists were open to creating these systems. In 2010, nearly 10 million e-prs had already been created in 18,000 pharmacies. However, obstacles to this initiative have been identified, and patient reticence is

the most important. The patient has the right to refuse the creation of their e-pr. This is consistent with results of a recent study [28], which gathered the opinions of patients, GPs and community pharmacists on the development of an electronic transfer system for prescription-related information between GPs and community pharmacies. All groups acknowledged the potential benefits of a full, primary-care information system, but GPs and patients had reservations about allowing community pharmacists to access parts of their medical records that did not concern medications. Technical problems (such as slow internet connections and lack of standardized materials and software) and time were also cited as major obstacles to developing the e-pr. Our respondents also referred to other obstacles, such as patients opting out of the e-pr and deciding on what data to include in it. These obstacles and the technical issues contribute greatly to the time constraints on e-pr development. This would explain why, unlike with other practices, the time constraint was not accompanied by the issue of remuneration.

Pharmaceutical opinion is a procedure from Quebec. In 1984, the *Ordre des Pharmaciens du Québec* defined this as "a pharmacist's judgment on the value of a medication or medicinal treatment following his or her analysis of the patient's e-pr " [29]. Therefore, it is based on the development of an e-pr. Since 1978, pharmacists have been reimbursed for this development by the *Régie de l'Assurance-Maladie du Québec* (Quebec provincial drug plan) [30]. In France, pharmacists often contact prescribing doctors to revise a prescription (regarding dosage, appropriateness, or errors), but there are no formal procedures for transmitting such information. These are considered telephone contacts and are not billed by the pharmacist. This concept of pharmaceutical opinion is nevertheless the subject of a whole chapter in the French practical training guide for final-year pharmacy students [31]. Moreover, in our study, we found that respondents supported expanding this procedure but reported that the practice of pharmaceutical opinion faced major obstacles in terms of the time this would require (independently of remuneration) and the technical problems. Kröger et al had already discussed these obstacles in their 2000 study that aimed to identify factors that influenced Quebec community pharmacists to bill for a pharmaceutical opinion or for a refusal to dispense. The typical pharmacist who billed for opinions or refusals in Quebec was < 45 years of age, had attended a continuing education program on this topic and believed that billing for interventions was important. He or she handled a mean daily volume of 100-250 prescriptions, used a decision-support computer program and had sufficient technical staff assistance [32].

Pharmacist-prescribed medication

One important finding in our research was that our respondents wantcd to increase their status as pharmacist-prescribers for minor ailments (82.6%) but not to increase their sales of OTC drugs (34.3%). This reflects the recent debate in France over selling medications in supermarkets [33]. The majority of tomorrow's pharmacists think that pharmacies are not drugstores. This is consistent with the position of the professional association in defending its monopoly. France is one of the last European countries along with Spain, Italy and Greece where pharmacies have a monopoly over all medications (the sale and distribution of all medications whether or not they require a prescription) [34]. In our study, the problem of competing with doctors for pharmacy-prescribed medications echoes the debate over the recognition of pharmacists prescribing for minor ailments. Thus, even if the official representatives of the profession are ready to implement this, a survey reported in 2005 in the *Quotidien du médecin* showed that 6 out of 10 GPs were still opposed to pharmacists prescribing for low-risk ailments [35]. Since 2005, pharmacists have been authorized to dispense medications for contraception and for breaking tobacco addiction.

Participation in health-care networks

The practice of direct collaborations between pharmacists and other health-care professionals (particularly GPs) to discuss a patient's clinical case has been borrowed from the "pharmacotherapeutic consultation groups" (FTOs) in the Netherlands [8], where these collaborations began in the 1990s to improve co-ordination between health professionals. In France, such practices appear to occur infrequently, but they are, nevertheless, developing through the extension of health-care networks and the increased participation of pharmacists in these networks [36]. Time and remuneration, according to our respondents, were the principal obstacles to developing this practice.

Limitations

This study has several limitations. First, the respondents were young Parisian pharmacy students, and their opinions may not reflect those of pharmacists throughout France, given the urban setting of their practices; however, even if Paris is not one of the areas most exposed to problems of proximity and access to health care, the respondents were in favor of (or strongly in favor of) to developing the new practices included in our study. Second, the results of this opinion survey would have been very different, particularly with respect to the obstacles to developing new practices, if the respondents had already been established pharmacists. Our choice of final-year pharmacy students, in addition to the fact that

they were accessible, was justified because all respondents would soon be affected by the current reform. Third, this is a study of opinions from the pharmacist's perspective, and the results cannot be seen as predictors of the adoption and application of the reform. They have to be considered alongside the opinions of the two other major protagonists: doctors and patients. This merits subsequent research.

Conclusions

Overall, the final-year pharmacy students participating in this study, who are tomorrow's pharmacists, held favorable opinions toward developing new practices that are more focused on the patient. However, they saw many obstacles for themselves in the diffusion of these practices. The most significant obstacles were remuneration, working time and organizational and technical problems. The *Ordre des Pharmaciens* has proposed solutions to these problems based on the experiences of other countries. However, nothing can be achieved without creating cooperation contracts with other health-care professionals, particularly doctors, to provide care for chronic ailments. The patient's consent must also be obtained. The opinions of doctors and patients remain as open questions.

Acknowledgements

The authors warmly thank all the pharmacy students of the University Paris Descartes who were kind enough to participate in the survey.

Author details

[1]Faculté de Médecine Paris-Sud Paris XI, Le Kremlin-Bicêtre, France. [2]Institut National de la Santé et de la Recherche Médicale (INSERM) Unité 988, Villejuif, France. [3]Centre National de la Recherche Scientifique (CNRS) UMR 8211, Villejuif, France. [4]Ecole des Hautes Etudes en Sciences Sociales (EHESS), Paris, France. [5]Faculté de Pharmacie, Université Paris Descartes, France. [6]APHP Hôpital Robert Debré, Paris, France.

Authors' contributions

CP led the design of the study, collected the data, performed the statistical analysis and wrote the manuscript. FB and OB contributed to the revising of the questionnaire and the manuscript and acquisition of data. NPF led the design of the study and wrote the manuscript. All authors read and approved the final manuscript.

Competing interests

The authors declare that they have no competing interests.

References

1. Ordre National des Pharmaciens: *Pharmaciens: panorama au 1er janvier 2010* 2010.
2. Coulomb A, Baumelou A: Situation de l'automédication en France et perspectives d'évolution: marché, comportements, positions des acteurs. Ministère de la santé et de la protection sociale; 2007.
3. Hepler CD, Strand LM: Opportunities and responsibilities in pharmaceutical care. *Am J Hosp Pharm* 1990, 47:533-543.
4. Edmunds J, Calnan MW: The reprofessionalisation of community pharmacy? An exploration of attitudes to extended roles for community pharmacists amongst pharmacists and General Practitioners in the United Kingdom. *Soc Sci Med* 2001, 53:943-955.

5. van Mil JW: Pharmaceutical care, the future of pharmacy: theory, research and practice. *PhD Thesis* University Center of Pharmacy in Groningen; 2000.

6. Grindrod KA, Marra CA, Colley L, Tsuyuki RT, Lynd LD: Pharmacists' preferences for providing patient-centered services: a discrete choice experiment to guide health policy. *Ann Pharmacother* 2010, 44:1554-1564.

7. Isetts BJ, Schondelmeyer SW, Artz MB, Lenarz LA, Heaton AH, Wadd WB, Brown LM, Cipolle RJ: Clinical and economic outcomes of medication therapy management services: the Minnesota experience. *J Am Pharm Assoc (2003)* 2008, 48:203-211.

8. van Mil JW: Pharmaceutical care in community pharmacy: practice and research in the Netherlands. *Ann Pharmacother* 2005, 39:1720-1725.

9. Hobson RJ, Sewell GJ: Supplementary prescribing by pharmacists in England. *Am J Health Syst Pharm* 2006, 63:244-253.

10. Hughes CM, Hawwa AF, Scullin C, Anderson C, Bernsten CB, Björnsdóttir I, Cordina MA, da Costa FA, De Wulf I, Eichenberger P, Foulon V, Henman MC, Hersberger KE, Schaefer MA, Søndergaard B, Tully MP, Westerlund T, McElnay JC: Provision of pharmaceutical care by community pharmacists: a comparison across Europe. *Pharm World Sci* 2010, 32:472-487.

11. Ducharne P, Mailhot C, Parent M: Adaptation de la définition de "Pharmaceutical care" dévelopée par Hepler et Strand. 1994.

12. *Le pharmacien peut maintenant vous dresser un plan de soins* , in La Presse 2004 Feb 28: Montréal..

13. René-Henri N, Khamla Y, Nadaira N, Ouellet C, Blais L, Lalonde L, Collin J, Beauchesne MF: Community pharmacists' interventions in asthma care: a descriptive study. *Ann Pharmacother* 2009, 43:104-111.

14. Association Québécoise des Pharmaciens Propriétaires. *Profession: Pharmacien 2010* 2010.

15. Zellmer WA: Collaborative drug therapy management. *Am J Health Syst Pharm* 1995, 52:1732.

16. *Québec: rémunération de la "consultation pharmaceutique"* Les Nouvelles Pharmaceutiques; 2004, Feb 13 n°272..

17. Rioli M, Groupe de travail pharmaciens d'officine: *Le pharmacien d'officine dans le parcours de soins* 2009.

18. Noyce PR: Providing patient care through community pharmacies in the UK: policy, practice, and research. *Ann Pharmacother* 2007, 41:861-868.

19. *AGF-Allianz et le CNGPO s'engagent pour l'évolution de l'automédication vers une médication officinale guidée, responsable et sécurisée* 2009 [http://www.collectif-groupements-pharmaciens.fr/images_bdd/presse/AGF-CNGPO_04_06_09.pdf].

20. World Health Organization and International Pharmaceutical Federation: *Developing pharmacy practice-A focus on patient care* , Edition 2006..

21. van Mil JW, Schulz M, Tromp TF: Pharmaceutical care, European developments in concepts, implementation, teaching, and research: a review. *Pharm World Sci* 2004, 26:303-311.

22. International Pharmaceutical Federation: *FIP Statement of professional standards continuing professional development* The Hague, The Netherlands; 2002.

23. *GIPHAR: Quand la prévention se fait dès l'officine. Présentation de la campagne de groupement GIPHAR* 2010 [http://www.santelog.com/modules/connaissances/actualite-sante-giphar-quand-la-preacutevention-se-fait-degraves-lofficine_2636_lirelasuite.htm].

24. Eickhoff C, Schulz M: Pharmaceutical care in community pharmacies: practice and research in Germany. *Ann Pharmacother* 2006, 40:729-735.

25. Ordre National des Pharmaciens: *Recommandations pour l'aménagement des locaux de l'officine établies par les conseils centraux A et E* 2006.

26. Rapport F, Doel MA, Jerzembek GS: "Convenience space" or "a tight squeeze": Insider views on the community pharmacy. *Health Place* 2009, 15:315-322.

27. Bourquard K: Dossier médical partagé ou personnel: situation internationale. *Prat Organ Soins* 2007, 38:55-67.

28. Porteous T, Bond C, Robertson R, Hannaford P, Reiter E: Electronic transfer of prescription-related information: comparing views of patients, general practitioners, and pharmacists. *Br J Gen Pract* 2003, 53:204-209.

29. Ordre des Pharmaciens du Québec: *Définitions d'actes pharmaceutiques* 1984.

30. Jones EJ, Mackinnon NJ, Tsuyuki RT: Pharmaceutical care in community pharmacies: practice and research in Canada. *Ann Pharmacother* 2005, 39:1527-1533.

31. Guide de stage pratique professionnelle en officine. 6ème année. 17ème édition. 2010 [http://www.ordre.pharmacien.fr/upload/Guidestage/guide-stage-6eme-annee.pdf].

32. Kröger E, Moisan J, Gregoire JP: Billing for cognitive services: understanding Québec pharmacists' behavior. *Ann Pharmacother* 2000, 34:309-316.

33. Attali J: In *Rapport de la Commission pour la libération de la croissance française* Edited by: La documentation française 245.

34. *DGEFP-CPNE de la pharmacie d'officine. Tome 1: Contrat d'études prospectives dans la pharmacie d'officine* Groupe INTERFACE Etudes Conseil & Formation; 2006, 263.

35. « Evolution des pratiques des professions de santé-59% des médecins opposés au pharmacien prescripteur » in. *Le quotidien du médecin* 2005.

36. Petit F: Réseaux diabète et implication du pharmacien d'officine: étude de trois réseaux diabète en région Centre. *PhD Thesis* Université Paris Descartes, Faculté des sciences pharmaceutiques et biologiques; 2006.

4

The association between drospirenone and hyperkalemia: a comparative-safety study

Steven T Bird[1,2*†], Salvatore R Pepe[1,2†], Mahyar Etminan[3†], Xinyue Liu[2†], James M Brophy[4†] and Joseph AC Delaney[2†]

Abstract

Background: Drospirenone/ethinyl-estradiol is an oral contraceptive (OC) that possesses unique antimineralocorticoid activity. It is conjectured that drospirenone, taken alone or concomitantly with spironolactone, may be associated with an increased risk of hyperkalemia.

Methods: A retrospective cohort study was conducted evaluating women between 18-46 years of age in the Lifelink™ Health Plan Claims Database. The study was restricted to new users of OCs between 1997-2009. Cox proportional hazards models were used to estimate the time to first occurrence of hyperkalemia diagnosis. The main analysis compared OCs containing drospirenone with OCs containing levonorgestrel, a second generation OC not known to impact potassium homeostasis. Logistic regression evaluated concomitant prescribing of drospirenone and spironolactone

Results: The cohort included 1,148,183 women, averaging 28.8 years of age and 280 days of OC therapy. 2325 cases of hyperkalemia were identified. The adjusted hazard ratio (HR) for hyperkalemia with drospirenone compared to levonorgestrel was 1.10 (95%CI 0.95-1.26). There was an increased risk of hyperkalemia with norethindrone HR 1.15 (95%CI: 1.00-1.33) and norgestimate HR 1.27 (95%CI: 1.11-1.46). Other OCs were unassociated with hyperkalemia. The odds of receiving spironolactone while taking drospirenone were 2.66 (95%CI 2.53-2.80) times higher than the odds of receiving spironolactone and levonorgestrel. Only 6.5% of patients taking drospirenone and spironolactone had a serum potassium assay within 180 days of starting concomitant therapy.

Conclusions: A clinically significant signal for hyperkalemia with drospirenone was not demonstrated in the current study. Despite the bolded warning for hyperkalemia with joint drospirenone and spironolactone administration, physicians are actually using them together preferentially, and are not following the recommended potassium monitoring requirements in the package insert.

Background

Drospirenone is a novel synthetic progestin approved in combination with ethinyl estradiol as an oral contraceptive (OC) [1]. Marketed as Yasmin® and Yaz®, drospirenone is one of the most popular oral contraceptives in the United States [2]. Drospirenone is a fourth generation OC and it possesses antimineralocorticoid effects not present in previous generations of OCs. Its antimineralocorticoid potency is approximately eight times greater than spironolactone [3], thus a 3 mg tablet of drospirenone has a similar effect to 20-25 mg of spironolactone [4]. This activity enhances sodium, chloride, and water excretion, while reducing the excretion of potassium, ammonium, and phosphate [5]. The similarity in chemical structure between drospirenone and spironolactone and the known association between spironolactone and hyperkalemia both strengthen the plausibility that clinically significant hyperkalemia might result from drospirenone use.

In May of 2001, when drospirenone/ethinyl estradiol (Yasmin®) was first approved, the package insert included a bolded warning for hyperkalemia, stating that "Yasmin should not be used in patients with conditions that predispose to hyperkalemia" [1]. The warning also

---

* Correspondence: steven.bird@fda.hhs.gov
† Contributed equally
[1]Department of Health and Human Services/Food and Drug Administration/ Center for Drug Evaluation and Research (CDER)/Office of Management/ CDER Academic Collaboration Program, Bldg 22, 10903 New Hampshire Avenue, Silver Spring, MD USA 20993
Full list of author information is available at the end of the article

instructs physicians to monitor potassium levels during the first cycle of treatment in patients taking concomitant medications known to cause hyperkalemia. Clinical evidence however has not shown a strong association between drospirenone and hyperkalemia [6-13]. Several studies have evaluated for hyperkalemia in postmenopausal women with hypertension or diabetes who use drospirenone to treat vasomotor spasms. These studies found no association between drospirenone and hyperkalemia in women with hypertension [6,7] or type 2 diabetes mellitus [8]; however, all three studies were twelve or fewer weeks in duration. Larger trials designed to evaluate the safety and efficacy of drospirenone either do not evaluate hyperkalemia or are not powered to detect it [9-12]. Only one large study, mandated by the FDA at approval, has been performed evaluating drospirenone for hyperkalemia in younger women, and it found no association between drospirenone and hyperkalemia [13].

Hyperkalemia is a potentially serious condition that may be associated with numerous pathophysiological conditions. Clinically significant hyperkalemia reduces membrane excitability and disturbs the acid-base balance, manifesting as weakness, flaccid paralysis, hypoventilation, and metabolic acidosis. Hyperkalemia can also result in cardiac toxicity with electrocardiographic changes, which in severe cases may lead to the terminal events of ventricular fibrillation or asystole [5].

The primary objective of the current study is to investigate the association between drospirenone and the diagnosis of hyperkalemia in a large unselected population. A secondary objective is to evaluate the impact of the package insert on medical prescribing as assessed by an examination of the 1) concomitant use of drospirenone and spironolactone and 2) respect for the stated potassium monitoring requirements.

Methods
Data Source
The IMS Lifelink™ Health Plan Claims Database contains paid claims data from over 102 managed care plans in the United States. The database contains fully adjudicated medical and pharmacy claims for over 68 million patients, including inpatient and outpatient diagnoses and procedures (*International Classification of Diseases, 9th Revision, Clinical Modification format*) in addition to retail and mail order prescription records. The data is representative of US residents with private health insurance in terms of geography, age, and gender. The Lifelink™ database is subject to quality checks to ensure data quality and to minimize error rates [14].

Cohort description
A retrospective cohort was developed, evaluating women in the Lifelink™ Claims database between January 1st,

1997 and December 31st, 2009. All women between 18-46 years of age with the first prescription for an OC containing ethinyl estradiol (0.35 ug or less) and one of the following progestins were included in the cohort: *desogestrel, drospirenone, ethynodiol diacetate, levonorgestrel, norethindrone acetate, norethindrone, norgestimate, and norgestrel.* All patients who met these inclusion criteria were analyzed in the utilization portion of the study.

For the hyperkalemia analysis, in order to include only new users, patients were excluded if they did not have at least 180 days of enrollment history prior to their first claim for an OC. Patients were also excluded if they had a prior diagnosis of hyperkalemia. Censoring was performed if a patient switched to another OC during the study period, on the final day of OC possession (determined from the final prescription date and day supply), before a gap in OC possession of 30 or more days, at the event of hyperkalemia, and at the end of the study period, December 31st, 2009. Evaluation of hyperkalemia was performed using a diagnostic ICD-9 code (276.7).

Statistical analysis
OCs and hyperkalemia
Cox proportional hazard models were used to estimate the time to first occurrence of hyperkalemia. The primary analysis used a new user design and compared OCs containing drospirenone with OCs containing levonorgestrel. Levonorgestrel was chosen *a priori* as a reference based on its high utilization, lack of association with hyperkalemia, and use as a reference in previous OC comparative-safety studies [15-21]. All estimates were adjusted by age, calendar time, chronic kidney disease, diabetes mellitus, hypertension, inflammatory bowel disease, obesity [22], polycystic ovary syndrome, premenstrual tension syndrome (premenstrual syndrome and premenstrual dysphoric disorder), smoking status, and concomitant medications known to cause hyperkalemia. The following medications were adjusted for: angiotensin-converting enzyme inhibitors (ACE)/angiotensin receptor blockers (ARB), non-steroidal anti-inflammatory drugs (NSAID), spironolactone, and other medications (cyclosporine, diuretics, heparin, penicillin G, tacrolimus, and trimethoprim).

Utilization
Concomitant utilization of drospirenone and spironolactone was analyzed during the entire study period. Logistic regression was used to form odds ratios (OR) comparing the odds for receiving concomitant spironolactone and drospirenone therapy against the odds of receiving concomitant spironolactone and levonorgestrel therapy. ORs were also formed calculating the odds of receiving spironolactone while on other progestin-

containing OCs compared to levonorgestrel. To evaluate compliance with potassium monitoring for patients taking concomitant drospirenone and spironolactone, the percentage of patients who had a blood serum potassium assay (CPT-4 84132) during the first 180 days of concomitant therapy was calculated.

This study was approved by the University of Florida IRB. All calculations were performed in SAS software version 9.2.

Results

OCs and hyperkalemia

The cohort included 1,148,183 women exposed to a progestin-based OC and 880,014 person-years of follow-up time. Patients in the study averaged 28.8 years of age and had a mean follow up time of 280 days. There were 2325 cases of hyperkalemia, representing 0.20% of the population. Baseline characteristics are shown in Table 1.

The adjusted hazard ratio (HR) for a recorded diagnosis of hyperkalemia while exposed to drospirenone compared to levonorgestrel was 1.10 (95% CI 0.95-1.26). Other OCs were unassociated with hyperkalemia: desogestrel HR 1.00 (95%CI: 0.85-1.17), ethynodiol diacetate HR 0.71 (95%CI: 0.49-1.02), norethindrone acetate HR 1.08 (95%CI: 0.91-1.29), norgestrel HR 1.00 (95%CI: 0.76-1.33), although there was an unexpected signal with norethindrone HR 1.15 (95%CI: 1.00-1.33) and norgestimate HR 1.27 (95%CI: 1.11-1.46) (Table 2). Additionally, the analysis found no interaction between drospirenone and spironolactone for hyperkalemia in the regression model (HR 1.08, 95%CI: 0.78-1.49). Other interactions with drospirenone in the regression model were as follows: ACEI/ARB HR 0.78 (95%CI 0.55-1.10) and NSAID HR 1.09 (95%CI 0.80-1.48).

Utilization

The utilization study evaluated all 2,925,407 patients that met the initial study inclusion criteria. 18,869 patients in this population were taking both spironolactone and an OC. The odds of receiving spironolactone while on drospirenone were 2.66 (95%CI 2.53-2.80) times higher than the odds of receiving spironolactone while on levonorgestrel. The ORs for receiving spironolactone while on other progestin-based OCs compared to levonorgestrel are as follows: desogestrel 1.46 (95%CI 1.38-1.55), ethynodiol diacetate 2.85 (95%CI 2.62-3.11),

Table 1 Characteristics of women included in the study cohort by type of progestin oral contraceptive used (n = 1,148,183)

	Desogestrel	Drospirenone	Ethynodiol Diacetate	Levonorgestrel	Norethindrone Acetate	Norethindrone	Norgestimate	Norgestrel
Number of patients	139,871	224,408	17,295	180,720	93,818	234,105	228,276	29,690
Age	28.7	29.0	28.8	29.0	30.5	29.7	26.9	29.7
Mean follow up (days)	327	272	327	304	240	230	307	249
Number of cases	267	488	33	349	200	433	499	56
Covariates (%)								
CKD †	0.15	0.09	0.08	0.09	0.12	0.15	0.08	0.19
Diabetes	4.10	4.10	4.41	3.93	4.13	4.12	3.37	5.43
Hypertension	8.34	8.47	8.53	8.62	9.78	8.89	6.55	10.82
IBD*	0.94	1.03	1.22	1.00	1.03	0.85	0.75	0.98
Obesity	11.59	12.53	12.44	11.22	10.75	10.08	9.50	13.60
PCOS □	4.47	5.78	5.00	2.11	2.80	2.81	2.21	3.48
PTS (PMS/ PMDD) ‡	3.63	5.53	3.04	3.01	3.26	1.95	1.69	2.73
Smoking	6.62	5.94	8.48	7.36	6.43	6.49	6.97	9.00
ACEI/ARB §	0.50	0.47	0.56	0.60	0.75	0.67	0.42	0.80
NSAIDS ς	5.67	4.84	5.79	5.56	5.13	5.90	4.77	6.09
Spironolactone	0.43	0.74	0.84	0.28	0.32	0.19	0.32	0.29
Other Medications ℥	0.46	0.36	0.56	0.46	0.37	0.35	0.27	0.44

*Inflammatory bowel disease

† CKD = Chronic Kidney Disease

□ PCOS = Polycystic Ovary Syndrome

‡ PTS (PMS/PMDD) = premenstrual tension syndrome (premenstrual syndrome and premenstrual dysphoric disorder)

§ ACE/ARB = angiotensin-converting enzyme inhibitors/angiotensin receptor blockers

ς NSAID = non-steroidal anti-inflammatory drugs

℥ Other medications = diuretics, heparin, cyclosporine, tacrolimus, trimethoprim, and penicillin G

Table 2 Risk for hyperkalemia* with use of commonly used oral contraceptives

	Crude HR (95% CI)	Adjusted HR† (95%CI)
Levonorgestrel	1.0 (reference)	1.0
Desogestrel	0.93 (0.79-1.09)	1.00 (0.85-1.17)
Drospirenone	1.26 (1.10-1.44)	1.10 (0.95-1.26)
Ethynodiol diacetate	0.96 (0.67-1.38)	0.71 (0.49-1.02)
Norethindrone acetate	1.41 (1.18-1.68)	1.08 (0.91-1.29)
Norethindrone	1.27 (1.11-1.47)	1.15 (1.00-1.33)
Norgestimate	1.13 (0.98-1.29)	1.27 (1.11-1.46)
Norgestrel	1.13 (0.85-1.49)	1.00 (0.76-1.33)

*Hyperkalemia determined from a diagnostic ICD-9 code (276.7)

† Adjusted by age, calendar time, chronic kidney disease, diabetes mellitus, hypertension, inflammatory bowel disease, obesity, polycystic ovary syndrome, premenstrual tension syndrome (premenstrual syndrome and premenstrual dysphoric disorder), smoking status, angiotensin-converting enzyme inhibitors/angiotensin receptor blockers, non-steroidal anti-inflammatory drugs, spironolactone, and other medications known to cause hyperkalemia (cyclosporine, diuretics, heparin, penicillin G, tacrolimus, and trimethoprim).

norethindrone acetate 1.01 (95%CI 0.93-1.08), norethindrone 0.78 (95%CI 0.74-0.83), norgestimate 1.34 (95%CI 1.27-1.41), and norgestrel 0.98 (95%CI 0.89-1.08). The Yasmin® and Yaz® package inserts recommend potassium monitoring within the first treatment cycle for patient taking other medications known to cause hyperkalemia. Of the 5,752 patients who took drospirenone and spironolactone concomitantly, only 376 (6.5%) patients underwent a serum potassium assay within 180 days of starting concomitant therapy.

Discussion

The current study did not find a substantial and meaningful association between drospirenone use and hyperkalemia compared to patients taking levonorgestrel. It is interesting to note that norethindrone and norgestimate are both associated with a higher risk for hyperkalemia compared to levonorgestrel. These however were not *a priori* hypotheses and may be chance findings due to multiple testing. These results must also be taken into context with the low absolute risk for hyperkalemia in OC users. The increased HR for norethindrone of 1.16 results in a number need to harm (NNH) of 3086 patients, while the HR for norgestimate of 1.27 results in a NNH of 1829 patients.

The null association between drospirenone and hyperkalemia is concordant with the results from previous studies [13,23]. To our knowledge, only one prior cohort study has been conducted with the primary aim to evaluate drospirenone and hyperkalemia [13]. This study had 67,287 OC users, identified 378 cases of hyperkalemia, and found a RR comparing drospirenone to other OCs of 0.9 (95%CI 0.7-1.1). Our study population has approximately seventeen times the OC user population of this prior analysis, allowing greater detection for

hyperkalemia and providing increased statistical precision. Another study identified 102 cases of drug-associated hyperkalemia and did not attribute any cases to use of drospirenone [23]. In our study, the comparison among OC users in our analysis minimizes the risk of confounding by indication, and the new user design eliminates the survivor effect that long term OC users are tolerant to the therapy and healthier than short term users. The totality of the evidence suggests that hyperkalemia while on drospirenone is not of clinical importance.

Utilization

We found that drospirenone users are 2.66 times more likely to receive spironolactone compared with levonorgestrel users. An OR of this magnitude suggests that physicians are not avoiding the concomitant use of drospirenone and spironolactone, but prescribing them together. This is a particularly interesting finding because drospirenone is the only OC with a bolded warning for hyperkalemia. These medications have no overlap in labeled indications; however, drospirenone does have an indication for acne vulgaris, while spironolactone has an off-label use for its treatment. Another likely explanation in the recent literature is that drospirenone and spironolactone are both seen as beneficial for treatment of weight gain and bloating experienced by patients with postmenstrual dysphoric disorder and in reducing hirsutism and acne in patients with polycystic ovarian syndrome (PCOS) [24-28].

It was recently reported that, among 11,019 drospirenone users, 17.6% of patients are taking another medication known to induce hyperkalemia [29]. In this study, spironolactone accounted for 11.1% of this concomitant utilization. Our study found that only 6.5% of patients taking drospirenone and spironolactone underwent potassium monitoring. This raises concern that few physicians are following the recommendations for monitoring serum potassium as stated in the package insert.

Although we found a non-significant interaction for hyperkalemia with concomitant use of drospirenone and spironolactone, this does not assure the safe combined use of these two medications. Particularly, patients with PCOS generally express characteristics of metabolic syndrome, are at an increased risk for drug induced liver injury [30], and warrant careful monitoring.

Limitations

The use of ICD-9-CM codes for the detection of hyperkalemia provides a high specificity for diagnosed cases because this diagnosis is made from an assay of serum potassium. This measurement however lacks sensitivity due to a lack of potassium testing in the general population. Inadequacies in documenting ICD-9-CM codes could also lead to underreporting of hyperkalemia. To determine if this was likely to be problematic, we interrogated the Lifelink™ database to investigate control drugs with known associations to hyperkalemia. Amiloride, a potassium-sparing diuretic, spironolactone, an aldosterone antagonist, and all ACE inhibitors were selected as positive controls. The Lifelink™ database was able to replicate three known positive associations: amiloride HR 7.94 (95%CI 1.96-32.08), spironolactone HR 3.46 (95%CI 2.97-4.02), and ACE inhibitors HR 1.90 (95%CI 1.70-2.11). Negative controls selected were loratadine, a non-drowsy antihistamine, topical hydrocortisone, and all statins. All negative associations were replicated: loratadine HR 0.84 (95%CI 0.60-1.20), topical hydrocortisone HR 1.37 (95%CI 0.92-2.05), and statins HR 1.06 (95%CI 0.92-1.22). A positive association was not found between NSAIDS and hyperkalemia (HR 0.93 (95%CI 0.81-1.06)). The above positive and negative controls are reassuring for the ability of this claims database to detect clinically relevant hyperkalemia and to find a null result when no association is known.

The bolded warning for drospirenone and hyperkalemia also has the potential to introduce a measurement bias. This warning makes potassium monitoring in the drospirenone group more likely, inducing a bias away from the null. This anti-conservative bias provides additional confidence in our null result. If channeling bias is present in our study population, steering patients at high risk for hyperkalemia away from drospirenone would provide a bias toward the null. Another interpretation of the study results is that, based on the regulatory framework, current clinical practice is sufficient to mitigate the risk of hyperkalemia in this population.

Due to the nature of a claims database, residual confounding is always present. Alcohol consumption, ethnicity, and diet are all potential unadjusted confounders in our study. Two covariates in the analysis, smoking and obesity, are reported only to justify treatment (such as bariatric surgery or smoking cessation therapy) and are not completely controlled.

Future implications
Although a clinically significant increase in the diagnosis of hyperkalemia was not found in our analysis, a subclinical increase in serum potassium in this population cannot be ruled out. Increased utilization of spironolactone in patients taking drospirenone and poor compliance with the requirement for potassium monitoring in the package insert suggests a lack of attention to the possibility of hyperkalemia. Spironolactone however has a strong association with hyperkalemia, and, for patients taking both spironolactone and drospirenone, it is concerning that so few physicians follow the package insert monitoring recommendations. This

suggests that package inserts may not be an effective mechanism for the communication of drug safety information. If an increase in hyperkalemia had been found in patients taking drospirenone, this current monitoring practice may not have been sufficient to detect it.

Conclusions
In a large cohort of young women, drospirenone did not cause a clinically significant increase in risk for hyperkalemia when compared with other progestin-containing OCs. It is however concerning that, despite the bolded warning for hyperkalemia, drospirenone and spironolactone are used together preferentially. This likely demonstrates a channeling of patients with premenstrual dysphoric disorder and polycystic ovary syndrome to use of drospirenone. Furthermore, physicians are not following the monitoring requirements for serum potassium assays in the package insert for patients taking these two medications.

Author detail
STB and SRP work at the Center for Drug Evaluation and Research in the Food and Drug Administration. JMB is a professor of medicine and epidemiology at McGill University; ME is an assistant professor of medicine in the Pharmaceutical Outcomes Programme at the University of British Columbia; and JACD is an assistant professor of Pharmaceutical Outcomes & Policy at the University of Florida. XL is a graduate student in the department of Pharmaceutical Outcomes & Policy at the University of Florida.

Acknowledgements
This study was supported by an unrestricted operating grant, funded in part by the McGill University Health Center, Fonds de la Recherche en Santé du Québec, and the Ministère de la Santé et des Services Sociaux. The sources of funding had no role in the collection, analysis, and interpretation of data; in the writing of the manuscript; and in the decision to submit the manuscript for publication. Publication of this article was funded in part by the University of Florida Open-Access Publishing Fund.

Author details
[1]Department of Health and Human Services/Food and Drug Administration/ Center for Drug Evaluation and Research (CDER)/Office of Management/ CDER Academic Collaboration Program, Bldg 22, 10903 New Hampshire Avenue, Silver Spring, MD USA 20993. [2]University of Florida, College of Pharmacy, Pharmaceutical Outcomes & Policy, 101 S. Newell Drive (HPNP), PO Box 100496, Gainesville FL, USA 32611. [3]University of British Columbia, Pharmaceutical Outcomes Programme, 709-828 West 10th Avenue, Vancouver, British Columbia, Canada V5Z1M9. [4]McGill University, Royal Victoria Hospital, 687 Pine Street West, Montreal, Quebec H3A 1A1, Canada.

Authors' contributions
JMB, JACD, and ME acquired data for this analysis. All authors contributed to the study design. The statistical analysis was completed by STB and JACD, and all authors contributed to the interpretation of the data. STB wrote the draft manuscript and all authors contributed to critical revision of the manuscript for important intellectual content. JACD is the study guarantor. All authors read and approved the final manuscript for publication.

Competing interests

This manuscript represents the opinions of the authors and not those of the Food and Drug Administration. JMB is a physician scientist who receives peer review financial support from le Fonds de la Recherche en Santé du Québec. The authors have no other competing interests.

References

1. Yasmin [package insert], Wayne NJ: Bayer Healthcare Pharmaceuticals, Inc.; 2010.
2. The World Health Organization: **Cardiovascular disease and steroid hormone contraception.** *Technical Report Series 877* Geneva: The Organization; 1998.
3. Muhn P, Fuhrmann U, Fritzemeier KH, Krattenmacher R, Schillinger E: **Drospirenone: a novel progestogen with antimineralocorticoid and antiandrogenic activity.** *Ann N Y Acad Sci* 1995, **761**:311-335.
4. Heinemann LA, Dinger J: **Safety of a new oral contraceptive containing drospirenone.** *Drug Saf* 2004, **27**(13):1001-1018.
5. **Disorders of the adrenal cortex.** In *Harrison's principles of internal medicine.. 18 edition. Edited by: Longo DL, Kasper DL, Jameson JL, Fauci AS, Hauser SL, Loscalzo J. New York: McGraw-Hill; 2011:.
6. White WB, Pitt B, Preston RA, Hanes V: **Antihypertensive effects of drospirenone with 17β-estradiol, a novel hormone treatment in postmenopausal women with stage 1 hypertension.** *Circulation* 2005, **112**(13):1979-1984.
7. White WB, Hanes V, Chauhan V, Pitt B: **Effects of a new hormone therapy, drospirenone and 17-β-estradiol, in postmenopausal women with hypertension.** *Hypertension* 2006, **48**(2):246-253.
8. Preston RA, White WB, Pitt B, Bakris G, Norris PM, Hanes V: **Effects of drospirenone/17-β estradiol on blood pressure and potassium balance in hypertensive postmenopausal women.** *Am J Hypertens* 2005, **18**(6):797-804.
9. Parsey KS, Pong A: **An open-label, multicenter study to evaluate yasmin, a low-dose combination oral contraceptive containing drospirenone, a new progestogen.** *Contraception* 2000, **61**(2):105-111.
10. Freeman EQ, Kroll R, Rapkin A, Pearlstein T, Brown C, Parsey K, Zhang P, Patel H, Foegh M: **Evaluation of a unique oral contraceptive in the treatment of premenstrual dysphoric disorder.** *J Womens Health Gend Based Med* 2001, **10**(6):561-569.
11. Lüdicke F, Johannisson E, Helmerhorst FM, Campana A, Foidart J, Heithecker R: **Effect of a combined oral contraceptive containing 3 mg of drospirenone and 30 μg of ethinyl estradiol on the human endometrium.** *Fertil Steril* 2001, **76**(1):102-107.
12. Gaspard U, Endrikat J, Desager JP, Buicu C, Gerlinger C, Heithecker R: **A randomized study on the influence of oral contraceptives containing ethinylestradiol combine with drospirenone or desogestrel on lipid and lipoprotein metabolism over a period of 13 cycles.** *Contraception* 2004, **69**(4):271-278.
13. Loughlin J, Seeger JD, Eng PM, Foegh M, Clifford CR, Cutone J, Walker AM: **Risk of hyperkalemia in women taking ethinylestradiol/drospirenone and other oral contraceptives.** *Contraception* 2008, **78**(5):377-383.
14. IMS Health: **LifeLink health plan claims database: overview and study design issues.** [http://uams.edu/cctr/hsrcore/ Lifelink_Health_Plan_Claims_Data_DesignIssues_wcost_April2010%5B1%5D. pdf].
15. Dinger JC, Heinemann LAJ, Kühl-Habich D: **The safety of a drospirenone-containing oral contraceptive: final results from the European active surveillance study on oral contraceptives based on 142,475 women-years of observation.** *Contraception* 2007, **75**(5):344-354.
16. World Health Organization Collaborative Study of Cardiovascular Disease and Steroid Hormone Contraception: **Effect of different progestagens in low oestrogen oral contraceptives on venous thromboembolic disease.** *Lancet* 1995, **346**(8990):1582-1588.
17. Jick H, Jick SS, Gurewich V, Myers MW, Vasilakis C: **Risk of idiopathic cardiovascular death and nonfatal venous thromboembolism in women using oral contraceptives with differing progestagen components.** *Lancet* 1995, **346**(8990):1589-1593.
18. Bloemankamp KW, Rosendaal FR, Helmerhorst FM, Büller HR, Vandenbroucke JP: **Enhancement by factor V leiden mutation of risk of**

19. deep-vein thrombosis associated with oral contraceptives containing a third-generation progestagen. *Lancet* 1995, **346**(8990):1593-1596.
19. Jick H, Kaye JA, Vasilakis-Scaramozza C, Jick SS: **Risk of venous thromboembolism among users of third generation oral contraceptives compared with users of oral contraceptives with levonorgestrel before and after 1995: cohort and case-control analysis.** *BMJ* 2000, **321**(7270):1190-1195.
20. Jick SS, Kaye JA, Russmann S, Jick H: **Risk of nonfatal venous thromboembolism with oral contraceptives containing norgestimate or desogestrel compared with oral contraceptives containing levonorgestrel.** *Contraception* 2006, **73**(6):566-570.
21. Kemmeren JM, Algra A, Grobbee DE: **Third generation oral contraceptives and risk of venous thrombosis: meta-analysis.** *BMJ* 2001, **323**(7305):131-134.
22. Gillessen S, Templeton A, Marra G, Kuo YF, Valtrta E, Shahinian VB: **Risk of colorectal cancer in men on long-term androgen deprivation therapy for prostate cancer.** *J Natl Cancer Inst* 2010, **102**(23):1760-1770.
23. Noize P, Bagheri H, Durrieu G, Haramburo F, Moore N, Giraud P, Galinier M, Pourrat J, Montastruc JL: **Life-threatening drug-associated hyperkalemia: a retrospective study from laboratory signals.** *Pharmacoepidemiol and Drug Saf* .
24. Jarvis CI, Lynch AM, Morin AK: **Management strategies for premenstrual syndrome/premenstrual dysphoric disorder.** *Ann Pharmacother* 2008, **42**(7):967-978.
25. De Berardis D, Serroni N, Salerno RM, Ferro FM: **Treatment of premenstrual dysphoric disorder (PMDD) with a novel formulation of drospirenone and ethinyl estradiol.** *Ther Clin Risk Manag* 2007, **3**(4):585-590.
26. Freeman EW, Kroll R, Rapkin A, Pearlstein T, Brown C, Parsey K, Zhang P, Patel H, Foegh M: **Evaluation of a unique oral contraceptive in the treatment of premenstrual dysphoric disorder.** *J Womens Health Gend Based Med* 2001, **10**(6):561-569.
27. Wang M, Hammarback S, Lindhe BA, Bäckström T: **Treatment of premenstrual syndrome by spironolactone: a double-blind, placebo-controlled study.** *Acta Obstet Gynecol Scand* 1995, **74**(10):803-808.
28. Saha L, Kaur S, Saha PK: **Pharmacotherapy of polycystic ovary syndrome-an update.** *Fundam Clin Pharmacol* .
29. McAdams M, Staffa JA, Dal Pan GJ: **The concomitant prescribing of ethinyl estradiol/drospirenone and potentially interacting drugs.** *Contraception* 2007, **76**(4):278-281.
30. Tarantino G, Conca P, Basile V, Gentile A, Capone D, Polichetti G, Leo E: **A prospective study of acute drug-induced liver injury in patients suffering from non-alcoholic fatty liver disease.** *Hepatol Res* 2007, **37**(6):410-415.

5

Public perception on the role of community pharmacists in self-medication and self-care in Hong Kong

Joyce H You[1], Fiona Y Wong[2], Frank W Chan[2*], Eliza L Wong[2] and Eng-kiong Yeoh[2]

Abstract

Background: The choices for self-medication in Hong Kong are much diversified, including western and Chinese medicines and food supplements. This study was to examine Hong Kong public knowledge, attitudes and behaviours regarding self-medication, self-care and the role of pharmacists in self-care.

Methods: A cross-sectional phone survey was conducted, inviting people aged 18 or older to complete a 37-item questionnaire that was developed based on the Thematic Household surveys in Hong Kong, findings of the health prorfessional focus group discussions on pharmacist-led patient self management and literature. Telephone numbers were randomly selected from residential phone directories. Trained interviewers invited eligible persons to participate using the "last birthday method". Associations of demographic characteristics with knowledge, attitudes and beliefs on self-medication, self-care and role of pharmacists, and spending on over-the-counter (OTC) products were analysed statistically.

Results: A total of 1, 560 phone calls were successfully made and 1, 104 respondents completed the survey which indicated a response rate of 70.8%. 63.1% had adequate knowledge on using OTC products. Those who had no formal education/had attended primary education (OR = 3.19, 95%CI 1.78-5.72; p < 0.001), had attended secondary education (OR = 1.50, 95%CI 1.03-2.19; p = 0.035), and aged ≥60 years (OR = 1.82, 95% CI 1.02-3.26; p = 0.042) were more likely to have inadequate knowledge on self-medication. People with chronic disease also tended to spend more than HKD100 on western (OR = 3.58, 95%CI 1.58-8.09; p = 0.002) and Chinese OTC products (OR = 2.94, 95%CI 1.08-7.95; p = 0.034). 94.6% believed that patients with chronic illnesses should self-manage their diseases. 68% agreed that they would consult a pharmacist before using OTC product but only 45% agreed that pharmacists could play a leading role in self-care. Most common reasons against pharmacist consultation on self-medication and self-care were uncertainty over the role of pharmacists and low acceptance level of pharmacists.

Conclusions: The majority of respondents supported patients with chronic illness to self-manage their diseases but less than half agreed to use a pharmacist-led approach in self-care. The government should consider developing doctors-pharmacists partnership programs in the community, enhancing the role of pharmacists in primary care and providing education to patients to improve their awareness on the role of pharmacists in self-medication and self-care.

Background

Self-care is defined by World Health Organization (WHO) as activities that individuals, families and communities undertake with the intention of enhancing health, preventing disease, limiting illness, and restoring health [1]. Self-care and self-medication have attracted considerable international healthcare policy interest, because they do not only effectively reduce the burden on health services, but also improve compliance and disease outcome [2,3]. These have significant implications to the health system and society at large, as poor adherence to drug regimes among patients would lead to considerable economic and social costs [4]. Evidence suggests that self-care skill-orientated programmes may be more effective than information-only patient education in improving clinical outcomes and reducing health

* Correspondence: cwkfrank@cuhk.edu.hk
[2]School of Public Health and Primary Care, The Chinese University of Hong Kong, Prince of Wales Hospital, Shatin, N.T., Hong Kong
Full list of author information is available at the end of the article

care costs [2]. In the United Kingdom, it had been a new approach to Chronic Disease Management for the 21st Century. The Expert Patient Programme, which aims to introduce lay led self-care training for patients, is expected to become one of a range of integrated self-care options in health and social care for people with long-term conditions [5].

Medication compliance is one of the important elements in self-care. It is common for patients to use over-the-counter (OTC) medicines without the supervision of healthcare professionals, which can limit the opportunity for ongoing patient follow-up and safety monitoring. The establishment of a robust pharmacovigilance system is therefore advocated, in which pharmacists play an important role in providing advice to patients when they purchase OTC drugs [6]. In the UK, there is also a move to promote the role of pharmacists and develop a broader concept of the primary care team [7-9]. Pharmacist's role has been extended to tobacco cessation therapy, local health promotion, advice to family doctors and other health professionals, repeated prescription, advice to nursing and residential homes, health screening and diagnosis, etc [10]. Meanwhile, general practitioners have also become more supportive of pharmacists' extended role in western countries [11,12].

Of the seven-million population in Hong Kong, approximately 20.2% reported to have diseases that required long-term follow-up [13]. The care of patients with chronic illness is a substantial burden to the Hong Kong health system as well as to their care-givers [14]. The choices for self-medication in Hong Kong are much diversified, including western medicines, Chinese medicines and food supplements. The wide spectrum of OTC products potentiates adverse drug events and undesirable drug interactions, particularly in patients receiving chronic drug therapy. The role of pharmacists in Hong Kong, however, mainly focuses on medication management and is much more limited compared to many western countries. To better understand the public perspective on these issues and to develop a policy framework on pharmacist-led self-management in the future, we therefore examined public knowledge, attitudes and behaviour regarding self-medication and self-care of chronic illness as well as the role of community pharmacists in patient self-care and self-medication in Hong Kong.

Methods
Study design and setting
This study was based a cross-sectional phone survey on a random sample of approximately 1, 100 non-institutionalized Hong Kong residents. The survey was conducted by trained interviewers from the telephone survey service team based at the School of Public Health and Primary Care, CUHK. The interviewers had experiences in

conducting numbers of telephone surveys and they were supervised by a project coordinator to ensure survey quality. All phone calls were made between 6:30 pm and 10 pm, during the period of June to July, 2009. Hong Kong permanent residents aged ≥18 years who were able to communicate in Cantonese were eligible to participate in the survey. Telephone numbers were randomly selected from residential phone directories. Interviewers, after briefing the purpose of the study, invited eligible persons to participate in the survey using "the last birthday method". Household member at least 18 years of age, whose birthday was closest to the date of the interview, was invited to complete the survey. Verbal consent was obtained in advance.

The interview was conducted in Cantonese for about 10-15 minutes. Those who were in the city for vacation, or were incapable of responding to survey questions because of psychiatric or neurological disorders were excluded. The interview was pre-tested with 10 subjects. Appropriate adjustments were made before it was administered in the main study.

Instruments
Since a validated pre-developed questionnaire could not be identified, the questionnaire was developed based on the Thematic Household Surveys in Hong Kong [15,16], health professional focus group discussions and literature. It consisted of a total of 37 questions divided into 5 sections: (1) knowledge and attitude on self-medication, (2) utilization and expenses on OTC products including western medicine, Chinese medicine and food supplement, (3) behaviour and attitude on self-care of chronic illnesses, (4) role of pharmacist in patient self-care of chronic illnesses and self-medication, and (5) respondent's demographics. Questions on knowledge and attitude were responded with three choices: agree, no comment/don't know, and disagree. Open-ended questions to explore the reasons of agreeing, no comment and disagreeing of self-care of chronic illnesses, and role of pharmacist in self-care and self-medication, were also developed. The reasons given were further categorized in the analysis. There were a total of six questions on knowledge. "One" point was given for answering each question correctly which gave a full score of 6. OTC products were described as western and Chinese medications and supplements which could be purchased without physicians' prescription. The tasks of pharmacists in pharmacist-led patient self-care of chronic diseases were described as handling of drug-related issues, monitoring the effectiveness and safety of drug treatment, providing information/education on drug therapy and life-style modification, and performing medical triage services. Chronic diseases were explained to the respondents as long-term diseases diagnosed by physicians. They were asked to name the chronic disease(s) they were diagnosed

of. A total of 19 common chronic diseases were listed on the questionnaire. If the disease mentioned was not on the list, the interviewers would mark it down and investigators of this project, who were clinicians, would judge whether the disease was a chronic one.

The questionnaire had been commented and revised by experts and pilot-tested before implementation in the main study.

The study protocol was approved by the Joint CUHK-NTEC Clinical Research Ethics Committee and was performed in accordance with the World Medical Association's Declaration of Helsinki.

Statistical analysis

Descriptive statistics were reported by mean ± standard deviation or percentage, as appropriate. The Hong Kong population size was 6.8 million in mid-2006 [17]. Assuming a prevalence rate of 50%, a sample size of 1100 would provide a precision of 3% from the true values at 95% confidence level. Associations of socio-demographic variables with knowledge, attitudes/beliefs on self-medication, self-care and role of pharmacists, and spending on OTC products were first evaluated using univariate analysis by logistic regression. Factors with significant association in the univariate analysis were further analyzed by stepwise multiple logistic regression analysis. A p-value of < 0.05 was considered as statistically significant.

Results

Characteristics of the study population

A total of 1, 560 phone calls were successfully made and 1, 104 (70.8%) respondents met the selection criteria and completed the survey. Socio-demographic data of the respondents were shown in Table 1. There were 532 (48.2%) male respondents and the largest age group was 30 to 49 years (39.7%).

Knowledge and attitude on self-medication

A majority of respondents had correct knowledge on the need to seek medical care when symptoms continues despite the use of OTC products (98.5%), awareness of drug-food interactions (86.8%) and not to share medications with others who have similar symptoms (84.5%). Over half of the respondents agreed that the OTC products may mask the symptoms of severe underlying diseases (65.2%). Only 23.1% of respondents were correct about Chinese OTC products not necessarily cause less adverse effects than western OTC products. Few respondents (12.6%) agreed that western OTC products can be concurrently used with Chinese OTC products. A total of 1093 respondents completed all the six knowledge questions and 690 (63.1%) scored 4 or above. A cut-off point of 4 was chosen as the mean of knowledge score was 3.71 ± 0.99. Multiple logistic regression analysis showed that lower

Table 1 Demographic characteristics of 1, 104 respondents

	Number
Age (years) (N = 1, 103)*	
18-29	218
30-49	438
50-69	334
≥70	113
Male	532
Presence of chronic disease(s)	215
Education (N = 1, 096)*	
Primary or below	164
Secondary	604
Tertiary or above	328
Family monthly income (HKD) (N = 823)# *	
≤ $5, 999	83 (10.1)
$6, 000- $9, 999	73 (8.9)
$10, 000-$29, 999	424 (51.5)
$30, 000-$59, 999	172 (20.9)
$60, 000 or above	71 (8.6)

*Total number < 1, 104 because of missing data; #HKD1 = USD0.128

education level, including no schooling/primary education (OR = 3.19, 95%CI 1.78-5.72; p < 0.001) and secondary education (OR = 1.50, 95%CI 1.03-2.19; p = 0.035), and patients aged 60 years or above (OR = 1.82, 95% CI 1.02-3.26; p = 0.042) were associated with higher odds of inadequate knowledge score (less than 4) (Table 2).

Utilization and expenses on OTC products

Over the past three months, 363 of 1102 (32.9%) respondents had purchased OTC products. Among these 363 OTC product users, the numbers of people who used western OTC medications only, Chinese OTC products only and food supplement only including vitamins and minerals were 150 (41.3%), 43(11.8%) and 118 (32.5%), respectively. Besides, the numbers of people who used western and Chinese OTC products, western OTC products and food supplement, Chinese OTC products and food supplement, and western and Chinese OTC products and food supplement were 24 (6.6%), 16 (4.4%), 6 (1.7%) and 6 (1.7%), respectively. The most commonly used western OTC products were common cold medicines (108/196; 55.1%) and oral analgesics (73/196; 37.2%). The most commonly used Chinese OTC products were proprietary medicines (27/79; 34.2%) and herbal medicines (25/79; 31.56%). Most of the respondents spent HKD 100 or less in purchasing western OTC products (80.7%) and Chinese OTC products (48%), while 59.2% spent HKD 101-500 in food supplement including vitamins and minerals (HKD1 = USD0.128). As the proportion of spending HKD100 versus over HKD100 was approximately 50/50, therefore, the breakpoint of

Table 2 Factors affecting knowledge score on self-medication

	Univariate analysis (Chi-square) Knowledge Score				Multivariate analysis (Logistic regression) Knowledge Score < 4	
	< 4 n (%)	≥4 n (%)	X^2	P	OR (95% CI)	P
Age						
18-29	64 (15.9)	154 (22.4)	49.05	< 0.001	reference	
30-59	208 (51.6)	434 (63.0)			0.97 (0.64-1.47)	0.893
60 or above	131 (32.5)	101 (14.7)			1.82 (1.02-3.26)	0.042
Gender						
Male	191 (47.5)	340 (49.3)	0.316	0.616	0.91 (0.67-1.23)	0.529
Female	211 (52.5)	350 (50.7)			reference	
Education						
No schooling/primary	100 (25.1)	61 (8.9)	64.74	< 0.001	3.19 (1.78-5.72)	< 0.001
Secondary	218 (54.6)	379 (55.2)			1.50 (1.03-2.19)	0.035
Diploma/degree	81 (20.3)	246 (35.9)			reference	
Monthly household income (HK$)[#]						
< $2000-$5999	37 (13.4)	45 (8.3)	11.98	0.007	0.90 (0.48-1.68)	0.746
$6000-$9999	27 (9.8)	46 (8.5)			0.99 (0.55-1.78)	0.973
$10000-$24999	130 (47.1)	231 (42.5)			1.20 (0.83-1.73)	0.336
≥$25000	82 (29.7)	221 (40.7)			reference	
Presence of chronic illness						
Yes	309 (76.9)	571 (82.9)	5.88	0.017	1.03 (0.68-1.57)	0.877
No	93 (23.1)	118 (17.1)			reference	

[#]HKD1 = USD0.128

HKD100 was selected for the analysis. Multiple logistic regression analysis showed that the presence of chronic disease was a significant predictor of spending over HKD100 on western OTC products (OR = 3.58, 95%CI 1.58-8.09; p = 0.002) and Chinese OTC products (OR = 2.94, 95%CI 1.08-7.95; p = 0.034) (Table 3). No influential factor was identified on the spending of food supplement.

Questions on attitudes/beliefs of self-medication using OTC products indicated that 30.8% (339/1100) respondents believed that OTC products should be used at the occurrence of first sign/symptom. Less than half of the respondents believed that OTC products were effective (390/1098; 35.5%) or safe (490/1099; 44.6%). Most of respondents (983/1093; 89.8%) would follow instructions on package. Of 1, 098 respondents, 754 (68.3%) agreed that users should consult a pharmacist before using OTC product, whereas 238 (21.6%) disagree and 112 (10.1%) had no comment on consulting the pharmacist. Of the 347 respondents who either had no comment or disagreed to consulting pharmacists, their most common reasons were unsure about the role of pharmacists, not seeing the need to consult a pharmacist, and low level of acceptance/trust to pharmacists. Multiple logistic regression showed that female gender (OR = 1.62; 95%CI 1.18-2.17; p < 0.003) and aged 18-29 years (OR = 1.99; 95%CI 1.08-3.64; p = 0.026) were two demographic factors associated with positive attitude towards pharmacist consultation on OTC products.

Behaviour and attitude on self-care of chronic illnesses

Majority of the respondents (1024/1082; 94.6%) believed that patients with chronic illnesses should participate in self-management of their diseases, including life-style modification, routine monitoring of clinical parameters (e. g. blood pressure and blood glucose) and compliance to drug treatment. 19.5% (215/1102) respondents reported that they had chronic disease(s). The three most common chronic conditions were hypertension (n = 104; 49.1%), diabetes mellitus (n = 32; 15.1%) and hypercholesterolemia (n = 27; 12.7%). Among the respondents with chronic diseases, most of them always complied with medication (n = 188; 90.4%), complied with follow-up appointment (n = 187; 89.9%) and monitored own disease progress (n = 180, 84.5%) (Table 4). The mostly reported barriers against chronic disease self-care were lack of disease knowledge (n = 88; 43.1%), lack of monitoring equipment (n = 85; 41.5%) and unstable health status (n = 84; 40.6%) (Table 4). Patients under 60 years of age were less likely to participate in self-care of chronic diseases (OR = 0.30, 95%CI = 0.13-0.71; p = 0.006).

Role of pharmacist in patient self-care of chronic illnesses and self-medication

Less than half of the (497/1102; 45.1%) respondents agreed that pharmacists could play a leading role in patient self-care of chronic diseases, whereas 492 (44.6%) disagreed and 113 (10.3%) were neutral. The most common reasons for agreeing was that pharmacists facilitate medical service triage when needed (n = 206; 41.9%) and are able to monitor disease condition (n = 170, 34.6%). Those who did not agree believed that pharmacists should not take the leading role (n = 325; 67.1%) and were not familiar with the role of pharmacists (n = 80; 16.6%). Respondents in the age group of 18-29 years were more likely to support pharmacist-led patient self-care, showed by multiple logistic regression (OR = 1.6, 95%CI = 1.06-2.42; p = 0.027).

Discussion

It is inferred from our study that approximately 60% of population in the Hong Kong community had adequate knowledge on using OTC products, primarily on western OTC products (> 60%). However, those who were at lower education level and elderly were more likely to have inadequate knowledge on using OTC products. Almost one-third (32.6%) of the respondents had purchased OTC products over the past 3 months and the majority (89.8%) claimed to follow product package instructions, which were quite consistent with the findings of the study of Wazaify and her team [18]. Our study also showed that Chinese patients with chronic diseases tended to spend more money on western and Chinese OTC products than those without chronic diseases. A study in Australia also found that 80% of their patients with a chronic condition used OTC products and many of them were not using the right dose [19]. It is therefore anticipated that patients with chronic diseases would be prone to higher risk of drug interactions between prescription drugs for chronic diseases and OTC products [20]. Based on previous studies and our research findings, elderly who received lower education and with a chronic condition are at high risk of improper use of OTC products and they are the group which needs pharmacist counselling most.

The majority (94.6%) of the population supported the practice of self-care for chronic diseases, and over 80% of those with chronic diseases claimed to perform self-care tasks regularly. Community pharmacist-provided self-care programmes had demonstrated positive impact on chronic diseases. Doucette et al. conducted a randomized controlled trial in patients with diabetes to evaluate the effect of community pharmacist-provided extended diabetes care service on patients' self-care activities [21]. Patients in the intervention group increased the number of days per week significantly (1.25 versus 0.73 days/week) engaging in diabetes diet and self-care activities. Barbanel et al. also demonstrated that patients with asthma in a self-care programme delivered by a community pharmacist had significantly better improvement of

Table 3 Factors affecting amount spent in purchasing western and Chinese OTC products

| | Western OTC products | | | | Multivariate Analysis (Logistic Regression) | | Chinese OTC products | | | | Multivariate Analysis (Logistic Regression) | |
| | Univariate analysis (Chi-square) | | | | | | Univariate analysis (Chi-square) | | | | | |
	≤ $100 n (%)	$101 or above n (%)	X^2	P	$101 or above OR (95% CI)	P	≤ $100 n (%)	$101 or above n (%)	X^2	P	$101 or above OR (95% CI)	P
Age (yrs)												
18-29	34 (22.5)	5 (13.9)	1.61	0.446			5 (14.3)	4 (10.3)	0.28	0.868		
30-59	99 (65.6)	25 (69.4)					23 (65.7)	27 (69.2)				
60 or above	18 (11.9)	6 (16.7)					7 (20.0)	8 (20.5)				
Gender												
Male	74 (49.3)	12 (33.3)	2.99	0.096	0.54 (0.25-1.19)	0.126	18 (50.0)	12 (30.8)	0.29	0.104	0.50 (0.19-1.31)	0.157
Female	76 (50.7)	24 (66.7)			reference		18 (50.0)	27 (69.2)			reference	
Education												
No schooling/primary	14 (9.3)	3 (8.3)	0.11	0.949			5 (14.3)	8 (21.1)	0.86	0.651		
Secondary	79 (52.7)	20 (55.6)					18 (51.4)	20 (52.6)				
Diploma/degree	57 (38.0)	13 (36.1)					12 (34.3)	10 (26.3)				
Monthly household income (HK$)#												
< $2000-$5999	7 (5.4)	2 (8.0)	3.05	0.384			1 (3.8)	4 (14.8)	2.16	0.339		
$6000-$9999	12 (9.2)	0					0	0				
$10000-$24999	56 (43.1)	10 (40.0)					15 (57.7)	12 (44.4)				
≥$25000	55 (42.3)	13 (52.0)					10 (38.5)	11 (40.7)				
Presence of chronic illness												
Yes	22 (14.6)	14 (38.9)	11.06	0.002	3.58 (1.58-8.09)	0.002	9 (25.0)	20 (51.3)	5.45	0.032	2.94 (1.08-7.95)	0.034
No	129 (85.4)	22 (61.1)			reference		27 (75.0)	19 (48.7)			reference	

#HKD1 = USD0.128

Table 4 Behaviours related to self-care and the potential barriers of respondents with chronic conditions

	Frequency in performing behaviours related to self-care		
	Always/ Most of the time n (%)	Sometimes n (%)	Not very often/Never n (%)
Disease progress monitoring#	180 (84.5%)	12 (5.6%)	21 (9.9%)
Medication compliance	188 (90.4%)	8 (3.8%)	12 (5.8%)
Clinic follow-up compliance	187 (89.9%)	7 (3.4%)	14 (6.7%)
Lifestyle modification	158 (74.9%)	28 (13.3%)	25 (11.8%)
Obtain emotional support	84 (44.7%)	27 (14.4%)	77 (41.0%)
Obtain caregiver support	124 (63.9%)	23 (11.9%)	47 (24.2%)
Potential barriers inhibiting self-care of chronic conditions			
	n (%)		
Lack of disease knowledge (n = 204)	88 (43.1%)		
Lack of monitoring equipment (n = 205)	85 (41.5%)		
Unstable health status (n = 207)	84 (40.6%)		
Lack of family/friend's support (n = 212)	70 (33.0%)		
Lack of motivation (n = 203)	62 (30.5%)		

#Measurement of blood pressure or blood glucose

symptom scores (adjusted difference for baseline scores = 7.0 (95% CI = 4.4-9.5)) [22]. Self-care programmes provided by community pharmacists had established ground works in various chronic illnesses through health services research in western populations, yet such evidence is limited for populations in Hong Kong, China as well as other Asia regions. Though there is evidence to support the effectiveness of pharmacist-led self-care programme, only less than half (45.5%) of the population supported the pharmacist-led approach according to our study.

The evolution of the Hong Kong healthcare system and the health policy might explain why Hong Kong people have a low acceptance rate on pharmacist-led self-care management. In Hong Kong, patients receive health services from either private or public sectors seldom have the opportunity to consult community pharmacists as patients usually receive prescribed medications from private doctors directly or from government clinic pharmacies. Community pharmacists would only have the chance to provide consultation when patients visited them to buy drugs over the counter. Patients, therefore, are not familiar with the role of pharmacists besides dispensing drugs and not very supportive of pharmacist-led self-care management.

A study on the perspectives of physicians, pharmacists, traditional Chinese medicine practitioners and dispensers on patient self-care and roles of pharmacists indicated the importance of patients to self-care of their chronic conditions and they also supported pharmacists to be involved in patient self-care and take a major role in managing patients' medication issues. To provide successful continuity of care after patients return to the community, connectivity among patients, health professions and health services within the system is vital [23]. With the support

of medicine professionals [24] and approximately 45% of people agreed with the pharmacist-led approach in this study, there are a few strategies that can be considered to enhance the familiarity level of patients and people in the community with pharmacists.

Community pharmacists can undertake a more active role in health promotion campaign such as drug safety in order to increase their publicity. Besides, partnership programmes can be developed between doctors and pharmacists in the community so that patients can consult pharmacists when they are not able to make their appointments with doctors. In addition, it is also necessary for the government to enhance the involvement of pharmacists in primary care and promote the roles of pharmacists through patient education, so that people can have more opportunities to communicate and contact with pharmacists.

Limitations

The present study was limited by the relatively small number (total 37) of questions in the questionnaire. Our description of self-care activities in the survey might be inadequate. A case scenario would have provided more detailed requirements for self-care of chronic diseases and better described the role of pharmacists. The respondents therefore might have underestimated the complexity of self-care and the role of pharmacist for each common chronic disease, including hypertension, hyperlipidaemia and diabetes mellitus. In addition, those who responded to the survey could be more interested and knowledgeable about patient self-care and role of pharmacists. The views of people who refused to participate could have been neglected in this study.

Conclusions

Over 60% of the present cohort showed adequate knowledge on using OTC products and patients with chronic diseases tended to spend more on OTC products. The majority of respondents supported self-care for chronic diseases. However less that half supported pharmacist-led self- care programmes despite the fact that elderly people and those with lower education level and a chronic condition were at high risk of encountering problems with OTC products. To overcome these limitations, self-care programmes provided by pharmacists should be gradually developed with the support of the Hong Kong SAR Government.

Acknowledgements

We thank the Food and Health Bureau of the HKSAR Government for supporting this study and all interviewers and respondents who participated in the interview.

Author details

[1]School of Pharmacy, The Chinese University of Hong Kong, Shatin, N.T., Hong Kong. [2]School of Public Health and Primary Care, The Chinese University of Hong Kong, Prince of Wales Hospital, Shatin, N.T., Hong Kong.

Authors' contributions

JHY, FYW and FWC drafted the manuscripts. FYW performed data analysis. All authors were involved in the design of the study and approved the final manuscript.

Competing interests

The authors declare that they have no competing interests.

References

1. Global status report on noncommunicable diseases 2010. World Health Organization; 2011.
2. Bodenheimer T, Lorig K, Holman H, Grumbach K: Patient self-management of chronic disease in primary care. JAMA 2002, 288:2469-2475.
3. Chodosh J, Morton SC, Mojica W, Maglione M, Suttorp MJ, Hilton L, Rhodes S, Shekelle P: Meta-analysis: chronic disease self-management programs for older adults. Ann Intern Med 2005, 143:427-438.
4. Kinsey Quarterly: Getting patients to take their medicine.[http://www.mckinseyquarterly.com/article_abstract_visitor.aspx?ar=1872&l2=12&l3=62&srid=17&gp=0#registerNow].
5. Department of Health, NHS: The Expert Patients Programme: Introduction.[http://www.dh.gov.uk/en/Aboutus/MinistersandDepartmentLeaders/ChiefMedicalOfficer/ProgressOnPolicy/ProgressBrowsableDocument/DH_5380844].
6. Bergmann JF: Self-medication: from European regulatory directives to therapeutic strategy. Fundam Clin Pharmacol 2003, 17:275-280.
7. Department of Health, Pharmacy in the future-implementing the NHS plan: a programme for pharmacy in the National Health Services 2000. .
8. Hartnell NR, MacKinnon NJ, Sketris IS, Gass D: The roles of community pharmacists in managing patients with diabetes: Perceptions of health care professionals in Nova Scotia. Canadian Pharmacists Journal 2005, 138:46-53.
9. Dowell J, Cruikshank J, Bain J, Staines H: Repeat dispensing by community pharmacists: advantages for patients and practitioners. Br J Gen Pract 1998, 48:1858-1859.
10. King's Fund, United Kingdom: Developing Community Pharmacy [http://www.kingsfund.org.uk/document.rm?id=109].
11. Ford S, Jones K: Integrating pharmacy fully into the primary care team. BMJ 1995, 310:1620-1621.
12. Erwin J, Britten N, Jones R: General practitioners' views on over the counter sales by community pharmacists. BMJ 1996, 312:617-618.
13. Census and Statistics Department, Hong Kong Special Administrative Region: Thematic Household Survey 2007, July. Report No.:30.
14. You JHS, Ho SC, Sham A: Economic burden of informal caregivers for Chinese Elderly in Hong Kong. Journal of the American Geriatrics Society 2008, 56:1577-1578.
15. Census and Statistics Department, Hong Kong Special Administrative Region: Thematic Household Survey; 2000, December. Report No.:3.
16. Census and Statistics Department, Hong Kong Special Administrative Region: Thematic Household Survey; 2006, August. Report No.:26.
17. Census and Statistics Department, Hong Kong Special Administrative Region: 2006 Population by-census , Main report: Volume 1.
18. Wazaify M, Shields E, Hughes CM, McElnay JC: Society perspectives on over-the-counter (OTC) medicines. Family Practice 2005, 22:170-176.
19. Guirguis K: The use of nonprescription medicines among elderly patients with chronic illness and their need for pharmacist interventions. Consult Pharm 2010, 25:433-439.
20. Kaufman DW, Kelly JP, Rosenberg L, Anderson TE, Mitchell AA: Recent patterns of medication use in the ambulatory adult population of the United States: The Slone survey. JAMA 2002, 287:337-344.
21. Doucette WR, Witry MJ, Farris KB, McDonough RP: Community pharmacist-provided extended diabetes care. Ann Pharmacother 2009, 43:882-889.
22. Barbanel D, Eldridge S, Griffiths C: Can a self-management programme delivered by a community pharmacist improve asthma control? A randomized trial. Thorax 2003, 58:851-854.
23. Sparbel KJH, Anderson MA: Integrated literature review of continuity of care: Part 1, Conceptual issues. J Nursing Scholarship 2000, 32:17-24.
24. Wong FY, Chan FW, You JH, Wong EL, Yeoh EK: Patient Self-management and pharmacist-led patient self-management in Hong Kong: a focus group study from different healthcare professionals' perspectives. BMC Health Services Research 2011, 11:121.

6

Population prevalence of high dose paracetamol in dispensed paracetamol/opioid prescription combinations: an observational study

Roderick Clark[1], Judith E Fisher[2,3], Ingrid S Sketris[2*] and Grace M Johnston[4]

Abstract

Background: Paracetamol (acetaminophen) is generally considered a safe medication, but is associated with hepatotoxicity at doses above doses of 4.0 g/day, and even below this daily dose in certain populations.

Methods: The Nova Scotia Prescription Monitoring Program (NSPMP) in the Canadian province of Nova Scotia is a legislated organization that collects dispensing information on all out-of-hospital prescription controlled drugs dispensed for all Nova Scotia residents. The NSPMP provided data to track all paracetamol/opioids redeemed by adults in Nova Scotia, from July 1, 2005 to June 30, 2010. Trends in the number of adults dispensed these prescriptions and the numbers of prescriptions and tablets dispensed over this period were determined. The numbers and proportions of adults who filled prescriptions exceeding 4.0 g/day and 3.25 g/day were determined for the one-year period July 1, 2009 to June 30, 2010. Data were stratified by sex and age (<65 versus 65+).

Results: Both the number of prescriptions filled and the number of tablets dispensed increased over the study period, although the proportion of the adult population who filled at least one paracetamol/opioid prescription was lower in each successive one-year period. From July 2009 to June 2010, one in 12 adults (n = 59,197) filled prescriptions for over 13 million paracetamol/opioid tablets. Six percent (n = 3,786) filled prescriptions that exceeded 4.0 g/day and 18.6% (n = 11,008) exceeded 3.25 g/day of paracetamol at least once. These findings exclude non-prescription paracetamol and paracetamol–only prescribed medications.

Conclusions: A substantial number of individuals who redeem prescriptions for paracetamol/opioid combinations may be at risk of paracetamol-related hepatotoxicity. Healthcare professionals must be vigilant when prescribing and dispensing these medications in order to reduce the associated risks.

Background

Paracetamol (acetaminophen) is a commonly used analgesic that has been considered safe at doses below 4.0 grams per day. [1-3] However, acute overdose [4], chronic doses over 4–6 g/day [5] and lower doses in certain populations [3,6-8], may be associated with hepatotoxicity. The Acute Liver Failure Study Group found that the median dose among American patients with unintentional overdose causing acute liver failure was 7.5 g per day, range of 1.0-78 g. [4] Paracetamol-related hepatotoxicity occurs through a complex sequence.[9,10] In high single doses (15 g or more), paracetamol causes hepatic injury through a toxic metabolite, NAPQI (N-acetyl-p-benzoquinone imine) [11,12]. Acetaminophen has been postulated to cause liver injury by mechanisms including glutathione depletion, oxidative stress and mitochondrial dysfunction leading to loss of adenosine triphosphate (ATP). Factors that induce cytochrome P-450, such as alcohol consumption and possibly, malnutrition, increase NAPQI synthesis and contribute to glutathione depletion, enhancing paracetamol-related hepatotoxicity [3,11,12].

Paracetamol-induced hepatotoxicity as a result of intentional or unintentional overdose is the most common drug-related cause of acute liver failure (ALF) in the USA, UK, Canada and most European countries, accounting for about one-half of all cases in the USA. [4,8,12-15] In the USA, about 150,000 poisoning cases

* Correspondence: ingrid.sketris@dal.ca
[2]College of Pharmacy, Faculty of Health Professions, Dalhousie University, Halifax, NS, Canada
Full list of author information is available at the end of the article

were attributed to paracetamol in 2009, according to the Annual Report of the American Association of Poison Control Center's National Poison Data System. [16] An estimated 70,000 cases occur annually in the UK [17,18]; in Canada, the estimated annual incidence of paracetamol overdose between 1997 and 2002 was about 46 per 100,000 population[13]. A substantial proportion of these cases may be unintentional or 'therapeutic misadventures'. Two American studies report that respectively one-half [4] and two-thirds [19] of identified paracetamol-related overdose cases were unintentional. In 2011 in Nova Scotia, there were 62 calls to the Nova Scotia Poison Centre with unintentional paracetamol (or paracetamol combination product) poisonings in people over 18 years of age. Of these, 23 were paracetamol/opioid combination products (Kim Sheppard R.N., B.ScN., CSPI. Clinical Leader IWK Regional Poison Centre. Personal Communication, April 13th 2012). Paracetamol toxicity can be difficult to diagnose, however; one study suggests that 18% of indeterminate cases of liver failure referred to an American tertiary care centre were due to unrecognized paracetamol toxicity [20].

A large number of paracetamol-containing products are available as both non-prescription and prescription medications. For example, as of August 2011, there were 434 paracetamol-containing medications available on the Canadian market.[21] Non-prescription products include cough and cold preparations, and analgesics and antipyretics. The high rates of paracetamol use may be due in part to recommendations that persons using acetylsalicylic acid for arthritis or other painful conditions consider taking paracetamol, to reduce the potential for gastrointestinal side effects [22].

Prescription medications include combinations with opioid analgesics such as hydrocodone, oxycodone and codeine. Paracetamol/opioid compounds are implicated in a substantial proportion of paracetamol-induced hepatotoxicity cases.[4,23] For example, an American study found that 44% of individuals in a cohort of 275 consecutive patients with paracetamol-related ALF reported taking a prescription paracetamol/opioid combination. [4] These medications are very commonly prescribed in both the USA and Canada. In 2010, 131 million prescriptions for acetaminophen (paracetamol) in combination with hydrocodone were filled in the USA, making this medication the most commonly dispensed prescription drug.[24] This combination is not available in Canada; however, Canadians filled about 8.3 million prescriptions in 2010 for paracetamol/opioid compounds, such as acetaminophen (paracetamol)/caffeine/codeine combinations (~5.5 million) and acetaminophen (paracetamol)/oxycodone (~2.7 million).[25] Because these products are fixed dose combinations, increasing the opioid dose results in an increase in the paracetamol

dose also. Therefore, such fixed dose combinations may not be appropriate for all patients; for some patients, the paracetamol and opioid should be titrated separately. [26] Further, the relative contribution of the opioid to the hepatotoxicity is unknown [27].

Professional and public education initiatives and legislation to limit paracetamol use are increasingly being suggested, in order to limit the potential harm from overuse of paracetamol. [20,28-30] However, only a few population level studies, all using American data, [31,32] have documented the prevalence of paracetamol use exceeding the dosage limits recommended by regulatory bodies. The objective of this study is to provide population-based Canadian data on the prevalence of high-dose paracetamol use from prescribed paracetamol/opioid combinations.

Methods

Data were extracted from the electronic database of the Nova Scotia Prescription Monitoring Program (NSPMP). Paracetamol/opioid combinations are "controlled substances" under Canadian federal [33] and provincial legislation. In the province of Nova Scotia, the monitoring of prescribed controlled substances dispensed in the community is the legislated responsibility of the NSPMP.[34,35] The NSPMP collects dispensing information on all controlled drugs for all people dispensed in NS community pharmacies within an electronic database, and reviews and investigates use patterns that suggest potentially inappropriate use.[34,35] This database does not include medications dispensed while a person is in hospital, but it does include medications prescribed for nursing home residents.

The study population included all Nova Scotia residents age 19+ years eligible for provincial health benefits who were dispensed any paracetamol/opioid combination (World Health Organization (WHO) Anatomical Therapeutic Chemical (ATC) Classification: N02AA59, N02BE51)[36] in community pharmacies from July 1, 2005 to June 30, 2010. In Nova Scotia, virtually all residents are eligible for provincial health benefits.[37] The adult population of Nova Scotia increased from 751,000 to 768,000 over this period.[38]

For each one-year period, July 1, 2005 to June 30, 2010, three totals were extracted: individuals filling at least one paracetamol/opioid prescription; paracetamol/opioid prescriptions dispensed; and tablets dispensed. The trend over time (2005–2010) was examined using the Cochran-Armitage test [39].

The average paracetamol daily dose was calculated for each individual who filled a paracetamol/opioid prescription from July 1, 2009 to June 30, 2010 (mg paracetamol per tablet X quantity of tablets dispensed/days' supply). These products contain either 300 mg or 325 mg paracetamol per tablet.[21] Provincial regulations [40] require prescribers to include the intended days' supply on the prescription. The numbers of individuals who filled prescriptions supplying average daily doses exceeding 3.25 g and 4.0 g during this period at least once and more than once were determined.

The data were stratified by sex and age (<65 years, 65+). Differences by sex and age for each one-year period were examined using chi square tests with Microsoft Excel 2010^{TM}.

Dalhousie Health Sciences Ethics Review Board approved the research protocol.

Results

Both the number of prescriptions filled and the number of tablets dispensed increased over the study period (Figure 1). Tests for trend showed an annual increase from July 2005 through June 2010 in the total prescriptions by age and sex and in total tablets by age. However, as shown in Figures 1 and 2, the number of individuals and the proportion of the adult population who filled at least one paracetamol/opioid prescription was lower in each successive one-year period from 2005 to 2010 [e.g. 64,567 (8.6%) in 2005/06 versus 59,197 (7.7%) in 2009/10].

In each one-year period, a greater proportion of women than men filled at least one prescription for paracetamol/opioid combinations [e.g. 8.9% versus. 8.3% in 2005/06, and 8.0% versus 7.4% in 2009/10,   p < .001]. A greater proportion of individuals age 65 and older, than those younger than 65, filled at least one prescription.

Among the 7.7% of adult Nova Scotians who filled at least one prescription for paracetamol/opioids in 2009/10, 18.6% (n = 11,008) filled prescriptions providing an average daily paracetamol dose over 3.25 g at least once and 6.4% (n = 3,786) over 4.0 g/day (Table 1). Individuals exceeded these respective dose limits more than once at rates of 21% (n = 2,307) and 10% (n = 395), respectively.

A greater proportion of women than men filled prescriptions exceeding 4.0 g/day [6.7% versus 6.0%,   p < .001] and 3.25 g/day [19.1% versus 18.0%, p = .001] at least once during this one-year period. A larger percentage of women than men exceeded 3.25 g/day more than once [26.1% versus 14.6%, p < .001].

Compared with those age 65 and older, a greater proportion of younger individuals filled prescriptions exceeding 4.0 g/day [6.9% versus 4.9%, p < .001] at least once. However, a similar proportion of younger and older individuals filled prescriptions exceeding 3.25 g/day [18.5% versus 18.9%, ns]. A larger percentage of those age 65 and older filled prescriptions exceeding these daily limits more than once [14.2% (65+) versus 9.5% (<65), p < .001 (4.0 g/day); 25.9% versus 19.3%, p < .001 (3.25 g/day)].

Discussion

Of the approximately 760,000 adults in Nova Scotia from 2005–2009, almost 60,000 (7.9%) adults, redeemed an out-of-hospital prescription for paracetamol/opioid combinations over a one-year period (July 2009/2010). Of this 60,000, almost 4,000 (6.7%) filled prescriptions at least once that provided daily doses exceeding the usual

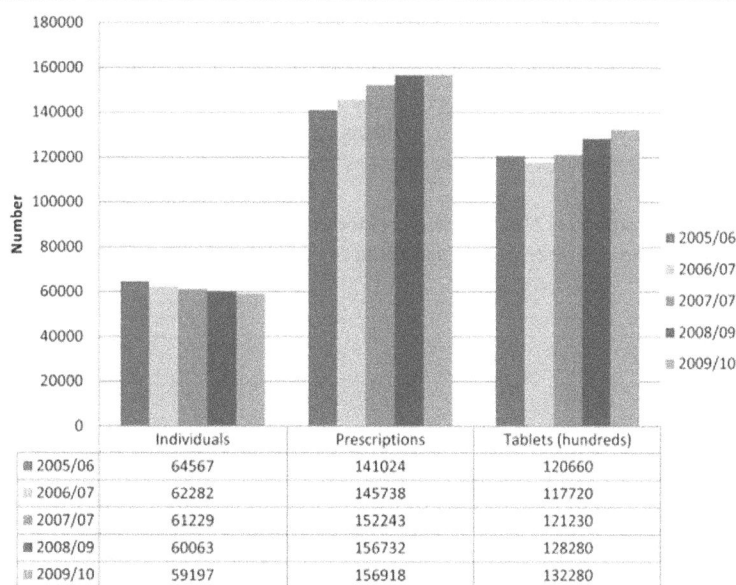

	Individuals	Prescriptions	Tablets (hundreds)
2005/06	64567	141024	120660
2006/07	62282	145738	117720
2007/07	61229	152243	121230
2008/09	60063	156732	128280
2009/10	59197	156918	132280

Figure 1 The number of adult (age 19+) Nova Scotia residents who filled at least one paracetamol/opioid prescription, prescriptions filled and tablets dispensed (in hundreds) in each one-year period from July 1, 2005 to June 30, 2010.

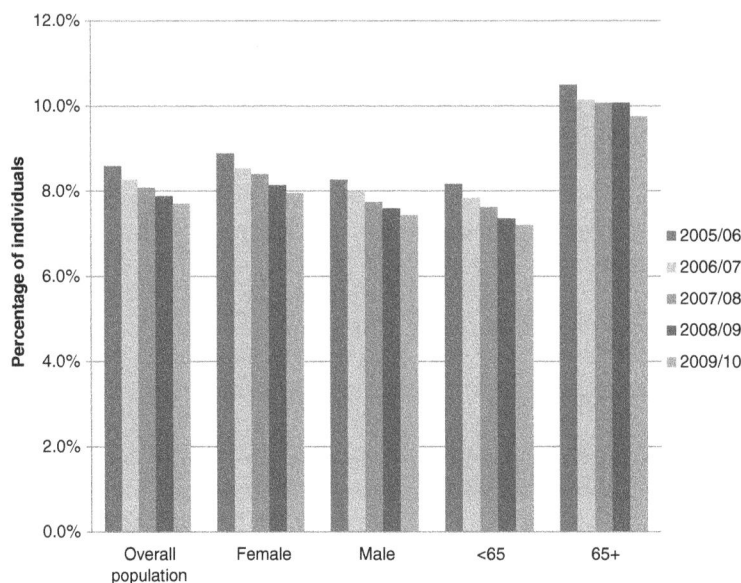

Figure 2 Percentage of adult (age 19+) Nova Scotia residents who filled at least one prescription for paracetamol/opioid, by sex and age, and overall, per one-year period: July 1, 2005 to June 30, 2010. Denominator is adult population of Nova Scotia for each year, based on data from Statistics Canada.

Health Canada recommended maximum (4.0 g). This finding is consistent with the findings of Mort et al. [41] and Albertson et al. [32] who report rates of 8.1% and 5.9% respectively, but lower than the rate (23.3%) observed in other studies [31]. The Nova Scotia and other study findings are considered underestimates because they exclude medications dispensed in-hospital, non-prescription paracetamol containing products and paracetamol–only prescriptions. However, an advantage of the Nova Scotia study over previously published population studies is that this study includes virtually all persons in a geographic area and is not limited by the enrollment criteria of US-based health insurance programs.

One in five, more than 10,000 individuals, filled at least one prescription with a daily paracetamol dose greater than 3.25 g. Further, the number and percentage of adults redeeming out-of-hospital prescriptions for paracetamol/opioid combinations decreased in each year from 2005 through 2010, despite a slight population increase, but the numbers of prescriptions filled and tablets dispensed increased. This finding suggests that fewer individuals filled more prescriptions for more tablets over this period. Taken together, these findings raise concerns regarding the potential for a substantial number of adults to be at risk for paracetamol-induced hepatotoxicity due to the unintentional ingestion of high doses of paracetamol.

Table 1 Number and Percent of adult (age 19+) Nova Scotia residents who fill at least one prescription for an acetaminophen/opioid product and whose prescriptions are filled for over 3.25 g/day and 4.0 g/day (July 1st 2009 to June 30th 2010)

		Individuals who filled at least one prescription	Average prescriptions per individual[1]	> 3.25 g/day(%)	> 4.0 g/day(%)
Sex	Male	27,384	2.53	4,939 (18 %)	2,145(7.8%)
	Female	31,813	2.80	6,069 (19.0%)	1,641 (5.1%)
Age	<65	44,443	2.62	8,216 (18.4%)	3,062 (6.8%)
	65+	14,754	2.75	2,792 (18.9%)	724 (4.9%)
Total		59,197	2.68	11,008 (18.6 %)	3,786 (6.4 %)

1. "Average prescriptions" was computed based on the total number of individuals who filled at least one prescription divided by the total number of prescriptions dispensed during this time period.
2. The denominator for the percentage is individuals who filled at least one prescription during this time period.

Certain sub-populations may be particularly vulnerable to accidental overdose. The findings suggest that older persons, i.e. those age 65 and over, may fill more prescriptions for these combinations than younger persons, and for larger quantities of tablets. Older persons may be particularly likely to consume paracetamol-containing medications long-term because of their high prevalence of painful conditions such as osteoarthritis.[42] The finding that among those who filled prescriptions exceeding 4.0 g/day or 3.25 g/day, older persons were significantly more likely to do so multiple times raises concerns that they may be at increased risk of chronically consuming high-dose paracetamol.

Similarly, women may be at higher risk than men, given that a greater percentage of women than men filled any prescription and filled prescriptions that exceeded 4.0 g/day (7%) and 3.25 g/day (19%). Li and Martin [2011] observed a higher rate of paracetamol overdose among females presenting in emergency departments that provide care to children, youth and adults. [43] The authors speculated that compared with males, females use more non-prescription analgesics for longer durations, and are more likely to use these medications in suicide attempts. [43] In contrast, Mort et al. [41] observed a significantly higher rate of paracetamol use among male beneficiaries of three insurance programs. The possibility of an interaction between sex and age was not examined in any of these studies, and the population characteristics varied markedly.

More than one-quarter of women and one-quarter of persons age 65 and over who filled prescriptions that provided more than 3.25 g/day did so multiple times. These patterns of use, together with the widespread availability and use of non-prescribed paracetamol-containing products raise the potential for the unintentional consumption of high – and potentially hepatotoxic – doses of paracetamol. Individuals may take paracetamol-containing products such as a cough and cold preparation or plain non-prescription paracetamol in addition to their prescribed analgesic and be unaware of the actual amount of paracetamol that they are consuming.

The use of paracetamol/opioid compounds may place patients at increased risk of unintentional paracetamol overdose because they are fixed-dose combinations. Increasing the opioid dose – in order to achieve adequate analgesia - also increases the dose of paracetamol, possibly over the recommended daily maximum dose. In Canada, there is a high consumption of codeine-paracetamol compounds. [44] The analgesic efficacy of codeine is potentially unreliable because of its unpredictable pharmacokinetics. [45,46] Codeine is a prodrug that must be converted to morphine. This conversion depends on the polymorphic cytochrome P4502D6

(CYP2D6) pathway. Genetic polymorphisms result in three phenotypes, poor, extensive and ultra-rapid metabolizers. A poor metabolizer may receive almost no analgesic effect from a standard dose of codeine. [47,48] Prescribers need to evaluate the role of these compounds compared with other analgesics and determine the risks and benefits for individual patients.

An American, multicentre, prospective study of 275 identified paracetamol-induced cases of acute liver failure, 48% of cases were unintentional or 'therapeutic misadventures'. [4] Most (79%) of these individuals reported taking paracetamol for pain, almost two-thirds (63%) reported taking a prescription paracetamol/opioid combination and 38% were consuming two paracetamol-containing products concurrently. Of particular concern was the fact that these persons have poorer outcomes than those with intentional overdoses; a significantly greater percentage presented with severe (grades 3 and 4) hepatic encephalopathy, possibly because of a delay in seeking medical care.[4] Two Canadian studies found lower proportions of unintentional overdoses, 25% [14] and 13% [13] respectively. However, while paracetamol overdose-related hospitalisations declined from 1995 to 2004 among persons younger than 50 years, the rate increased for those ages 50 and over, as did their rate of hospitalisation.

Various strategies have been proposed or implemented in an effort to reduce paracetamol-related harms. The UK introduced legislation that limits the quantity of paracetamol sold without prescription and required these products to be blister-packed. In 2009, the US Food and Drug Administration (FDA) convened an internal working group from the Center for Drug Evaluation and Research (CDER) to prepare a report on the issue of paracetamol-related hepatotoxicity in preparation for the joint meeting of three Advisory Committees: Drug Safety and Risk Management; Nonprescription Drug; and Anesthetic and Life Support Drugs.[29,30,49] Upon discussion of the working group's report, the Advisory Committees accepted some, but not all, of the working group's recommendations. The Committees recommended: the elimination of prescription paracetamol combinations; reduction of the maximum daily dose to 3.25 g and the maximum individual dose to 650 mg; designating 500 mg tablets as prescription-only; and a single concentration for all liquid products. The Committees also voted to encourage the FDA to promote awareness among health professionals by including a black box warning in product information and to encourage patient-education regarding the potential risks.[29,30,49] In Canada, the National Opioid Guideline Group recommends that paracetamol doses not exceed 3.20 g/day for the management of chronic non-cancer pain.[50,51] Health Canada issued an advisory in January 2011 reminding Canadians about using paracetamol wisely [52] and referencing the labelling requirements for over-the-counter products that include a maximum daily dose of 4.0 g for adults and children 12 years and older [2].

Healthcare professionals must be vigilant when prescribing and dispensing paracetamol/opioid combinations and educate their patients about paracetamol-containing products and their potential toxicity. The need for greater public education has been recognized.[41] Persons who receive care from multiple health care prescribers such as physicians (primary care and specialists), dentists, pharmacists and nurse practitioners may be particularly at risk. In the future, computer generated alerts in decision support systems might be helpful in determining maximum doses for over-the-counter and prescription paracetamol-containing medications.

A limitation to our study is that patient level information was not available. For example, data were not available regarding patient weight, ethnicity, type and severity of pain or adequacy of pain control, comorbidities, patient preferences or specific risk factors for hepatotoxicity such as the presence of non-alcoholic fatty liver disease, or the concomitant use of other drugs or herbal therapies.[3,7,32,53-56] In addition, we were unable to determine the rates of genetic polymorphisms of the CYP2D6 pathway in our population.[45,46] Further, the extent to which the population was at a palliative stage is unknown; stratified analysis by this time period of need for increased pain management is warranted.

Research is required to provide a more extensive understanding of the number of high risk individuals, treatment appropriateness and methods employed to optimize treatment, and the relationship between therapeutic doses of paracetamol and acute liver failure. In addition, investigation of the sex-based differences in patterns of use is warranted. Further, as government regulators and clinical practice guidelines adopt lower maximum doses, it will be important to determine if the application of these guidelines results in increased use of non-steroidal anti-inflammatory drugs (NSAIDS) and increased NSAID-related adverse events [28].

Comprehensive evidence on the extent of paracetamol use and the relationship between therapeutic doses of paracteamol and acute liver failure is sparse as yet, as is the value of interventions that attempt to reduce harm [57]. Further population-based studies are needed to better understand the role of paracetamol in the etiology of acute liver failure and to monitor changes over time as multifaceted interventions are introduced in an attempt to limit harm from pain medications.

Conclusions

About one in 12 adults in Nova Scotia filled at least one prescription for paracetamol/opioid combination drugs during a one-year period starting July 2009. Of these

individuals, six percent filled prescriptions that supply paracetamol doses greater than the usual recommended daily dose of 4.0 g and one in five exceeded 3.25 g/day. These individuals may be at risk for paracetamol-related hepatotoxicity. Given the widespread use of paracetamol-containing products, including non-prescription products, the potential exists for unintentional paracetamol overdose. Health professionals, policy makers, patients and caregivers must be made aware of the many products containing paracetamol, their potential for toxicity, and approaches to minimize the risks.

Competing interests

Dr. Ingrid Sketris has received compensation from Green Shield Canada and Health Canada. Other authors declare they have no competing interests.

Acknowledgements

The authors wish to thank Dawn Frail (Manager, Pharmaceutical Services, the Nova Scotia Department of Health and Wellness), the Drug Evaluation Alliance of Nova Scotia, and the Nova Scotia Prescription Monitoring Program, in particular Denise Pellerin (Manager, Nova Scotia Prescription Monitoring Program) and Kirstin Crabtree and Lori Etsell (Medavie Blue Cross and NSPMP analysts) for their support of this project, and Dr. Pantelis Andreou (Biostatistical Consulting Unit, Community Health and Epidemiology, Faculty of Medicine, Dalhousie University).

Funding and support

Roderick Clark was a resident in the Drug Use Management and Policy Residency Program funded by the Canadian Health Services Research Foundation (CHSRF), Canadian Institutes of Health Research (CIHR), and the Nova Scotia Health Research Foundation (NSHRF).
This work was completed while Dr. Judith Fisher was a post-doctoral fellow at the College of Pharmacy, Dalhousie University where she received post-doctoral funding through the Network for End of Life Studies Interdisciplinary Capacity Enhancement (NELS ICE), funded by Canadian Institutes for Health Research (CIHR) through a strategic initiative grant (#HOA-80067), 2006–2011.
Ingrid Sketris held a Canadian Health Services Research Foundation and Canadian Institutes of Health Research Chair in Health Services Research, cosponsored by Nova Scotia Health Research Foundation (Halifax, Nova Scotia).

Author details

[1]Department of Community Health and Epidemiology, Dalhousie University, Halifax, NS, Canada. [2]College of Pharmacy, Faculty of Health Professions, Dalhousie University, Halifax, NS, Canada. [3]Pharmaceutical Services, Department of Health and Wellness, Halifax, NS, Canada. [4]School of Health Administration, Faculty of Health Professions Dalhousie University, Halifax, NS, Canada.

Authors' contributions

JF, RC and IS contributed to conception and design, JF and RC in data analysis and all authors participated in interpretation of the data and drafting or critical review of the manuscript. All authors read and approved the final manuscript.

References

1. Barozzi N, Tett SE: Perceived barriers to paracetamol (acetaminophen) prescribing, especially following rofecoxib withdrawal from the market. *Clin Rheumatol* 2009, **28**(5):509–519.
2. http://www.hc-sc.gc.ca/dhp-mps/prodpharma/applic-demande/guide-ld/label_stand_guide_ld-eng.php.
3. Schilling A, Corey R, Leonard M, Eghtesad B: Acetaminophen: old drug, new warnings. *Cleve Clin J Med* 2010, **77**(1):19–27.

4. Larson AM, Polson J, Fontana RJ, Davern TJ, Lalani E, Hynan LS, Reisch JS, Schiodt FV, Ostapowicz G, Shakil AO, Lee WM, Acute Liver Failure Study Group: **Acetaminophen-induced acute liver failure: results of a United States multicenter, prospective study.** *Hepatology* 2005, **42**(6):1364–1372.

5. Bolesta S, Haber SL: **Hepatotoxicity associated with chronic acetaminophen administration in patients without risk factors.** *Ann Pharmacother* 2002, **36**(2):331–333.

6. Claridge LC, Eksteen B, Smith A, Shah T, Holt AP: **Acute liver failure after administration of paracetamol at the maximum recommended daily dose in adults.** *BMJ* 2010, **341**:c6764.

7. Jickling G, Heino A, Ahmed SN: **Acetaminophen toxicity with concomitant use of carbamazepine.** *Epileptic Disord* 2009, **11**(4):329–332.

8. Moling O, Cairon E, Rimenti G, Rizza F, Pristera R, Mian P: **Severe hepatotoxicity after therapeutic doses of acetaminophen.** *Clin Ther* 2006, **28**(5):755–760.

9. Hinson JA, Roberts DW, James LP: **Mechanisms of acetaminophen-induced liver necrosis.** *Handb Exp Pharmacol* 2010, **196**:369–405.

10. James LP, Mayeux PR, Hinson JA: **Acetaminophen-induced hepatotoxicity.** *Drug Metabolism and Disposition* 2003, **31**(12):1499–1506.

11. McClain CJ, Price S, Barve S, Devalarja R, Shedlofsky S: **Acetaminophen hepatotoxicity: An update.** *Curr Gastroenterol Rep* 1999, **1**(1):42–49.

12. Sabate M, Ibanez L, Perez E, Vidal X, Buti M, Xiol X, Mas A, Guarner C, Forne M, Sola R, Castellote J, Rigau J, Laporte JR: **Paracetamol in therapeutic dosages and acute liver injury: causality assessment in a prospective case series.** *BMC Gastroenterol* 2011, **11**:80.

13. Myers RP, Li B, Fong A, Shaheen AA, Quan H: **Hospitalizations for acetaminophen overdose: a Canadian population-based study from 1995 to 2004.** *BMC Public Health* 2007, **7**:143.

14. Myers RP, Li B, Shaheen AA: **Emergency department visits for acetaminophen overdose: a Canadian population-based epidemiologic study (1997–2002).** *CJEM* 2007, **9**(4):267–274.

15. Lee WM, Squires RH Jr, Nyberg SL, Doo E, Hoofnagle JH: **Acute liver failure: Summary of a workshop.** *Hepatology* 2008, **47**(4):1401–1415.

16. Bronstein AC, Spyker DA, Cantilena LR Jr, Green JL, Rumack BH, Giffin SL: **2009 Annual Report of the American Association of Poison Control Centers' National Poison Data System (NPDS): 27th Annual Report.** *Clin Toxicol (Phila)* 2010, **48**(10):979–1178.

17. Bond GR, Novak JE: **The human and economic cost of paracetamol (acetaminophen) overdose.** *Pharmacoeconomics* 1995, **8**(3):177–181.

18. Fagan E, Wannan G: **Reducing paracetamol overdoses.** *BMJ* 1996, **313** (7070):1417–1418.

19. Ostapowicz G, Fontana RJ, Schiodt FV, Larson A, Davern TJ, Han SH, McCashland TM, Shakil AO, Hay JE, Hynan L, Crippin JS, Blei AT, Samuel G, Reisch J, Lee WM. US Acute Liver Failure Study Group: **Results of a prospective study of acute liver failure at 17 tertiary care centers in the United States.** *Ann Intern Med* 2002, **137**(12):947–954.

20. Khandelwal N, James LP, Sanders C, Larson AM, Lee WM, Acute Liver Failure Study Group: **Unrecognized acetaminophen toxicity as a cause of indeterminate acute liver failure.** *Hepatology* 2011, **53**(2):567–576.

21. http://webprod.hc-sc.gc.ca/dpd-bdpp/index-eng.jsp.

22. Anonymous: **Is acetaminophen safe? Accidental overdoses are common, but avoidable.** *Mayo Clin Womens Healthsource* 2010, **14**(1):1–2.

23. Bower WA, Johns M, Margolis HS, Williams IT, Bell BP: **Population-based surveillance for acute liver failure.** *Am J Gastroenterol* 2007, **102**(11):2459–2463.

24. IMS Institute for Healthcare Informatics: *The Use of Medicines in the United States*, Review of 2010. 2011.

25. Campeau L: *Top Rx drugs of 2010*, Pharmacy Practice 2011. 2011.

26. Fishman SM, Gilson AM: **Commentary to Michna et al.: The elephant in the room: hydrocodone/acetaminophen combination compounds and the substitution effect.** *Pain Med* 2010, **11**(3):379–381.

27. Ho V, Stewart M, Boyd P: **Cholestatic hepatitis as a possible new side-effect of oxycodone: a case report.** *J Med Case Reports* 2008, **2**:140.

28. Michna E, Duh MS, Korves C, Dahl JL: **Removal of opioid/acetaminophen combination prescription pain medications: assessing the evidence for hepatotoxicity and consequences of removal of these medications.** *Pain Med* 2010, **11**(3):369–378.

29. Anonymous: *Summary Minutes of the Joint Meeting of the Drug Safety and Risk Management Advisory Committee, Nonprescription Drugs Advisory Committee, and the Anesthetic and Life Support Drugs Advisory Committee.* 2009.

30. Anonymous: *Joint Meeting of the Drug Safety and Risk Management Advisory Committee with the Anesthetic and Life Support Drugs Advisory Committee and the Nonprescription Drugs Advisory Committee: Meeting Announcement.* 2009.

31. Mort JR: **High dose acetaminophen in narcotic combinations: should there be concern?** *S D Med* 2008, **61**(8):294–295.

32. Albertson TE, Walker VM Jr, Stebbins MR, Ashton EW, Owen KP, Sutter ME: **A population study of the frequency of high-dose acetaminophen prescribing and dispensing.** *Ann Pharmacother* 2010, **44**(7–8):1191–1195.

33. Minister of Justice, Government of Canada: *Controlled Drugs and Substances Act. S.C.* 1996:19.

34. Nova Scotia Prescription Monitoring Program: **Nova Scotia Prescription Monitoring Program Operational Policies.** In *Nova Scotia Prescription Monitoring Program: Policy and Reference Materials.* Edited by Anonymous Halifax. Nova Scotia: Nova Scotia Prescription Monitoring Program; 2008:17–21.

35. http://www.nspmp.ca/history.php.

36. http://www.whocc.no/ddd/definition_and_general_considera/.

37. http://cansim2.statcan.ca/cgi-win/cnsmcgi.exe?Lang=E&CNSM-Fi=CII/CII_1-eng.htm.

38. http://www.gov.ns.ca/health/msi/eligibility.asp.

39. Armitage P: **Tests for linear trends in proportions and frequencies.** *Biometrics* 1955, **11**(3):375–386.

40. Province of Nova Scotia: Regulations Act. R.S., c. 393, s. 1; 2005:132.

41. Mort JR, Shiyanbola OO, Ndehi LN, Xu Y, Stacy JN: **Opioid-paracetamol prescription patterns and liver dysfunction: a retrospective cohort study in a population served by a US health benefits organization.** *Drug Saf* 2011, **34**(11):1079–1088.

42. Buckwalter JA, Martin JA: **Osteoarthritis.** *Adv Drug Deliv Rev* 2006, **58**(2):150–167.

43. Li C, Martin BC: **Trends in emergency department visits attributable to acetaminophen overdoses in the United States: 1993–2007.** *Pharmacoepidemiol Drug Saf* 2011, **20**(8):810–818.

44. http://www.imshealth.com/deployedfiles/imshealth/Global/Americas/North%20America/Canada/StaticFile/Top10DispensedTherapeutic_En_11.pdf.

45. MacDonald N, MacLeod SM: **Has the time come to phase out codeine?** *CMAJ* 2010, **182**(17):1825.

46. Kelly LE, Rieder M, van den Anker J, Malkin B, Ross C, Neely MN, Carleton B, Hayden MR, Madadi P, Koren G: **More Codeine Fatalities After Tonsillectomy in North American Children.** *Pediatrics* 2012, **129**(5):e1343–e1347.

47. Kirchheiner J, Schmidt H, Tzvetkov M, Keulen JT, Lotsch J, Roots I, Brockmoller J: **Pharmacokinetics of codeine and its metabolite morphine in ultra-rapid metabolizers due to CYP2D6 duplication.** *Pharmacogenomics J* 2007, **7**(4):257–265.

48. Gaedigk A, Simon SD, Pearce RE, Bradford LD, Kennedy MJ, Leeder JS: **The CYP2D6 activity score: translating genotype information into a qualitative measure of phenotype.** *Clin Pharmacol Ther* 2008, **83**(2):234–242.

49. Krenzelok EP: **The FDA Acetaminophen Advisory Committee Meeting - what is the future of acetaminophen in the United States? The perspective of a committee member.** *Clin Toxicol (Phila)* 2009, **47**(8):784–789.

50. Furlan AD, Reardon R, Weppler C: National Opioid Use Guideline Group: **Opioids for chronic noncancer pain: a new Canadian practice guideline.** *CMAJ* 2010, **182**(9):923–930.

51. National Opioid Use Guideline Group (NOUGG): *Canadian Guideline for Safe and Effective Use of Opioids for Chronic Non-Cancer Pain© 2010.*: National Opioid Use Guideline Group (NOUGG); 2010:5–6.

52. http://www.hc-sc.gc.ca/ahc-asc/media/advisories-avis/_2011/2011_05-eng.php.

53. Prior MJ, Cooper K, Cummins P, Bowen D: **Acetaminophen availability increases in Canada with no increase in the incidence of reports of inpatient hospitalizations with acetaminophen overdose and acute liver toxicity.** *Am J Ther* 2004, **11**(6):443–452.

54. Tarantino G, Conca P, Basile V, Gentile A, Capone D, Polichetti G, Leo E: **A prospective study of acute drug-induced liver injury in patients suffering from non-alcoholic fatty liver disease.** *Hepatol Res* 2007, **37**(6):410–415.

55. Tarantino G, Di Minno MN, Capone D: **Drug-induced liver injury: is it somehow foreseeable?** *World J Gastroenterol* 2009, **15**(23):2817–2833.

56. Barshop NJ, Capparelli EV, Sirlin CB, Schwimmer JB, Lavine JE: **Acetaminophen pharmacokinetics in children with nonalcoholic fatty liver disease.** *J Pediatr Gastroenterol Nutr* 2011, **52**(2):198–202.

57. Graham GG, Day RO, Graudins A, Mohamudally A: **FDA proposals to limit the hepatotoxicity of paracetamol (acetaminophen): are they reasonable?** *Inflammopharmacology* 2010, **18**(2):47–55.

7

Attitudes among healthcare professionals to the reporting of adverse drug reactions in Nepal

Santosh KC[1,2], Pramote Tragulpiankit[1*], Sarun Gorsanan[3] and I Ralph Edwards[4]

Abstract

Background: Healthcare professional's knowledge and attitudes to adverse drug reaction (ADR) and ADR reporting play vital role to report any cases of ADR. Positive attitudes may favour ADR reporting by healthcare professionals. This study was aimed to investigate the attitudes towards and ways to improve adverse drug reaction (ADR) reporting among healthcare professionals working at four Regional Pharmacovigilance Centres (RPCs) of Nepal.

Methods: A cross sectional study was done by survey using a self-administered structured questionnaire. The questionnaire was distributed to 450 healthcare professionals working at four RPCs.

Results: The overall response rate was 74.0%. There were 74.8% of healthcare professionals who had seen patient experiencing an ADR; however, only 20.1% had reported. Reporting form not available (48.1%) and other colleagues not reporting ADR cases (46.9%) would significantly discourage the ADR reporting among healthcare professionals working at four RPCs. Healthcare professionals perceived that seriousness of the reaction (75.6%); unusual reaction (64.6%); reaction to new product (71.2%); new reaction to existing product (70.2%); and confidence in diagnosis of ADR (60.8%) were important factors on the decision to report ADR. Awareness among healthcare professionals (85.9%), training (76.0%), collaboration (67.0%), and involve pharmacist for ADR reporting (63.1%) were mostly recognized ways to improve reporting. Regular newsletter on current awareness in drug safety (71.2%), information on new ADR (65.8%), and international drug safety information (64.0%) were the identified feedbacks they would like to receive from the Nepal pharmacovigilance programme.

Conclusion: Healthcare professionals working at four RPCs of Nepal have positive attitudes towards ADR reporting. Awareness among healthcare professionals, training and collaboration would likely improve reporting provided they would receive appropriate feedback from the national pharamcovigilance programme.

Keywords: Adverse drug reaction, Attitudes, Healthcare professional, Nepal

Background

Spontaneous reporting system (SRS) still remains as the most common method to report adverse drug reaction (ADR) even though under reporting is estimated higher than 90–95% [1-4]. Healthcare professionals are the primary reporter of the ADR cases either to national centre or to Pharma Company. There are different factors which encourage healthcare professionals to report ADRs. Among all, healthcare professionals' knowledge about and attitudes towards ADR and ADR reporting debate more frequently as an influential factors [5-8]. Reporting of each and every cases of ADR is important;

however, reporting of previously unknown ADR, rare ADR and serious unlabeled ADR is more important to generate new signal and new knowledge. Healthcare professionals are reluctant to report ADR when the ADR is common, too trivial and uncertainty about the association [9-11]. But it is interesting that some healthcare professionals especially doctors report ADR because of their professional interest to inform others [12]. Overall, knowledge about and attitudes towards ADR plays vital role in terms of ADR reporting.

In Nepal, ADR reporting is not mandatory for healthcare professionals. The Department of Drug Administration (DDA), the national drug regulatory authority, was established in 1979 to enforce the Drug Act 1978. After its establishment it had banned several drugs and its

---

* Correspondence: pramote.tra@mahidol.ac.th
[1]Faculty of Pharmacy, Mahidol University, Bangkok, Thailand
Full list of author information is available at the end of the article

combinations on the ground of irrational combination, potential toxicity, doubtful efficacy, and potential for irrational use [13]. Though the need of pharmacovigilance has been identified early; however, it is started several years after its establishment. The DDA took the initiatives to set up a pharmacovigilance programme in 2002. In 2004, DDA was designated as a National Pharmacovigilance Centre (NPC). Two years later, it became full member of World Health Organization (WHO) collaborating Centre for International Drug Monitoring. Immediately after its establishment, NPC facilitated the operation of Regional Pharmacovigilance Centre (RPC) in different part of the country. Currently there are six RPCs operating in the country based on Kathmandu, Lalitpur, Pokhara and Biratnagar. Though the NPC is encouraging the RPCs to report more ADR, the current reporting trend suggests high under reporting. There was only total of 304 ADR cases reported during the year 2006 to 2009 by four RPCs [14]. Therefore, the purpose of this study is to investigate the knowledge and attitudes of healthcare professionals to report ADR working at four RPCs of Nepal and to suggest possible ways to improve the ADR reporting based on the findings. The findings of knowledge about ADR and ADR reporting among healthcare professionals will be presented elsewhere.

Methods

Study design and setting

This study was conducted in the four RPCs of Nepal. The four RPCs were Manipal Teaching Hospital (MTH), Pokhara, Tribhuvan University Teaching Hospital (TUTH), Kathmandu, Nepal Medical College Hospital (NMCH), Kathmandu and KIST Medical College Hospital (KISTMCH), Lalitpur. All those RPCs are teaching hospital in nature.

A cross sectional study was done by survey using a self-administered structured questionnaire. The attitude components of the questionnaire are presented in Additional file 1. There were 450 self-administered structured questionnaires distributed to all potential healthcare professionals (doctors, nurses and pharmacists) working at four RPCs. The questionnaire was structured to obtain the demographics of healthcare professionals, factors discouraging ADR reporting, factors that they perceived may influence reporting, ways to improve ADR reporting and feedbacks they would like to receive from NPC. Questionnaire was designed to five level likert scale (1 = strongly disagree and 5 = strongly agree) and single choice. The questionnaire was attached with the covering letter, which had aimed to provide the information of the research to the participants. The participant information sheet contained the objective of the research, the number of participants expected to include in the research, the

way to response the questionnaire, their right to decide about whether or not to participate in the research and confidentiality of the response. The questionnaire so designed was tested for content validity by consensus of the expert's panel comprising Prof. Ralph Edwards and Assist. Prof. Pramote Tragulpiankit. Objectivity test was done by distributing to 10 of the principal investigator's colleagues and instructors of Mahidol University, Bangkok, Thailand. The comments made were incorporated and questionnaire was modified accordingly. Finally, pilot study was conducted at two hospitals of Nepal, which were Alka Hospital Pvt. Ltd., Lalitpur and Civil Service Hospital, Kathmandu, for the reliability of the questionnaire. There were 50 questionnaires randomly distributed among doctors, nurses and pharmacists working at two hospitals. The reliability of the questionnaire was evaluated by calculating Cronbach alpha. The alpha score for the attitudes towards ADR was calculated 0.81 and was considered good.

Data collection

The self-administered structured questionnaires were distributed among healthcare professional through different departments of the four RPCs. The first response was collected within 3 weeks of the distribution. After that reminder was sent to all respondents with apologize to the ones who have already answered the questionnaire. The second response was collected within 3 weeks of the reminder. Targeted follow up was also done after this reminder to the respondents by personal visit or telephone call. This study was approved by Mahidol University, Faculty of Dentistry/ Faculty of Pharmacy, Institutional Review Board (MU-DT/PY-IRB) and, Institutional Review Board of the four hospitals before starting the data collection.

Statistical analysis

The SPSS statistical programme for Windows, version 17.0 was used for the analysis of the data. The coded data was systematically verified and checked for errors. Results were presented as mean ± standard deviation for quantitative variables and number with percentage or graphic presentation for categorical variables, where applicable. Percentage on each category, median and mode was presented for the likert scale. The chi-square test was performed to find out the association between ADR occurrence and ADR reporting among healthcare professionals. The comparison of the attitudes among different category of healthcare professionals was analyzed by Kruskal Wallis test. Significance level of $P < 0.05$ was used, where the test was relevant.

Results

Out of 450 questionnaires distributed, 333 were received back with an overall response rate of 74.0%. There were

Table 1 Demography details and characteristic features of the respondents

Category	Sub-category	Number (%)
Gender	Male	128 (38.4)
	Female	201 (60.4)
	Data missing	4 (1.2)
Age (years)	Up to 20	9 (2.7)
	21–30	221 (66.4)
	31–40	69 (20.7)
	41–50	19 (5.7)
	51–60	3 (0.9)
	Above 60	6 (1.8)
	Mean	29.5
	Minimum	19
	Maximum	72
	Data missing	6 (1.8)
Professional qualification	Doctor	162 (48.6)
	Nurse	135 (40.5)
	Pharmacist	32 (9.6)
	Data missing	4 (1.2)
Work experience (years)	Less than 1	9 (2.7)
	1–5	226 (67.9)
	6–10	44 (13.2)
	11–15	10 (3.0)
	16–20	11 (3.3)
	21–25	7 (2.1)
	26–30	4 (1.2)
	Above 30	6 (1.8)
	Mean	5.4
	Minimum	0
	Maximum	40
	Data missing	16 (4.8)

Category	Sub-category*	Number (%)
Doctor	MD/MS	70 (21.0)
	MBBS	86 (25.8)
	MDS	3 (0.9)
	BDS	2 (0.6)
Nurse	MN	2 (0.6)
	BN	36 (10.8)
	PCL	97 (29.1)
Pharmacist	PhD and Master	9 (2.7)
	BPharm	6 (1.8)
	PCL/Diploma	17 (5.1)
Country of undergraduate study	Nepal	163 (75.8)
	India	26 (12.1)
	Bangladesh	11 (5.1)

Table 1 Demography details and characteristic features of the respondents (Continued)

China	5 (2.3)
Philippines	2 (1.6)
Russia	1 (0.5)
Ukraine	1 (0.5)
Data missing	6 (2.8)

*Note: *MD*: Doctor of medicine, *MS*: Master of surgery, *MBBS*: Bachelor of medicine and surgery, *MDS*: Master of dental surgery, *BDS*: Bachelor of dental surgery, *MN*: Master in nursing, *BN*: Bachelor in nursing, *PCL*: Proficiency certificate level, *PhD*: Doctor of Philosophy, *BPharm*: Bachelor of Pharmacy.

128 males and 201 females. Among the respondents, 4 did not mention about their gender and profession. There were 162 doctors, 135 nurses and 32 pharmacists. Among the respondents, 66.4% were in the age group 21–30 years and 67.9% of them had experiences of 1–5 years followed by 13.2% who had experiences of 6–10 years. The mean age and the experience were 29.5 years and 5.4 years, respectively. The characteristic features of the respondents are shown in Table 1.

Two hundred and forty six healthcare professionals (74.8%) had seen patient experiencing an ADR. Among them, 82.7% of doctors, 67.4% of nurses and 65.6% of pharmacists had seen ADR during their routine work (P = 0.005). In contrast, only 66 respondents (20.1%) had ever reported an ADR to the pharmacovigilance centre/unit of their hospital. There were 21.6% of doctors, 17.0% of nurses and 25.0% of pharmacists who had ever reported ADR (P = 0.440). The details are shown in Table 2. There were 38.3% of doctors, 40.7% of nurses, and 28.1% of pharmacists provided reasons for ADR not reported. Among the respondents, 28.4% of doctors, 26.7% of nurses, and 9.4% of pharmacists were unaware about the existence of PV centre/unit in the hospital.

Two hundred and forty five respondents (75.6%) agreed (score 4 or 5 on the likert scale) on seriousness of the reaction, 230 (71.2%) agreed on reaction to new product, 226 (70.2%) agreed on new reaction to existing product, 208 (64.6%) agreed on unusual reaction, and 196 (60.8%) agreed on confidence in diagnosis of ADR as an important factors on the decision to report ADR. In contrast, ADR reporting form not available 155 (48.1%) and other colleagues not reporting ADR cases 151 (46.9%) were the major discouraging factors. Among the respondents, 167 (51.8%) disagreed (score 1 or 2 on the likert scale) on ADR reporting as a guilt of causing patient harm and 165 (51.2%) disagreed on ambition to publish case report personally as a factor discouraging ADR reporting. Similarly, 151 (46.9%) disagreed on ADR reporting will generate extra work, 141 (43.8%) disagreed on fear of legal liability, 141 (43.8%) disagreed on belief of only safe drugs are marketed, and 129 (40.1%) disagreed on lack of time to actively look for an ADR (Table 3).

Table 2 Experience of ADR occurrence and ADR reporting among healthcare professionals

Category	Profession	Yes (%)	No (%)	P-value*
Even seen any patient experiencing an ADR	**Total**	**246 (74.8)**	**83 (25.2)**	
	Doctor	134 (82.7)	28 (17.3)	P=0.005
	Nurse	91 (67.4)	44 (32.6)	
	Pharmacist	21 (65.6)	11 (34.4)	
Ever reported an ADR to the Pharmacovigilance Centre/ Unit of his/her hospital	**Total**	**66 (20.1)**	**263 (79.9)**	
	Doctor	35 (21.6)	127 (78.4)	P=0.440
	Nurse	23 (17.0)	112 (83.0)	
	Pharmacist	8 (25.0)	24 (75.0)	

* Chi-square test.

Two hundred and eighty six respondents (85.9%) suggested awareness among healthcare professionals, training for healthcare professionals 253 (76.0%), collaboration among other healthcare professionals 223 (67.0%), involve pharmacists for ADR reporting 210 (63.1%), and make reporting a professional obligation 184 (55.5%) as possible ways to improve ADR reporting in the context of Nepal. Majority of the respondents would like to receive feedbacks from the national pharmacovigilance programme. The identified mode of feedbacks were regular newsletter on current awareness on drug safety 237 (71.2%), information of new ADR by newsletter 219 (65.8%), international drug safety information 213 (64.0%), annual national statistics 196 (58.9%), and individual response to report 146 (43.8%).

Discussion

This study identified the attitudes towards ADR and ADR reporting among healthcare professionals working

at four RPCs of Nepal. Among six RPCs, we did not include two RPCs in this study as they recognized after this study was started. This study found that healthcare professionals have positive attitudes towards ADR and ADR reporting. The overall response rate of 74.0% was acceptable. The higher percentage of female respondents compared to male is because of nurses as a segmented group included in this research. Nursing practitioners in Nepal are female only. While looking at experiences and ages of the respondents, mostly the young and beginner healthcare professionals were participated in this research. In Nepal, the clinical role of pharmacist is in infancy, mostly involved in dispensing and counseling, rather than direct pharmaceutical care. Two hundred and six healthcare professionals participated in this research had only first degree qualification to practice. One hundred and sixty three had perused the qualification in Nepal. In the curricula of Bachelor of Medicine and Surgery (MBBS) and Bachelor of Pharmacy (BPharm) in

Table 3 Factors discouraging ADR reporting

Factors	n	Response (%)					Median	Mode
		1a	2b	3c	4d	5e		
Concern that the report may be wrong	323	68 (21.1)	58 (18.0)	85 (26.3)	64 (19.8)	48 (14.9)	3.0	3
Lack of time to fill in a report and a single unreported case may not affect ADR database	322	65 (20.2)	54 (16.8)	86 (26.7)	74 (23.0)	43 (13.4)	3.0	3
Not confident to decide whether or not an ADR has occurred	322	72 (22.4)	48 (14.9)	91 (28.3)	70 (21.7)	41 (12.7)	3.0	3
Lack of time to actively look for an ADR while at work	322	74 (23.0)	55 (17.1)	77 (23.9)	70 (21.7)	46 (14.3)	3.0	3
Fear of legal liability by reporting adverse reaction	322	87 (27.0)	54 (16.8)	88 (27.3)	51 (15.8)	42 (13.0)	3.0	3
Concern that a report will generate an extra work	322	97 (30.1)	54 (16.8)	87 (27.0)	56 (17.4)	28 (8.7)	3.0	1
Belief that only safe drugs are marketed	322	74 (23.0)	67 (20.8)	74 (23.0)	66 (20.5)	41 (12.7)	3.0	1*
Think that you may have caused a patient harm	322	99 (30.7)	68 (21.1)	76 (23.6)	46 (14.3)	33 (10.2)	2.0	1
Ambition to publish case report personally	322	99 (30.7)	66 (20.5)	89 (27.6)	39 (12.1)	29 (9.0)	2.0	1
Reporting forms are not available when needed	322	40 (12.4)	46 (14.3)	81 (25.2)	71 (22.0)	84 (26.1)	3.0	5
Other colleagues are not reporting ADR cases	322	54 (16.8)	43 (13.4)	74 (23.0)	79 (24.5)	72 (22.4)	3.0	4

a 1 = strongly disagree.
b 2 = moderately disagree.
c 3 = neutral.
d 4 = moderately agree.
e 5 = strongly agree.
* More than one mode exists, the lowest is presented.

Nepal, the content of ADR and ADR reporting is not adequately covered. However, as a part of MBBS course in some institutions students are trained to ADR reporting and causality assessments [15]. But in UK, majority of the medical schools have included yellow card scheme in the undergraduate syllabuses and most of them assess student knowledge on the scheme [16]. The healthcare professionals, doctors, nurses and pharmacists, are the main reporter of the ADR case which they encountered on their routine work in general; however, involvement of nurses as a reporter is not well accepted by hospital physicians [17]. In Nepal, nurses are allowed to report ADR; however, they are not encouraged enough to report.

Different studies reported that all the ADRs encountered by healthcare professionals during their work are never reported [8,11,17-19], even though, majority of them felt ADR reporting is important in principle. This study also showed the same trend in terms of ADR encountered and ADR reporting. Two hundred and forty six (74.8%) healthcare professionals who had seen patient experiencing an ADR. However, only 66 (20.1%) of them had reported to the pharmacovigilance centre/unit of their hospital. But in the countries where ADR monitoring system is well established for example UK, France, Netherland and Sweden the ADR reporting rates among physicians estimate 40–70% [6-8,17,20]. This might be because ADR reporting is mandatory in all those countries. In 2006, the reporting rate in Sweden was 563 per million inhabitants [17]. The main reason for not reported ADR cases in this study were healthcare professionals did not know about existence of pharmacovigilance centre/unit in their hospitals. The other reasons for not reporting ADR were, reactions were not serious, did not know how to report, reported to concern doctors, did not think necessary to report.

This study showed positive attitudes to ADR reporting among healthcare professionals working at four RPCs of Nepal. Out of 11 discouraging factors to report ADR provided to rate, most had neutral response. The median of 9 factors was 3. Due to lack of practice of ADR reporting most of the respondents might have chosen neutral response. We found that reporting form not available and other colleagues not reporting ADR cases would significantly influence the ADR reporting among healthcare professional. Reporting form not available identified as a discouraging factor to report ADRs by other studies too [19,21,22]. On the other hand, lack of time to actively look for an ADR while at work, fear of legal liability, ADR reporting will generate extra work, belief of only safe drugs are marketed, think that they may have caused patient harm and ambition to publish case report personally were not significant factors to discourage ADR reporting among healthcare professionals. Even though, 119 (36.0%) of the healthcare professionals

agreed on lack of time to actively look for an ADR while at work and 107 (33.2%) believed that only safe drug are marketed. This is suggestive for train healthcare professionals by including ADR reporting and causality assessment in undergraduate syllabuses. This study showed that healthcare professionals working at four RPCs perceived that seriousness of the reaction, unusual reaction, reaction to new product, new reaction to existing product and, confidence in diagnosis of ADR are important factors on the decision to report ADR. Seriousness, unusual reaction, reaction to new product and certainty were also identified as important factors to report ADR among physicians in different studies [7,8,17,18].

Awareness among healthcare professionals, collaboration among other healthcare professionals and training for healthcare professionals were the highly suggested ways to improve ADR reporting. Healthcare professionals believed that making ADR reporting, a professional obligation and involved pharmacists for ADR reporting can also improve ADR reporting. Previous studies have also identified ADR reporting as a professional obligation [21,23]. In some countries for example Sweden, France, ADR reporting by healthcare professionals is compulsory, even though, the impact to counter underreporting is still controversial [24]. ADR reporting as a professional obligation will have moral binding to healthcare professionals and ethical issues. Studies have shown that pharmacist involvement can improve the number and quality of ADR reports along with substantial role in maintenance of drug safety monitoring programme [25-27]. The feedbacks they would like to receive from the national pharmacovigilance programme as regular newsletters on current awareness in drug safety, information on new drug adverse reactions by newsletters, annual national statistics and international drug safety information can be incorporate in a single newsletter. DDA is publishing Drug Bulletin of Nepal (BDN) on a regular basis [28]. The scope of the bulletin is wide. It can be updated with a regular column related to national and international drug safety information, even though; it has regular information related to current awareness in drug safety. The feedback from the national centre ensures two way communications between healthcare professionals and the national centre. In Sweden, feedback letters along with result of causality assessment of the reported ADR case is sent to the reporter concerned [17]. This is supposed to be one of the possible reasons of the high reporting rate in Sweden and elsewhere.

There are some limitations of this study. First, the sample does not represent the whole population of healthcare professionals of Nepal as it was conducted only on the four RPCs of Nepal, where the ADR monitoring is already in place. Second, questionnaires were distributed through different departments of the hospitals, responding by the aid of relevant books/publications or contemporary colleagues could not be excluded.

Conclusion

This study showed that healthcare professionals working at four RPCs of Nepal have positive attitudes about ADR reporting; however, the reporting culture is not well developed as reflected by the huge gap between the ADR encountered and ADR reporting trend among healthcare professionals. The unavailability of ADR reporting form and colleague's negative reporting nature are significantly discouraging them to report ADRs. However, awareness among healthcare professionals, training and collaboration would likely improve ADR reporting provided they would receive appropriate feedbacks from the national pharmacovigilance programme preferably as regular newsletter on current awareness in drug safety, information on new ADR and international drug safety information.

Additional file

Additional file 1: Questionnaire for evaluating healthcare professionals' attitudes towards ADR reporting in Nepal.

Abbreviations

ADR: Adverse drug reaction; RPC: Regional Pharmacovigilance Centre; SRS: Spontaneous reporting system; DDA: Department of Drug Administration; NPC: National Pharmacovigilance Centre; WHO: World Health Organization; MTH: Manipal Teaching Hospital; TUTH: Tribhuvan University Teaching Hospital; NMCH: Nepal Medical College Hospital; KISTMCH: KIST Medical College Hospital; MU-DT/PY-IRB: Mahidol University, Faculty of Dentistry/ Faculty of Pharmacy, Institutional Review Board; MBBS: Bachelor of medicine and surgery; BPharm: Bachelor of Pharmacy; PCL: Proficiency certificate level; MD: Doctor of medicine; MS: Master of surgery; MDS: Master of dental surgery; BDS: Bachelor of dental surgery; MN: Master in nursing; BN: Bachelor in nursing; PhD: Doctor of Philosophy, DBN, Drug Bulletin of Nepal; DTC: Drug and Therapeutic Committe.

Competing interests

The authors have no competing interests to report.

Authors' contributions

SKC and PT designed the study and draft questionnaire. SKC collected data of the study. PT, SG and IRE suggested the data analysis and sequence of draft manuscript. All the authors participated in the critical review of the draft manuscript, editing and approval for submission.

Acknowledgements

We thank all the participating healthcare professionals of four RPCs for responding the questionnaire, Mrs. Sabina K.C. Basnyat for support on pilot study, and Thailand International Development Cooperation Agency (TICA) for substantial financial support for data collection.

Author details

[1]Faculty of Pharmacy, Mahidol University, Bangkok, Thailand. [2]Bir Hospital, Kathmandu, Nepal. [3]Faculty of Pharmacy, Siam University, Bangkok, Thailand. [4]Uppsala Monitoring Centre, Uppsala, Sweden.

References

1. Harmark L, van Grootheest AC: Pharmacovigilance: methods, recent developments and future perspectives. Eur J Clin Pharmacol 2008, 64:743–752.
2. Montastruc JL, Sommet A, Lacroix I, Olivier P, Durrieu G, Damase-Michel C, et al: Pharmacovigilance for evaluating adverse drug reactions: value, organization, and methods. Joint Bone Spine 2006, 73:629–632.
3. Wise L, Parkinson J, Raine J, Breckenridge A: New approaches to drug safety: a pharmacovigilance tool kit. Nat Rev Drug Discov 2009, 8:779–782.
4. Hazell L, Shakir SA: Under-reporting of adverse drug reactions: a systematic review. Drug Saf 2006, 29:385–396.
5. Lopez-Gonzalez E, Herdeiro MT, Figueiras A: Determinants of under-reporting of adverse drug reactions: a systematic review. Drug Saf 2009, 32:19–31.
6. Belton KJ, Lewis SC, Payne S, Rawlins MD, Wood SM: Attitudinal survey of adverse drug reaction reporting by medical practitioners in the United Kingdom. Br J Clin Pharmacol 1995, 39:223–226.
7. Belton KJ: Attitude survey of adverse drug-reaction reporting by health care professionals across the European Union. The European Pharmacovigilance Research Group. Eur J Clin Pharmacol 1997, 52:423–427.
8. Oshikoya KA, Awobusuyi JO: Perceptions of doctors to adverse drug reaction reporting in a teaching hospital in Lagos, Nigeria. BMC Clin Pharmacol 2009, 9:14.
9. Hasford J, Goettler M, Munter KH, Muller-Oerlinghausen B: Physicians' knowledge and attitudes regarding the spontaneous reporting system for adverse drug reactions. J Clin Epidemiol 2002, 55:945–950.
10. Williams D, Feely J: Underreporting of adverse drug reactions: attitudes of Irish doctors. Ir J MedSc 1999, 168:257–261.
11. Chatterjee S, Lyle N, Ghosh S: A survey of the knowledge, attitude and practice of adverse drug reaction reporting by clinicians in eastern India. Drug Saf 2006, 29:641–642.
12. Biriell C, Edwards IR: Reasons for reporting adverse drug reactions-some thoughts based on an international review. Pharmacoepidemiol Drug Saf 1997, 6:21–26.
13. Department of Drug Administration: http://www.dda.gov.np/band_drugs.php.
14. KC S, Bhuju GB, Tragulpiankit P: Pattern of adverse drug reactions reported by Nepal regional pharmacovigilance centers [abstract]. Drug Saf 2010, 33(10):940.
15. Ravi Shankar P, Subish P, Mishra P, Dubey AK: Teaching pharmacovigilance to medical students and doctors. Indian J Pharmacol 2006, 38:316–319.
16. Cox AR, Marriott JF, Wilson KA, Ferner RE: Adverse drug reaction teaching in UK undergraduate medical and pharmacy programmes. J Clin Pharm Ther 2004, 29:31–35.
17. Ekman E, Backstrom M: Attitudes among hospital physicians to the reporting of adverse drug reactions in Sweden. Eur J Clin Pharmacol 2009, 65:43–46.
18. Backstrom M, Mjorndal T, Dahlqvist R, Nordkvist-Olsson T: Attitudes to reporting adverse drug reactions in northern Sweden. Eur J Clin Pharmacol 2000, 56:729–732.
19. Li Q, Zhang SM, Chen HT, Fang SP, Yu X, Liu D, et al: Awareness and attitudes of healthcare professionals in Wuhan, China to the reporting of adverse drug reactions. Chin Med J (Engl) 2004, 117:856–861.
20. Eland IA, Belton KJ, van Grootheest AC, Meiners AP, Rawlins MD, Stricker BH: Attitudinal survey of voluntary reporting of adverse drug reactions. Br J Clin Pharmacol 1999, 48:623–627.
21. Vessal G, Mardani Z, Mollai M: Knowledge, attitudes, and perceptions of pharmacists to adverse drug reaction reporting in Iran. Pharm World Sci 2009, 31:183–187.
22. Ohaju-Obodo JO, Iribhogbe OI: Extent of pharmacovigilance among resident doctors in Edo and Lagos states of Nigeria. Pharmacoepidemiol Drug Saf 2010, 19:191–195.
23. Green CF, Mottram DR, Rowe PH, Pirmohamed M: Attitudes and knowledge of hospital pharmacists to adverse drug reaction reporting. Br J Clin Pharmacol 2001, 51:81–86.
24. Backstrom M, Mjorndal T, Dahlqvist R: Under-reporting of serious adverse drug reactions in Sweden. Pharmacoepidemiol Drug Saf 2004, 13:483–487.
25. van Grootheest AC, van Puijenbroek EP, de Jong-van den Berg LT: Contribution of pharmacists to the reporting of adverse drug reactions. Pharmacoepidemiol Drug Saf 2002, 11:205–210.

26. van Grootheest K, Olsson S, Couper M, De Jong-van den Berg L: **Pharmacists' role in reporting adverse drug reactions in an international perspective.** *Pharmacoepidemiol Drug Saf* 2004, **13**:457–464.

27. van Grootheest AC, de Jong-van den Berg LT: **The role of hospital and community pharmacists in pharmacovigilance.** *Res Social Adm Pharm* 2005, **1**:126–133.

28. Drug Bulletin of Nepal: http://www.dda.gov.np/publication.php.

8

Statin therapy in critical illness: an international survey of intensive care physicians' opinions, attitudes and practice

Manu Shankar-Hari[1,2,3]*, Peter S Kruger[4,5], Stefania Di Gangi[1,3], Damon C Scales[6,7], Gavin D Perkins[8], Danny F McAuley[9] and Marius Terblanche[1,2,3]

Abstract

Background: Pleotropic effects of statins on inflammation are hypothesised to attenuate the severity of and possibly prevent the occurrence of the host inflammatory response to pathogen and infection-related acute organ failure. We conducted an international survey of intensive care physicians in Australia, New Zealand (ANZ) and United Kingdom (UK). The aims of the survey were to assess the current prescribing practice patterns, attitudes towards prescribing statin therapy in critically ill patients and opinions on the need for an interventional trial of statin therapy in critically ill patients.

Methods: Survey questions were developed through an iterative process. An expert group reviewed the resulting 26 items for face and content validity and clarity. The questions were further refined following pilot testing by ICU physicians from Australia, Canada and the UK. We used the online Smart Survey™ software to administer the survey.

Results: Of 239 respondents (62 from ANZ and 177 from UK) 58% worked in teaching hospitals; most (78.2%) practised in 'closed' units with a mixed medical and surgical case mix (71.0%). The most frequently prescribed statins were simvastatin (77.6%) in the UK and atorvastatin (66.1%) in ANZ. The main reasons cited to explain the choice of statin were preadmission prescription and pharmacy availability. Most respondents reported never starting statins to prevent (65.3%) or treat (89.1%) organ dysfunction. Only a minority (10%) disagreed with a statement that the risks of major side effects of statins when prescribed in critically ill patients were low. The majority (84.5%) of respondents strongly agreed that a clinical trial of statins for prevention is needed. More than half (56.5%) favoured rates of organ failure as the primary outcome for such a trial, while a minority (40.6%) favoured mortality.

Conclusions: Despite differences in type of statins prescribed, critical care physicians in the UK and ANZ reported similar prescription practices. Respondents from both communities agreed that a trial is needed to test whether statins can prevent the onset of new organ failure in patients with sepsis.

Keywords: Survey, Statin, Sepsis, Critical care, Clinical trials

* Correspondence: manu.shankar-hari@kcl.ac.uk
[1]Division of Asthma, Allergy and Lung Biology, King's College London, London, UK
[2]Critical Care and Anesthesia Research Group, King's Health Partners Academic Health Sciences Centre, London, UK
Full list of author information is available at the end of the article

Background

Host immune and inflammatory response to infection manifests as sepsis syndromes [1]. Sepsis is common and its incidence appears to be increasing[2,3], accounting for 27% of United Kingdom (UK) and 12% of Australia-New Zealand (ANZ) critical care admissions [4]. Worryingly the reported case fatality rate from sepsis syndromes remains high (25%-50%) [5]. The estimated annual cost of treating sepsis in the United States was $16.7 billion [5], whilst the estimated cost of managing a patient with sepsis in the intensive care unit has been reported to vary between $19,000 to $28,000 [6]. Furthermore, interventions such as resuscitation of patient with sepsis further adds to the management cost [7].

The biology of sepsis syndrome is characterised by unregulated systemic inflammation and immune dysfunction involving multiple pathways [8]. Numerous studies have tested the efficacy and effectiveness of immune-modulating agents; so far all have failed to show benefit. One reason may be that modulating a single immune target, embedded in a complex system with multiple redundancy, is insufficient to effect a subsequent improvement in morbidity or mortality[9]. Testing agents with modulating effects at multiple points may therefore be a more successful strategy [10-14] to prevent the onset of acute organ failure.

Statins are 3-hydroxy-3-methylglutaryl coenzyme A (HMG-CoA) reductase inhibitors with an established role in primary and secondary prevention of cardiovascular events by lowering low-density lipoprotein cholesterol [15]. Recent mechanistic reviews show statins influence inflammatory pathways at multiple levels through effects on cellular signalling pathways independent of lipid lowering ability [16,17]. In addition to the potential role in treating critically ill patients with established organ dysfunction like sepsis syndromes [14] and acute lung injury [13], statins have also been proposed as a potential intervention to prevent new organ dysfunction in sepsis [18].

HMGCoA reductase catalyses the rate limiting step in the production of cholesterol by inhibiting the conversion of HMG CoA to mevalonate. As a consequence of this action, the intermediates of the mevalonate pathway are also reduced. Under normal circumstances the mevalonate pathway leads to the formation of isoprenoids which regulate the lipid modification of proteins necessary for interaction with cellular membranes which drive inflammatory responses. Inhibition of isoprenoid formation by statins therefore, has significant anti-inflammatory effects. These have been demonstrated in vitro and in vivo as well as in a human model of pulmonary inflammation induced by inhaled endotoxin [19]. Enzymes of the mevalonate pathways are also key

for gram positive bacterial infection pathogenesis and are considered potentially modifiable with statin therapy [20]. Statins could potentially improve bacterial clearance by neutrophils and macrophages via novel extracellular traps linked to sterol pathway inhibition [21]. Antibacterial activity of compounds is often reported in terms of minimum inhibitory concentrations (MIC). However, the MICs required for antibacterial activity of statins invitro is much higher (approximately 1000 times) than what is achieved during conventional dosing for lipid homeostasis [22,23]. Therefore, the current thinking is that the antibacterial bacterial effects of statins are minimal at conventional doses and they are likely to be concentration independent, complex and as yet not fully clarified [22,24].

The literature on statin and sepsis is predominantly comprised of observational studies with inconsistent results and characterized by methodological limitations [25-27]. A recently published systematic review and meta analysis identified a potential publication bias in the existing literature on statin therapy and infections, and suggested that such publication bias might explain the inconsistent results from previous research [28]. These findings serve to highlight the need for well-designed interventional trials of statins to clarify their potential benefits in modulating the response to infections [29].

There is paucity of published evidence on the current critical care practices of statin prescribing. We conducted an international survey of critical care units in the United Kingdom (UK) and Australia & New Zealand (ANZ) to study current practice patterns of statin prescription in the critical care setting and to obtain background information to help inform the design of an interventional trial testing the hypothesis that statin therapy can prevent new acute organ failure.

Methods

Study participants

We targeted critical care physicians in UK and Australia identified using mailing lists maintained by The Intensive Care Society in the UK and The Australian and New Zealand Intensive Care Society Clinical Trials Group.

Survey development

Study investigators generated potential items for the survey by reviewing the literature on sepsis and statins and by seeking expert opinions [16,30]. Item reduction was achieved using an iterative process involving all 7 study investigators, 5 other critical care physicians and 2 external appraisers. The survey questionnaire was pilot tested using a group of senior critical care physicians and researchers from Canada, UK and ANZ (n = 15) to further refine and finalise question stems and response formats, and to assess its content, face validity and clarity [31]. The final survey questionnaire consisted of 26 items arranged into 3 domains. The online Smart Survey^{TM} software was used to format the questionnaire prior to administration [32]. The research and ethics committee at Guy's and St Thomas' Hospital NHS Foundation Trust considered the study to pose minimal risk and waived the need for formal ethical review.

Survey administration

Potential respondents were initially contacted by email. The email included a cover letter explaining the purpose of the survey and a link to the web-based Smart survey tool. A follow up reminder was sent 4 weeks after the initial mailing. No incentives were provided for responding to the survey.

Survey overview

The 3 survey domains were aimed at (1) understanding the respondent demographics and the intensive care unit characteristics including management policy, (2) determining the current practice patterns of statin therapy in critical illness, and (3) gathering opinions on key design issues for a proposed interventional trial of statin therapy in early critical illness.

The intensive care units management policy was defined using the following terms: a) 'open' refers to the policy where the referring physician remains directly responsible for majority of day to day patient care; b) 'closed' refers to the policy where the referring physicians hand over care to critical care physicians who are responsible for majority of day to day patient care until critical care discharge; and c) hybrid refers a combination of open and closed.

The current practice patterns of statin therapy were evaluated using scenarios in two separate contexts: 1) *initiating* new statin prescriptions (i.e. patients who are statin-naive), and 2) continuing pre admission prescriptions following admission to critical care. The likelihood with which new statin prescriptions are initiated following critical care admission in patients' NOT previously receiving statins was evaluated using the following 3 clinical scenarios: (1) a new cardiac indication during critical care admission; (2) preventing organ dysfunction in sepsis; and (3) treating organ dysfunction in severe sepsis. The frequency with which pre admission statin prescriptions are continued following critical care admissions for patients who were previously receiving statins was evaluated using the following 4 clinical scenarios: (1) outpatient indication like hyperlipidaemia without a new acute cardiac indication; (2) a new acute cardiac indication during critical care admission (e.g. acute coronary syndrome); (3) for preventing organ dysfunction in

sepsis; and (4) for treating organ dysfunction in severe sepsis.

Statistical analysis

We report responses to survey questions overall and by country (UK and ANZ). Institutional and ICU characteristics are described using proportions. Likert format response items were used to evaluate the reported statin prescribing practice and opinions on trial design. Reported practice and opinions evaluated using 5-point Likert scales are graphically represented by grouping responses at the tails (i.e. 1 and 2 grouped, 4 and 5 grouped). The grouping 1/2 refers to 'frequently/always' and grouping 4/5 refers to 'infrequently/never'; the remaining value 3 refers to 'sometimes' in the 'Likert Scale' choices used to seek opinions. The Chi square test (and Fisher exact test when number of observations in any category was less than 5) was used to evaluate the differences between responses from UK and ANZ physicians.

Results

Survey respondents

We received a total of 239 responses (177 from UK and 62 from ANZ). More respondents (overall 58.2%; n = 139; UK: n = 86, ANZ: n = 53) practised at university or teaching hospitals than at district general or community hospitals whilst 3 respondents did not specify the hospital type (overall 40.6%; n = 97; UK: n = 88, ANZ: n = 9). The ICUs in these hospitals had a median (IQR) 16 (13) [UK = 15 (11) and ANZ 18 (12)] critical care beds admitting a median (IQR) 900 (870) [UK = 750 (700) and ANZ = 1225(1100)] patients annually. The management policy for treating patients was described as closed by 78.2% (overall n = 187; UK: n = 133, ANZ: n = 54) and as hybrid by 21% (overall n = 50; UK: n =42, ANZ: n = 8) of respondents. The case-mix of patients was described as 'predominantly medical' by 12.2%', and 'predominantly surgical' by 11% and as 'mixed medical and surgical' by 71.3% (overall n = 169; UK: n = 124 & ANZ: n = 45) of the respondents,

Current statin prescription practices in critical care setting

The most frequently prescribed statins were simvastatin (overall 65.2%; UK = 77.6% *vs.* ANZ = 28.8%; p < 0.001) and atorvastatin (overall 28.3%; UK = 15.5% *vs.* ANZ = 66.1%; p < 0.001). The most common reason cited for choosing a particular statin from both the UK and ANZ physicians was prior use (overall 56.1%; UK 54.9% *vs.* ANZ 60.0%; p = 0.423). Other reported reasons included availability from hospital pharmacy (23.6%), drug policy (6.3%) and cost (9.9%). There was no statistically significant difference when comparing responses from UK and ANZ (p = 0.682). Overall, nearly half of respondents agreed or strongly agreed that the risks of major side effects of statins (i.e. increase in hepatic transaminases, elevated creatine kinase, rhabdomyolysis) are low when prescribed in critically ill patients (UK 48.6% *vs.* ANZ 50.0%). There was no statistically significant difference between UK and ANZ physicians' opinions on statin safety (p = 0.291).

Initiating new statin prescription following critical care admission

Overall 34.3% of all respondents stated they would start a new statin prescription for a new cardiac indication during a patient's ICU admission (35.6% UK *vs.* 30.7% ANZ; p = 0.26). Respondents reported rarely starting a new statin prescriptions to prevent organ dysfunction in sepsis or to treat organ dysfunction in severe sepsis (overall 2.5%; 1.1% UK *vs.* 6.4% ANZ; p = 0.03) and overall 0.8%; 0.6% UK *vs.* 1.6% ANZ; p = 0.75 respectively) [Figure 1].

Continuing pre admission statin prescriptions following critical care admission

Most respondents stated they would continue preadmission statin prescription for outpatient indications even if there were no new cardiac indications in the current ICU admission(overall 77.4%; 83.6% UK *vs.* 59.7% ANZ; p < 0.001). Similarly, most respondents reported that they would continue pre admission statin prescriptions if there was a new cardiac indication in the current admission (overall 85.8%; 87.0% UK *vs.* 82.3%ANZ; p = 0.18). However, fewer respondents would continue pre admission statin prescriptions for preventing organ dysfunction in sepsis or for treating organ dysfunction in severe sepsis (overall 32.2%; 31.6% UK *vs.* 33.9% ANZ; p = 0.87 and overall 31.8%; 32.8% UK *vs.* 29.3% ANZ; p = 0.72 respectively) [Figure 2].

Statin interventional trial
Hypothesis and trial participation
Overall, most respondents stated that they 'neither agree or disagree' that statin therapy can prevent the onset of acute organ failure in critically ill patients (overall 81.2%; UK 80.8 *vs.* 82.3% ANZ; p = 0.11). Importantly, most respondents either agreed or strongly agreed that there is a need for a randomised clinical trial to test the hypothesis that statin therapy prevents acute organ failure in critical illness (overall 84.5%; UK 84.2% *vs.* ANZ 85.5%; p = 0.56). The majority of UK physicians (75.1%) indicated a willingness to participate in a therapeutic trial evaluating the effect of statins for preventing organ failure in critical illness. Although in contrast no ANZ physicians were willing at this stage to participate in the proposed study, the vast majority were undecided (overall 36.0%; 17.5% UK *vs.* 88.7% ANZ; p < 0.001). Overall, few were unwilling to participate in the proposed trial (8.4%; 7.3% UK *vs.* 11.3% ANZ).

Type of statin therapy and safety triggers
The preferred statins for a future interventional trial were simvastatin and atorvastatin (overall 31.9% and 29.8% respectively). Comparing the responses from physicians in the UK and ANZ, there were significant differences in the choice of statins for the proposed trial (simvastatin - 38.4% UK *vs.* 13.1% ANZ; p < 0.001 and atorvastatin - 21.5% UK *vs.* 54.1% ANZ; p < 0.001). Almost one-third (32.4%) of respondents did not report preference to a particular statin.

We ascertained respondents' views regarding the biochemical cut offs (i.e. an increase above the upper limit of normal in hepatic transaminases, creatine kinase and/ or bilirubin) below which they considered it safe to enrol patients in the proposed trial. Comparing the responses from physicians in the UK and ANZ, there were

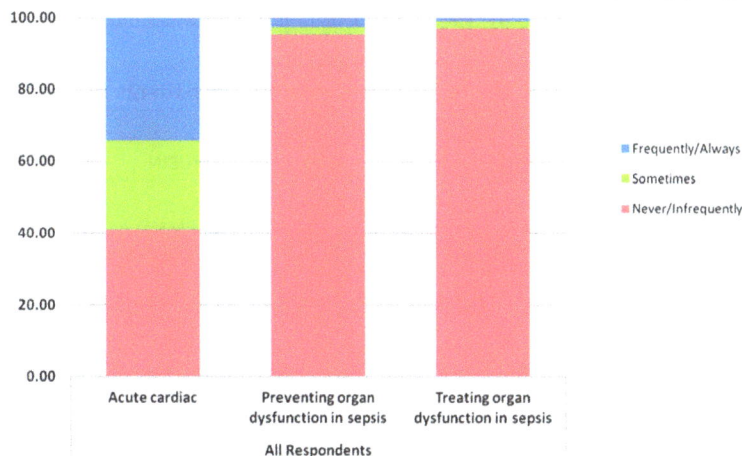

Figure 1 New statin prescription practice following critical care admission.

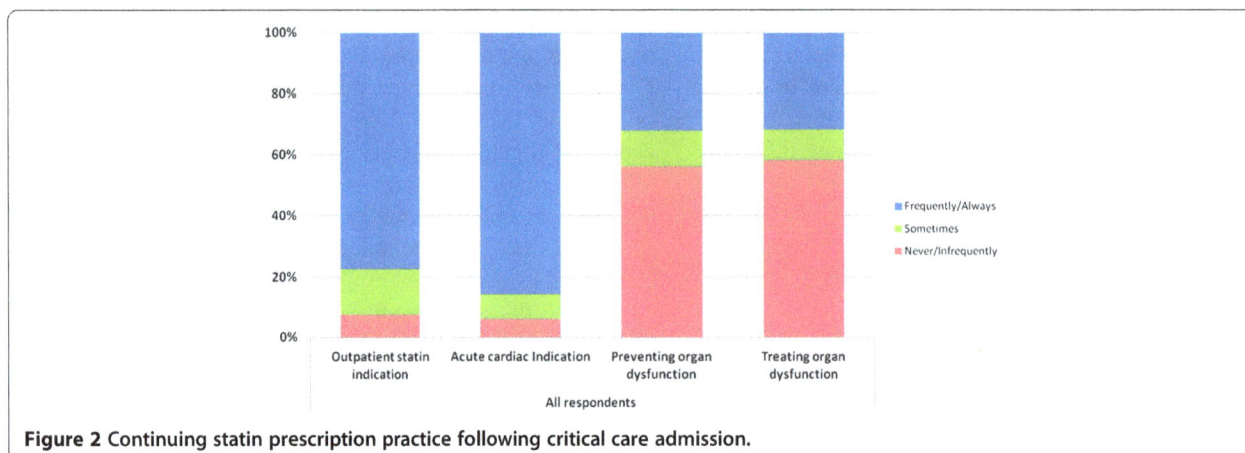

Figure 2 Continuing statin prescription practice following critical care admission.

statistically significant differences in the choice of cut offs for trial enrolment with higher biochemical cut-offs tolerated by physicians from ANZ (Table 1). Using three-times upper limit of normal as an example to demonstrate the heterogeneity in the choice of cut offs we observed for: 1) transaminase levels - overall 80.7%; UK = 83.5% *vs.* ANZ = 74.2%; p = 0.007; 2) serum creatine kinase levels – overall 79.2%; UK = 82.8% *vs.* ANZ = 71.0%; p < 0.001); and 3) serum total bilirubin levels – overall 82.6%; UK = 86.2% *vs.* ANZ = 74.2%; p = 0.003).

Trial end points

The majority of respondents (56.5%) preferred rates of new organ failure as the most appropriate primary outcome of choice for power calculations and there were no statistically significant differences when comparing responses between UK and ANZ (60.7% UK *vs.* 46.8% ANZ; p = 0.06). However, 40.6% of respondents felt that mortality was the most appropriate primary outcome of choice for power calculations and there were statistically significant differences when comparing responses between UK and ANZ (35.2% UK *vs.* 53.2% ANZ; p = 0.02). There were statistically significant differences in the

choice of follow up duration between the UK and ANZ (e.g. for 28 day follow up – overall 33.3%; UK = 37.9% *vs.* ANZ = 22.6%; p = 0.032) [Table 2].

Discussion

Key findings

We surveyed critical care physicians from a broad sample of critical care units in the UK and ANZ to obtain a cross section of statin prescribing practices in critically ill patients. The principal differences in reported statin prescription practices related to decisions to continue prior prescriptions, whether to initiate a new prescription, and about the degree of biochemical abnormalities physicians would tolerate when prescribing a statin. A significantly higher proportion of UK critical care physicians continued statins for outpatient indications in ICU, whereas more ANZ critical care physicians were likely to initiate new statin prescriptions to prevent organ dysfunction in sepsis. Interestingly, only a third of respondents would initiate a statin prescription for an acute cardiac indication in critically ill patients, whilst nearly a third of respondents would continue a pre existing statin

Table 1 Cut offs for biochemical tests below which the respondents would enrol patients into the proposed trial

THRESHOLD	OVERALL (%)			UK (%)			ANZ (%)		
	ALT/AST	CK	BILIRUBIN	ALT/AST	CK	BILIRUBIN	ALT/AST	CK	BILIRUBIN
ULN	27.6	34.7	33.9	31.6	41.8	38.4	16.1	14.5	21.0
3 ULN	42.3	33.9	37.7	36.7	26.0	32.2	58.1	56.5	53.2
5 ULN	13.8	13.4	12.1	11.3	10.7	8.5	21.0	21.0	22.6
10 ULN	2.5	2.9	1.7	2.3	2.8	1.7	3.2	3.2	1.6
>10 ULN	0.4	1.7	1.3	0	0.6	1.1	1.6	4.8	1.6
MISSING/NO RESPONSE	13.4	13.4	13.4	18.1	18.1	18.1	0	0	0
TOTAL	100	100	100	100	100	100	100	100	100

Shows the biochemical cut offs for hepatic transaminases (ALT/AST), creatine kinase (CK) and total bilirubin (bilirubin) below which the respondents would consider enrolling patients in the proposed statin interventional trial. Data are presented as proportions. ULN = upper limit of normal. p = 0.007 for ALT/AST; p < 0.001 for CK; p = 0.003 for Bilirubin (p-values when comparing the overall frequency distribution of the responses for ANZ and UK).

Table 2 Preferred follow up duration for the proposed statin interventional trial

follow up duration	overall - %	uk - %	anz - %	p*
1-7 days	1.9	1.4	3.2	0.585
8-14 days	3.4	4.1	1.6	0.677
15-21 days	2.4	2.8	1.6	1.000
21-28 days	33.3	37.9	22.6	0.032
3 months	29.0	22.8	43.6	0.003
6 months	26.1	28.3	21.0	0.304
other	3.9	2.8	6.5	0.244
total	100	100	100	

Shows respondents' preferred follow up duration for the proposed statin interventional trial. Data are presented as proportions. * p value for comparison of United Kingdom versus Australia and p = 0.024 when comparing the overall frequency distribution of the responses for ANZ and UK.

prescription for preventing or treating organ dysfunction secondary to sepsis syndromes.

Critical care physicians in both ANZ and UK agreed that a randomized controlled trial is needed to test the efficacy of statins for preventing organ dysfunction in early critical illness. However, while the majority of UK physicians would be willing to participate in such a trial, the majority of ANZ physicians were undecided based on the description of the trial that was provided. We can only speculate on the reasons for these differences, but one possibility is that ANZ physicians are more accustomed to focusing on large-scale pragmatic trials that aim to improve survival [33-35]. Indeed, more ANZ survey respondents wanted the interventional trial to be powered for mortality as the primary outcome, whereas more UK respondents preferred organ failure. The preferred statin for such an interventional trial was simvastatin in the UK and atorvastatin in ANZ, possible reflecting different prescribing practices between the two jurisdictions. Higher biomarker thresholds for stopping and initiating statin therapy were also reported by physicians in ANZ compared to those in the UK. These important differences must be considered when designing interventional trials of statin therapy in critical illness.

Strengths and weaknesses

The survey objectives were to evaluate opinions on an active area of critical care research in critical illness, i.e. the potential role of statins to attenuate or prevent organ dysfunction through the modulation of inflammation. This survey provides important information on the ICU community's views on this topic. The methodological rigour in the design of this survey, including careful sensibility testing and pilot testing, should reduce the potential for bias, a common problem in survey research [36]. We also targeted physicians in two large international regions to ensure

we had broad representation from the critical care community and to improve generalisability.

Our study has several limitations that are common to most surveys. First, as with most self-administered surveys, our response rate was incomplete. Although, we used the official mailing lists there are no data on completeness and accuracy of mailing lists. Furthermore, these mailing lists include non physician health care staff and trainee doctors who were not our target population. Although these groups were actively excluded the total number at any one time is variable. However, the survey responses represent replies from 74.6% of UK adult general critical units and 37.1% of ANZ critical care units. Second, our results reflect the reported practice of respondents, and may not reflect actual practice. Third, we are unable to rule out response bias, and some of the non-responding physicians may have provided different responses to survey questions.

Conclusions

Significant variability exists in the reported statin prescription practices in decisions to continue prior prescriptions, to initiate a new prescription, and in the degree of biochemical abnormalities physicians would tolerate when prescribing a statin. Our results, reflecting the opinions of critical care physicians across UK and ANZ, confirm that equipoise exists around the utility of statins to prevent and/or treat organ dysfunction in the critically ill patient population. Critical care physicians from both regions agreed that a clinical trial is needed to clarify the role of statins in this patient population.

Abbreviations
UK: United Kingdom; ANZ: Australia and New Zealand; ICU: Intensive care unit; RCT: Randomised controlled trial.

Competing interests
The authors declare that they have no competing interests.

Authors' contributions
All authors contributed equally to the conception and design of the study, interpretation of data, and critical revision of the manuscript. SG and MS-H developed the analysis plan and participated in the analysis. All authors read and approved the final manuscript.

Financial support
DCS is supported by a New Investigator Award from the Canadian Institutes for Health Research.
MT acknowledges the support of the UK NIHR Biomedical Research Centre scheme.

Acknowledgements
The Intensive Care Society, United Kingdom and The Australia and New Zealand Critical Care Trials Group.

Author details
[1]Division of Asthma, Allergy and Lung Biology, King's College London, London, UK. [2]Critical Care and Anesthesia Research Group, King's Health Partners Academic Health Sciences Centre, London, UK. [3]Department of Critical Care Medicine, Guy's and St Thomas' NHS Foundation Trust, London, UK. [4]Princess Alexandra Hospital, Wooloongabba, Brisbane, Australia.

[5]University of Queensland, Brisbane, Australia. [6]Interdepartmental Division of Critical Care, University of Toronto, Toronto, Canada. [7]Department of Critical Care Medicine, Sunnybrook Health Sciences Centre, Toronto, Canada. [8]Warwick Clinical Trials Unit, Warwick Medical, University of Warwick School, Warwick, UK. [9]Centre for Infection and Immunity, The Queen's University of Belfast, Belfast, UK.

References

1. Levy MM, Fink MP, Marshall JC, Abraham E, Angus D, Cook D, Cohen J, Opal SM, Vincent JL, Ramsay G: **2001 SCCM/ESICM/ACCP/ATS/SIS International Sepsis Definitions Conference.** *Crit Care Med* 2003, **31**(4):1250–1256.

2. Martin GS, Mannino DM, Eaton S, Moss M: **The epidemiology of sepsis in the United States from 1979 through 2000.** *N Engl J Med* 2003, **348** (16):1546–1554.

3. Harrison DA, Welch CA, Eddleston JM: **The epidemiology of severe sepsis in England, Wales and Northern Ireland, 1996 to 2004: secondary analysis of a high quality clinical database, the ICNARC Case Mix Programme Database.** *Crit Care* 2006, **10**(2):R42.

4. Linde-Zwirble WT, Angus DC: **Severe sepsis epidemiology: sampling, selection, and society.** *Crit Care* 2004, **8**(4):222–226.

5. Angus DC, Wax RS: **Epidemiology of sepsis: an update.** *Crit Care Med* 2001, **29**(7 Suppl):S109–S116.

6. Burchardi H, Schneider H: **Economic aspects of severe sepsis: a review of intensive care unit costs, cost of illness and cost effectiveness of therapy.** *Pharmacoeconomics* 2004, **22**(12):793–813.

7. Talmor D, Greenberg D, Howell MD, Lisbon A, Novack V, Shapiro N: **The costs and cost-effectiveness of an integrated sepsis treatment protocol.** *Crit Care Med* 2008, **36**(4):1168–1174.

8. Cinel I, Opal SM: **Molecular biology of inflammation and sepsis: a primer.** *Crit Care Med* 2009, **37**(1):291–304.

9. Phillip Dellinger R, Parrillo JE: **Mediator modulation therapy of severe sepsis and septic shock: does it work?** *Crit Care Med* 2004, **32**(1):282–286.

10. Bernard GR, Vincent JL, Laterre PF, LaRosa SP, Dhainaut JF, Lopez-Rodriguez A, Steingrub JS, Garber GE, Helterbrand JD, Ely EW, *et al*: **Efficacy and safety of recombinant human activated protein C for severe sepsis.** *N Engl J Med* 2001, **344**(10):699–709.

11. Van den Berghe G, Wilmer A, Hermans G, Meersseman W, Wouters PJ, Milants I, Van Wijngaerden E, Bobbaers H, Bouillon R: **Intensive insulin therapy in the medical ICU.** *New England Journal of Medicine* 2006, **354** (5):449–461.

12. Van den Berghe G, Wouters P, Weekers F, Verwaest C, Bruyninckx F, Schetz M, Vlasselaers D, Ferdinande P, Lauwers P, Bouillon R: **Intensive insulin therapy in critically Ill patients.** *New England Journal of Medicine* 2001, **345** (19):1359–1367.

13. Craig TR, Duffy MJ, Shyamsundar M, McDowell C, O'Kane CM, Elborn JS, McAuley DF: **A randomized clinical trial of hydroxymethylglutaryl-coenzyme a reductase inhibition for acute lung injury (The HARP Study).** *Am J Respir Crit Care Med* 2011, **183**(5):620–626.

14. Kruger PS, Harward ML, Jones MA, Joyce CJ, Kostner KM, Roberts MS, Venkatesh B: **Continuation of statin therapy in patients with presumed infection: a randomized controlled trial.** *Am J Respir Crit Care Med* 2011, **183**(6):774–781.

15. Lazar LD, Pletcher MJ, Coxson PG, Bibbins-Domingo K, Goldman L: **Cost-effectiveness of statin therapy for primary prevention in a low-cost statin era.** *Circulation* 2011, **124**(2):146–153.

16. Terblanche M, Almog Y, Rosenson RS, Smith TS, Hackam DG: **Statins and sepsis: multiple modifications at multiple levels.** *The Lancet Infectious Diseases* 2007, **7**(5):358–368.

17. Jasinska M, Owczarek J, Orszulak-Michalak D: **Statins: a new insight into their mechanisms of action and consequent pleiotropic effects.** *Pharmacol Rep* 2007, **59**(5):483–499.

18. Terblanche M, Smith TS, Adhikari NK: **Statins, bugs and prophylaxis: intriguing possibilities.** *Crit Care* 2006, **10**(5):168.

19. Shyamsundar M, McKeown STW, O'Kane CM, Craig TR, Brown V, Thickett DR, Matthay MA, Taggart CC, Backman JT, Elborn JS, *et al*: **Simvastatin decreases lipopolysaccharide-induced pulmonary inflammation in healthy volunteers.** *American Journal of Respiratory and Critical Care Medicine* 2009, **179**(12):1107–1114.

20. Wilding EI, Brown JR, Bryant AP, Chalker AF, Holmes DJ, Ingraham KA, Iordanescu S, So CY, Rosenberg M, Gwynn MN: **Identification, evolution, and essentiality of the mevalonate pathway for isopentenyl diphosphate biosynthesis in gram-positive cocci.** *J Bacteriol* 2000, **182**(15):4319–4327.

21. Chow OA, von Kockritz-Blickwede M, Bright AT, Hensler ME, Zinkernagel AS, Cogen AL, Gallo RL, Monestier M, Wang Y, Glass CK, *et al*: **Statins enhance formation of phagocyte extracellular traps.** *Cell Host Microbe* 2010, **8** (5):445–454.

22. Bergman P, Linde C, Putsep K, Pohanka A, Normark S, Henriques-Normark B, Andersson J, Bjorkhem-Bergman L: **Studies on the antibacterial effects of statins–in vitro and in vivo.** *PLoS ONE* 2011, **6**(8):e24394.

23. Masadeh M, Mhaidat N, Alzoubi K, Al-Azzam S, Alnasser Z: **Antibacterial activity of statins: a comparative study of Atorvastatin, Simvastatin, and Rosuvastatin.** *Ann Clin Microbiol Antimicrob* 2012, **11**(1):13.

24. Welsh AM, Kruger P, Faoagali J: **Antimicrobial action of atorvastatin and rosuvastatin.** *Pathology* 2009, **41**(7):689–691.

25. Falagas ME, Makris GC, Matthaiou DK, Rafailidis PI: **Statins for infection and sepsis: a systematic review of the clinical evidence.** *Journal of Antimicrobial Chemotherapy* 2008, **61**(4):774–785.

26. Tleyjeh IM, Kashour T, Hakim FA, Zimmerman VA, Erwin PJ, Sutton AJ, Ibrahim T: **Statins for the prevention and treatment of infections: a systematic review and meta-analysis.** *Arch Intern Med* 2009, **169**(18):1658–1667.

27. Douglas I, Evans S, Smeeth L: **Effect of statin treatment on short term mortality after pneumonia episode: cohort study.** *BMJ* 2011, **342**:d1642.

28. Björkhem-Bergman L, Bergman P, Andersson J, Lindh JD: **Statin treatment and mortality in bacterial infections – a systematic review and meta-analysis.** *PLoS ONE* 2010, **5**(5):e10702.

29. Truwit JD: **Statins: a role in infected critically ill patients?** *Crit Care* 2011, **15**(2):145.

30. Terblanche MJ, Pinto R, Whiteley C, Brett S, Beale R, Adhikari NK: **Statins do not prevent acute organ failure in ventilated ICU patients: single-centre retrospective cohort study.** *Crit Care* 2011, **15**(1):R74.

31. Feinstein AR: *Chapter 10: The Theory and Evaluation of Sensibility.* Yale University Press: Clinimetrics. New Haven; 1987.

32. *Smart-SurveyTM.* Smart-SurveyTM. http://www.smart-survey.co.uk.

33. Finfer S, Chittock DR, Su SY, Blair D, Foster D, Dhingra V, Bellomo R, Cook D, Dodek P, Henderson WR, *et al*: **Intensive versus conventional glucose control in critically ill patients.** *N Engl J Med* 2009, **360**(13):1283–1297.

34. Bellomo R, Cass A, Cole L, Finfer S, Gallagher M, Lo S, McArthur C, McGuinness S, Myburgh J, Norton R, *et al*: **Intensity of continuous renal-replacement therapy in critically ill patients.** *N Engl J Med* 2009, **361** (17):1627–1638.

35. Finfer S, Bellomo R, Boyce N, French J, Myburgh J, Norton R: **A comparison of albumin and saline for fluid resuscitation in the intensive care unit.** *N Engl J Med* 2004, **350**(22):2247–2256.

36. Burns KEA, Duffett M, Kho ME, Meade MO, Adhikari NKJ, Sinuff T, Cook DJ: **Group ftA: a guide for the design and conduct of self-administered surveys of clinicians.** *Canadian Medical Association Journal* 2008, **179** (3):245–252.

9

Adverse drug reaction monitoring: support for pharmacovigilance at a tertiary care hospital in Northern Brazil

Márcia Germana Alves de Araújo Lobo[1], Sandra Maria Botelho Pinheiro[2], José Gerley Díaz Castro[3], Valéria Gomes Momenté[4] and Maria-Cristina S Pranchevicius[2*]

Abstract

Background: Adverse drug reactions (ADRs) are recognised as a common cause of hospital admissions, and they constitute a significant economic burden for hospitals. Hospital-based ADR monitoring and reporting programmes aim to identify and quantify the risks associated with the use of drugs provided in a hospital setting. This information may be useful for identifying and minimising preventable ADRs and may enhance the ability of prescribers to manage ADRs more effectively. The main objectives of this study were to evaluate ADRs that occurred during inpatient stays at the Hospital Geral de Palmas (HGP) in Tocantins, Brazil, and to facilitate the development of a pharmacovigilance service.

Methods: A prospective study was conducted at HGP over a period of 8 months, from January 2009 to August 2009. This observational, cross-sectional, descriptive study was based on an analysis of medical records. Several parameters were utilised in the data evaluation, including patient demographics, drug and reaction characteristics, and reaction outcomes. The reaction severity and predisposing factors were also assessed.

Results: The overall incidence of ADRs in the patient population was 3.1%, and gender was not found to be a risk factor. The highest ADR rate (75.8%) was found in the adult age group 15 to 50 years, and the lowest ADR rate was found in children aged 3 to 13 years (7.4%). Because of the high frequency of ADRs in orthopaedic (25%), general medicine (22%), and oncology (16%) patients, improved control of the drugs used in these specialties is required. Additionally, the nurse team (52.7%) registered the most ADRs in medical records, most likely due to the job responsibilities of nurses. As expected, the most noticeable ADRs occurred in skin tissues, with such ADRs are more obvious to medical staff, with rashes being the most common reactions. Metamizole, tramadol, and vancomycin were responsible for 21, 11.6, and 8.4% of ADRs, respectively. The majority of ADRs had moderate severity (58.9%), thus requiring intervention. Type A reactions were the most common (82.1%). At least one predisposing factor was present in 79.9% of the reports examined, and the most common predisposing factor was polypharmacy.

Conclusions: The results obtained will contribute to the development of strategies for the pharmacovigilance service at HGP and other hospitals throughout the country, which will improve the quality of ADR reporting and ensure safer drug use in Brazilian hospitals.

* Correspondence: mcspranc@uft.edu.br
[2]Curso de Medicina, Universidade Federal do Tocantins, Av. NS 15 s/n (109 Norte), Palmas 77001-090, Brasil
Full list of author information is available at the end of the article

Background

An adverse drug reaction (ADR) is defined by the World Health Organization (WHO) as any noxious, unintended, or undesired effect of a drug that occurs at doses used in humans for prophylaxis, diagnosis, or therapy [1]. ADRs are a major cause of morbidity and place a substantial burden on limited healthcare resources [2]. Multiple factors influence ADR susceptibility, including multiple drug therapy, disease severity, age, and the type and number of drugs prescribed [3-8]. Several studies have shown that the proportion of patients admitted with ADRs ranges from approximately 2.0 to 21.4%, whereas between 1.7 and 25.1% of inpatients are reported to have developed an ADR during their hospital stay [9-12]. There are marked differences in disease prevalence, access to medicines, drug use patterns, and drug management systems between developed and developing countries, and such differences impact the frequency and nature of ADRs [13].

Reports of ADRs have become an important component of monitoring and evaluation activities performed in hospitals [14]. This information may be useful for identifying and minimising preventable ADRs while generally enhancing the ability of prescribers to manage ADRs more effectively [15,16].

Few reports are available regarding the incidence of ADRs in Brazilian hospitals. The Hospital Geral de Palmas (HGP) is a highly complex, 220-bed, tertiary care reference centre and teaching hospital located in the city of Palmas in Northern Brazil. An ADR reporting program has existed in HGP since July 2001 and is coordinated by the Hospital's Department of Pharmacy Practice. The ADR reporting unit of HGP is one of the reference centres of the National Pharmacovigilance Program.

The present study was undertaken to (1) determine the frequency of ADRs that occur in hospitalised patients and to classify the reactions according to the demographics of the affected patients and the preventability of the ADRs; (2) describe the types of drugs involved; (3) report the most common clinical manifestations associated with these ADRs and their severity; and (4) assess the predictive factors of ADRs.

Methods

Study design

A prospective study was conducted over a period of 8 months from January 2009 to August 2009 at HGP in Tocantins, Brazil. HGP is a 220-bed tertiary care hospital utilised by the entire state and its surrounding areas. The hospital's specialties are general medicine and surgery. The study was observational, non-interventional, and based on the ADRs reported by multiple departments of HGP; the reports were coordinated by clinical pharmacists. Male and female inpatients, except those in the Intensive Care Unit and Emergency Room, were included

in the study. HGP participates in standard pharmacovigilance and employs a system of spontaneous reporting, which was the form of reporting used in this study.

Functioning of the ADR reporting system at HGP

There was no organised pharmacovigilance program at the hospital prior to the study. Clinical meetings with allied hospital healthcare professionals raised awareness of ADR monitoring and its importance. Attendees were encouraged to report all suspected ADRs using various reporting modalities, such as using a printed ADR notification form (available at all nursing stations), reporting ADRs by telephone, or directly reporting ADRs to an attending clinical pharmacist in certain hospital departments. Nurses also completed notification forms. Many forms were designed for this study, including a notification form and a form to describe the ADR in detail. Notification forms were kept in the participating wards. All patients were assessed for ADRs during the study period. In suspected cases, patients' past medical history and medication history were collected. To provide complementary information concerning adverse reactions, especially unexpected reactions, ADRs were spontaneously reported as part of standard care. Patients were monitored daily throughout their hospital stay, and some their medical records were reviewed daily and others after discharge. The suspected ADRs were carefully analysed and documented. All relevant data, including all drugs that patients received prior to the reaction onset and their respective dosages, the most frequent routes of administration, the dates of the reaction onsets, and the patients' allergy status (to drugs and foods), were noted. Thus, the ADRs confirmed by the physicians and research pharmacists were classified and subjected to a severity assessment. Furthermore, information regarding the ADRs reported in the unit was published six times a year in a news bulletin of the Department of Pharmacovigilance (PHS) and was disseminated to all health care professionals at the hospital.

After initial notification of a suspected ADR, additional details were collected concerning previous allergies, concomitant medications, comorbidities, ADR management and outcome, and other details necessary for evaluation. These data were collected by reviewing patients' records and noting the reporters' comments. The collected data were recorded in separate ADR documents for further assessment. The physician responsible for the case was consulted when additional details and clarification were necessary.

Evaluation of data

Patient characteristics

The patients' age and gender were considered in the evaluation. In accordance with a previous paper, patients were divided into three age groups: children and teenagers (0–18 years old), adults (19–59 years old), and the elderly (over 60 years old).

Reaction characteristics

The ADRs were classified according to the Rawlins and Thompson classification system as type A or type B [17]. The severity of the reaction was determined according to the classification system of Hartwig et al. [18-20]. Mild reactions were those that were self-limiting, resolved over time without treatment, and did not extend a patient's hospital stay. Moderate ADRs were defined as those that required therapeutic intervention and prolongation of the hospital stay by one day but that resolved within 24 hours due to a change in drug therapy or the administration of a specific treatment to prevent further adverse outcomes. Severe ADRs threatened patients' lives, caused disability, led to hospitalisation, prolonged hospital stays, required intensive medical care, or led to death. Reactions were further classified depending on the organ system affected.

Drug characteristics

The drugs involved in the ADRs were categorised into various drug classes according to the anatomical therapeutic chemical (ATC) classification, based on the 2005 WHO-ATC Index [21].

Management and outcomes

Patients' outcomes were reported as death, fully recovered (during hospitalisation), recovering (but not fully recovered during hospitalisation), or unknown (not documented after the initial report in the chart). The management strategies used for the ADRs were categorised as drug withdrawal, dose reduction, additional treatment for the ADR, or no change in regimen with no additional treatment.

Predisposing factors

Factors with the potential to predispose patients to ADRs in the individual reports were evaluated. Predisposing factors were generally classified according to age, gender, multiple and intercurrent disease states, and polypharmacy [3-8]. Ages above 60 (geriatrics) and below 18 (paediatrics) were regarded as a predisposing factor under the age criterion. Polypharmacy was considered to be minor (2–3 drugs), moderate (4–5 drugs), or major (>5 drugs) based on the characterisation by Wong [6]. Gender was considered a factor only if there was previous information indicating that the patient's gender predisposed the patient to the reaction in question.

Statistical analysis

Student's t-test was used to compare means, and the χ^2 test was used for the other variables. A two-tailed P value of less than 0.05 was considered statistically significant.

Ethics and consent

The study was approved by the Institutional Human Ethics Committee of Centro Universitário Luterano de Palmas-Tocantins, filed under number 794/2008, and was conducted in accordance with the ethical guidelines of the Declaration of Helsinki (created in 1964 and revised in 2002). Permission to conduct the study was obtained from the Medical Superintendent of the Hospital Geral de Palmas.

Results

Throughout the 8-month study period, 95 ADRs were confirmed and reported in 81 inpatients. There were 2995 patient admissions at locations other than HGP, and the overall incidence of ADRs during hospitalisation in this patient group was 3.1%.

ADRs were more frequent in males (55.7%) than in females (44.3%). No significant difference was observed in the ADRs between males and females during the hospital stay (χ^2c = 1.05, P = 0.26). The rates of ADRs in paediatric (<18 years), geriatric (>60 years), and adult patients were 18.9, 20.0, and 61.0%, respectively. The rates of ADRs in adult patients were significantly higher than those in paediatric and geriatric patients ($\chi^2 = 33$; P = 0.0001). Details regarding the classification and assessment of ADRs are provided in Table 1.

Certain factors contributed to the occurrence of ADRs, such as the number of different drugs administered concomitantly. To assess contributing factors, we calculated the median number of prescriptions per patient that were suspected of causing ADRs, which was 6.8 medications/prescription. We also found that the risk of ADRs was higher in 7.4% of the patients who were using more than 6 medications.

The severity assessment of the ADRs showed that over half of the reactions reported were moderate (58.9%) ($\chi^2 = 29.3$, P = 0.00001), followed by mild (25.3%) and severe (15.8%) reactions. There were no fatal reactions. Complete recovery was achieved in 26.3% of patients with ADRs, 5.8% were in the recovery process, and 57.9% were classified as having 'unknown outcomes' (i.e., outcomes that could not be assessed due to a lack of recorded reports). Treatment with the offending drug was interrupted in 50.5% of patients. Another drug was substituted for the offending drug in 27.4% of patients, and other drugs were added to relieve the symptoms in 57.0% of patients; the drug dosage was not reduced in any patient to ameliorate symptoms. Treatment was unchanged in 37.8% of patients

Table 1 Patient characteristics

Age group	Number (%) of ADR reports (n = 95)	Gender group	Number (%) of ADR reports (n = 95)
Paediatric (0–18 years)	18 (19.0)	Male	53 (55.7)
Adult (19–59 years)	58 (61.0)	Female	42 (44.3)
Geriatric (>60 years)	19 (20.0)		
Total	95 (100.0)		95 (100.0)

(Table 2). The majority of reported reactions were type A reactions (82.1%).

The most common drugs causing ADRs and their reaction details are shown in Table 3. Analgesics (e.g., metamizole) were associated with approximately one-third of all ADRs reported (21.0%). Tramadol produced the highest number of reactions (11.6%), followed by vancomycin (8.4%), phenytoin (6.3%), and ceftriaxone (4.1%). Itching was the most common ADR reported (26.3%), followed by rashes and oedema (13.7%). The organ systems affected by the ADRs are shown in Table 4. The skin was found to be the most commonly affected organ system (34.5%), followed by the metabolic (16.5%) and gastrointestinal (14.2%) systems.

The minimum amount of time prior to ADR development was 1 day of hospitalisation, the median time was 6 days, and the maximum time was 180 days. The reactions that manifested during a period of 11 to 30 days of hospitalisation constituted 31.6% of the total number of reactions identified in this study, equivalent to the average percentage of reactions that occurred among inpatients in the Orthopaedics and General Medicine Departments.

Table 2 Management, outcomes, and severity of ADRs

Parameters	Number (%) of ADRs
Severity	
Mild	24 (25.3)
Moderate	56 (58.9)
Severe	15 (15.8)
Outcomes†	
Fatal	0
Fully Recovered	25 (26.3)
Recovering	15 (15.8)
Unknown	55 (57.9)
Treatment	
Stopped the medication	48 (50.5)
Reduced the dose	0
Added another drug to relieve the symptoms	54 (57.0)
Substituted another drug	26 (27.4)
No change	36 (37.8)

The highest ADR rate in young adults occurred in the Orthopaedics Department (25%). ADRs occurred in the General Medicine (22%) and Oncology (16%) Departments at the second and third greatest frequencies, respectively.

Discussion and conclusion

A total of 30-91% of ADRs could be avoided, thus saving health system resources and reducing harm to patients [22]. To work together toward ADR prevention, physicians, nurses, and pharmacists should be aware of potential clinical problems by assessing medicines that a patient has used recently; allergies or unusual reactions to any medicine, food, or product; special dietary or eating restrictions; and whether the patient is pregnant, breastfeeding, or planning pregnancy in the near future [23]. New drugs should also be closely monitored to avoid unknown and severe ADRs [24].

The fundamental role of pharmacovigilance centres is to collect and process data regarding ADRs and to support hospitals in the identification of these reactions [25]. The centres' actions serve to reduce risks related to medication usage, improve patients' quality of life, prevent iatrogenic diseases, and minimise health expenses.

The frequency of ADRs found in this study, which was based on inpatient records, was 3.1%. This value could have been greater if HGP had adopted intensive monitoring techniques or computer programs to supervise ADRs. The main reason for this low number is that our data were derived from spontaneous reporting. The ADR rate was low compared with the results of a meta-analysis conducted by Lazarou et al. [12], who reported that 15.1% of hospitalised patients develop an ADR. Other factors that may have contributed to this low number include the non-reporting of mild ADRs and the lack of guidelines and procedures for identification, registration, and notification. Reluctance to register ADRs persists, especially among nurses, as the registering of ADRs could signal medical mistakes or poor quality of care. This reluctance results in fewer ADR notifications and was also observed in Sobravime's study [13].

There is no agreement among studies regarding the incidence of ADRs with respect to gender. Certain authors [3,4] have reported that women are more susceptible to ADRs, possibly due to their high medication use, obstetric

Table 3 Drug classes and individual drugs most commonly associated with ADRs

Drug class	Drug (ATC)	Total number (%) (n = 95)
Antibiotics	Cefalexin (J01DB01)	1 (1.0)
	Cefalotin (J01DB03)	6 (6.3)
	Cefazolin (J01DB04)	1 (1.0)
	Cefepime (J01DE01)	3 (3.1)
	Ceftriaxone (J01DD04)	4 (4.2)
	Imipenem (J01DH51)	2 (2.1)
	Oxacillin (J01CF04)	1 (1.0)
	Rifampicin (J04AB02)	1 (1.0)
	Vancomycin (J01XA01)	8 (8.4)
Analgesics	Metamizole (N02BB02)	20 (21.0)
	Paracetamol (N02BE01)	1 (1.0)
Antipsychotics	Chlorpromazine (N05AA01)	1 (1.0)
	Olanzapine (N05AH03)	1 (1.0)
	Risperidone (N05AX08)	1 (1.0)
Opioids	Fentanyl (N01AH02)	1 (1.0)
	Tramadol (N02AX02)	11 (11.6)
Benzodiazepine	Diazepam (N05BA01)	1 (1.0)
	Midazolam (N05CD08)	1 (1.0)
ACE inhibitors	Captopril (C09BA01)	1 (1.0)
	Enalapril (C09AA02)	2 (2.1)
Antiarrhythmic	Amiodarone (C01BD01)	2 (2.1)
Local anaesthetic	Bupivacaine (N01BB01)	1 (1.0)
Anticonvulsant	Phenytoin (N03AB02)	6 (6.3)
Beta-blocker	Carvedilol (C07AG02)	1 (1.0)
Antiemetic	Metoclopramide (A03FA01)	2 (2.1)
H2 receptor antagonist	Ranitidine (A02BA02)	2 (2.1)
Antidiuretic	Furosemide (C03CA01)	4 (4.2)

complications, and metabolic alterations due to hormone levels. Other researchers [26-28] have found the incidence of ADRs to be unrelated to gender, which supports our finding that ADRs did not differ significantly between men and women.

Table 4 Organ systems affected by ADRs and the most commonly reported reactions

Organ system	Number (%) of ADRs (n = 133)
Skin	46 (34.5)
Gastrointestinal	19 (14.2)
Central nervous system	12 (9.0)
Cardiovascular	5 (3.7)
Eyes, ears, nose, and throat	3 (2.2
Musculoskeletal	9 (6.7)
Metabolic	22 (16.5)
Haematologic	4 (3.0)
Respiratory	2 (1.5)

Age is considered a risk factor for the occurrence of ADRs [29]. Therefore, children and the elderly, due to metabolic system alterations, require careful orientation and follow-up to avoid ADR occurrences and complications. However, in our study, the incidence of ADRs in adults (61.0%) was significantly higher than that in the other age groups [26,30]. These results seem to contradict those of Passarelli [4], who found that the elderly have a higher risk of ADRs. These conflicting results may be due to the dosage adjustments of paediatric and geriatric prescriptions as well as the higher number of young adults who are hospitalised at HGP.

The incidence of adverse reactions increases exponentially, but not necessarily simultaneously, with the number of drugs administered during a certain period [6]. Our study demonstrated that the usage of 6 to 10 medications per patient increased the risk of ADRs in 7.4% of cases.

Extension of hospital stay is also considered a risk factor for ADRs [26]. The highest ADR frequency (approximately 50%) occurred during the first five days of hospitalisation.

The minimum time prior to the development of ADRs was 1 day of hospitalisation, the median time was 6 days, and the maximum time was 180 days. The percentage of reactions that manifested during a period of 11 to 30 days of hospitalisation was 31.6%, which is equivalent to the average percentage of reactions among inpatients of the Orthopaedics and General Medicine Departments at HGP.

The higher ADR rate in young adults is related to the higher ADR frequency in the Orthopaedics Department (25%). These results revealed a correlation between the elevated number of young adults hospitalised and the number of traumas caused by motorcycle accidents, which are the second most common cause of hospitalisation at HGP. The second and third highest prevalence of ADRs occurred in the General Medicine (22%) and Oncology (16%) Departments, most likely due to the greater exposure to medication in the General Medicine Department and to the adverse effects of antineoplastic medications in the Oncology Department.

It was observed that several organ systems were affected by medications. However, in accordance with other studies [4,31], the highest frequency (48.4%) of adverse reactions occurred in the dermatological system, manifesting as formication, skin rashes, flushing, and dried skin. Eleven reactions were registered simply as allergic reactions with no further description in the records regarding the associated reaction manifestation, compromising the quality of the records and the notification process.

In our study, analgesics caused the highest rate of ADRs, followed by antibiotics. Our results are in accordance with those of a study by Bates [32], possibly due to the elevated consumption of such medications at HGP. Risperidone, olanzapine, ceftriaxone, vancomycin, and furosemide were responsible for severe ADRs (type B); although the medications' dose dependence and pharmacological properties were not indicated in the reports, severe ADR cases are frequently immune- or genetically related and usually prolong hospitalisation or require follow-up treatment. However, the majority of the ADRs studied were type A reactions (84.2%).

Due to intervention, the majority of ADRs were of moderate severity, and there was a significant difference in the degree of severity of the ADRs based on the records analysed.

A few doctors were able to control the ADRs by discontinuing the offending medication (50%). In other cases, clinical treatments were implemented using antihistamines, corticoids, antidotes, zinc dioxide, and vitamin creams to relieve symptoms, whereas no treatment was administered in some cases either due to the presence of only a mild ADR or because the offending medication was unknown (13%).

In conclusion, the ADRs that occurred at our hospital are comparable to those reported by other studies performed in Brazilian and foreign hospitals; nevertheless, certain aspects were different. The number of prescribed drugs and the length of drug use constitute risk factors for ADRs; monitoring these factors requires a review of clinical protocols, the quality of the prescription, and the therapeutic arsenal. Among the prescribed medications, metamizole, tramadol, and vancomycin caused the most ADRs due to their frequent usage and the inherent characteristics of these drugs. It is evident that pharmacovigilance systems are needed to facilitate ADR follow-ups by health professionals directly involved in patient care.

Competing interests

The authors have no competing interests to declare.

Authors' contributions

MGAAL and MCSP participated in the design of the study, analysed the data, and drafted the manuscript. SMBP analysed the data. JGDC participated in the design of the study and analysed the data. MCSP and VGM conceived the study. All authors read and approved the final manuscript.

Acknowledgements

We thank Paulo Faria Barbosa, Superintendent of the Hospital Geral de Palmas, for allowing us to conduct this study. We are grateful to the participating clinical pharmacists, namely, Vidal Gonzalez Mateos, Carlos Lacerda, Wanderley José Silva, and Léia Aires Cavalcante, as well as the volunteers who generously provided assistance at the hospital. Support for this study was provided by the authors.

Author details

[1]Hospital Geral de Palmas, Av NS1, s/n Conj. 02 - Lote 01, Palmas 77.054-970, Brasil. [2]Curso de Medicina, Universidade Federal do Tocantins, Av. NS 15 s/n (109 Norte), Palmas 77001-090, Brasil. [3]Curso de Enfermagem, Universidade Federal do Tocantins, Av. NS 15 s/n (109 Norte), Palmas 77001-090, Brasil. [4]Curso de Engenharia de Alimentos, Universidade Federal do Tocantins, Av. NS 15 s/n (109 Norte), Palmas 77001-090, Brasil.

References

1.   World Health Organization: International drug monitoring: the role of the hospital. In *Technical report series no. 425.* Geneva, Switzerland: World Health Organization; 1966:1–24.
2.   Juntti-Patinen L, Neuvoren PJ: Drug-related deaths in a university central hospital. *Eur J Clin Pharmacol* 2002, 58:479–482.
3.   Magalhães SMS, Carvalho WS: Reações Adversas a Medicamentos. In *Ciências Farmacêuticas. Uma Abordagem em Farmácia Hospitalar.* São Paulo: Atheneu; 2001:125–146.
4.   Passarelli MCG: *Reações adversas a medicamentos em uma população idosa hospitalizada. PhD thesis.* Universidade de São Paulo, Faculdade de Medicina; 2005.
5.   Lobstein R, Lakin A, Koren G: Pharmacokinetic Changes during pregnancy and Their clinical Relevance. *Clinical Pharmacokinet* 1997, 33:328–343.
6.   Wong A: Os usos inadequados e os efeitos adversos de medicamentos na prática clínica. *J Pediatr (Rio J)* 2003, 79:379–380.
7.   Tatro DS: *Textbook of therapeutics, drug and disease management.* Baltimore: William and Wilkins; 1996.
8.   May RJ: *Adverse drug reactions and interactions,* Pharmacoterapy: a pathophysiologic approach. Norwalk: Appleton & Lange; 1997:101–116.
9.   Laporte JR: *Famacovigilância Hospitalar.* http://www.cvs.saude.sp.gov.br/farde_hos.html.
10. Brandão A, Vasconcelos F: A tênue fronteira entre a cura e o malefício. *Pharmacia Brasileira* 2000, 22:36–39.
11. Einarson TR: Drug-related hospital admissions. *Ann Pharmacother* 1993, 27:832–840.

12. Lazarou J, Pomeranz BH, Corey PN: Incidence of adverse drug reactions in hospitalized patients: A meta-analysis of prospective studies. *JAMA* 1998, **279:**1200–1205.
13. Subravime: *Declaração de Berlim sobre Farmacovigilância*. São Paulo; 2005.
14. Van Grootheest K, Olsson S, Couper M, de Jong-van den Berg L: Pharmacists' role in reporting adverse drug reactions in an international perspective. *Pharmacoepidemiol Drug Saf* 2004, **3:**457–464.
15. Gallelli L, Ferreri G, Colosimo M, Pirritano D, Flocco MA, Pelaia G, *et al*: Retrospective analysis of adverse drug reactions to bronchodilatorsobserved in two pulmonary divisions of Catanzaro, Italy. *Pharmacol Res* 2003, **47**(Suppl 6):493–499.
16. Wu WK: Evaluation of outpatient adverse drug reactions leading to hospitalization. *Am J Health Syst Pharm* 2003, **60**(Suppl 3):253–259.
17. Rawlins MD, Thompson JW: Mechanisms of adverse drug reactions. In *Textbook of adverse drug reactions*. 4th edition. Oxford: Oxford University press; 1981:18–45.
18. Naranjo CA, Busto U, Sellers EM, Sandor P, Ruiz I, Robert EA, Ecek E, Domeck C, Greenblatt DJ: A method for estimating the probability of adverse drug reactions. *Clinic Pharmacological Therapeutic* 1981, **2:**239–245.
19. Pearson TF, Pittman D, Longley JM, Grapes T, Vigliotti DJ, Mullis SR: Factors associated with preventable adverse drug reactions. *Am J Hosp Pharm* 1994, **51:**2268–2271.
20. Sebastião ECO: *Intervenção farmacêutica na qualidade assistencial e nas reações adversas de amitriptilina prescrita para pacientes ambulatoriais do Sistema Único de Saúde de Ribeirão Preto. PhD thesis*. Universidade de São Paulo, Faculdade de Ciências Farmacêuticas; 2005.
21. *WHO Collaborating Centre for Drug Statistics Methodology: Completed ATC Index 2005*; [http://www.whocc.no/atcddd/].
22. Puerro MAP: *O custo das reações adversas medicamentosas em hospitais, MSc thesis*. Universidade de São Paulo, Faculdade de Saúde Pública; 2004.
23. Merck Sharp Dohme: Aspectos gerais dos medicamentos. In *Manual Merck. Saúde para a família*: Seção 2 – Medicamentos. Capítulo 5; [http://mmspf.msdonline.com.br/pacientes/manual_merck/secao_02/cap_005.html].
24. Harnik S: *Respostas nocivas a medicamentos podem ser evitadas, diminuindo custos*; [http://www.usp.br/agen/bols/2004/rede1426.htm].
25. Gomes MJV, Reis AAMM: *Ciências Farmacêuticas: Uma Abordagem em Farmácia Hospitalar*. São Paulo: Atheneu; 2001.
26. Rozenfeld S: Agravos provocados por medicamentos em hospitais do Estado do Rio de Janeiro. *Rev Saude Publica* 2006, **41:**1–8.
27. Gomes AP: *Incidência de reações adversas a medicamentos em Hospital de Ensino do Nordeste do Brasil. MSc thesis*. Universidade Federal do Ceará, Faculdade de Ciências Farmacêuticas; 2004.
28. Pfaffenbach G, Carvalho OM, Bergsten-Mendes G: Reações adversas a medicamentos como determinantes da admissão hospitalar. *Rev Assoc Med Bras* 2002, **48:**237–241.
29. Notteerman DA: *Farmacoterapia Pediátrica*, Farmacologia em Terapia Intensiva. Rio de Janeiro: Revinter; 1993:96–120.
30. Louro EO: Perfil de utilização de medicamentos e monitoração de reações adversas em pacientes pediátricos no Hospital Albert Sabin em São Paulo. *Rev Saude Publica* 2004, **41:**23–29.
31. Amaral FPM: *Avaliação do sistema de farmacovigilância do instituto de doenças tropicais Natan Portella em Teresina – PI. MSc Thesis.*: Universidade Federal do Ceará, Faculdade de Medicina; 2006.
32. Bates DW, Cullen DJ, Laird N: Incidence of adverse drug events and potential adverse drug events. *JAMA* 1995, **274:**29–34.

10

Price, familiarity, and availability determine the choice of drug - a population-based survey five years after generic substitution was introduced in Finland

Reeta Heikkilä[1*], Pekka Mäntyselkä[2,3†] and Riitta Ahonen[1†]

Abstract

Background: Mandatory generic substitution (GS) was introduced in Finland at the beginning of April 2003. However, individual patients or physicians may forbid the substitution. GS was a significant change for Finnish medicine users. It was thought it would confuse people when the names, colors, packages, etc., changed. The purpose of this study was to explore what medicine-related factors influence people's choice of prescription drugs five years after generic substitution was introduced in Finland.

Methods: A population survey was carried out during the autumn of 2008. A random sample was drawn from five mainland counties. A questionnaire was mailed to 3000 people at least 18 years old and living in Finland. The questionnaire consisted of both structured and open-ended questions. Factors that influenced the subjects' choice of medicines were asked with a structured question containing 11 propositions. Descriptive statistical analyses were performed.

Results: In total, 1844 questionnaires were returned (response rate, 62%). The percentage of female respondents was 55%. Price, availability, and familiarity were the three most important factors that influenced the choice of medicines. For the people who had refused GS, the familiarity of the medicine was the most important factor. For the subjects who had allowed GS and for those who had both refused and allowed GS, price was the most important factor.

Conclusions: The present study shows that price, familiarity, and availability were important factors in the choice of prescription medicines. The external characteristics of the medicines, for instance the color and shape of the tablet/capsule or the appearance of the package, were not significant characteristics for people.

Background

Generic substitution (GS) was introduced in Finland at the beginning of April 2003 with the aim of curbing the rise in medical expenses for society and individuals. The reform was preceded by heated public debate. For example, the Finnish Medical Association and the pharmaceutical industry (Pharma Industry Finland) objected to it because, for example, they were afraid of decreasing adherence [1,2]. It was thought that generic substitution would confuse people when the names, colors, packages and other physical appearance of drug products changed. It is certain that generic substitution was a considerable health policy reform for Finnish medicine users. People were not used to making decisions related to their medication. Before generic substitution, a medicine could be changed to another product in the pharmacy only after consultation with the physician. The reform places the dispensing pharmacy under an obligation to substitute a medical product, prescribed by a physician or dentist, with the cheapest, or close to the cheapest, interchangeable product. However, the prescriber or individual patients may forbid the substitution.

* Correspondence: Reeta.Heikkila@uef.fi
† Contributed equally
[1]University of Eastern Finland, Faculty of Health Sciences, School of Pharmacy, Social Pharmacy, P.O.Box 1627, FI-70211 Kuopio, Finland
Full list of author information is available at the end of the article

Individual patients can forbid GS at any time and the prescriber can forbid GS for medical or therapeutical reasons.

Previous studies have found some factors related to patient involvement in nonprescription medicine purchasing [3-6]. For example, higher educational level or higher family income has caused the lower involvement in nonprescription medicine purchase decisions [3]. Also a recommendation by pharmacists [5], effectiveness, familiarity with the name or brand and safety have influenced nonprescription medicines purchasing [4]. In addition, people's previous experiences of nonprescription medicines influence their decision later [6]. However, we did not know about medicine-related factors that influence patients' choice of prescription drugs.

Generic medicines have caused certain problems in many countries [7-14]. According to an Australian study (n = 204), patients (average age 72 years) were confused most frequently (56%) by generic and trade names, while poor adherence was reported by 53% [15]. Also, a new Swedish study reported that 40% of respondents reported at least one difficulty related to generic medicines and substitution. There was inconsistent information about the effects of generic substitution (GS) on adherence in patients who used antihypertensive drugs. According to a Netherlands study based on prescription data and hospital discharge records, generic substitution of hypertensive drugs did not lead to lower adherence compared with brand name drugs [16]. Neither was there any difference in hospitalizations for cardiovascular diseases in the six months after the substitutions were observed. In a Norwegian interview study, generic substitution affected adherence because patients were uncertain about the difference between old and new products [14].

This study was one part of a larger study exploring the risks and benefits of generic substitution in Finland. More details on generic substitution in Finland are described in our previous studies [17,18]. According to our best knowledge, there are no published population surveys dealing with factors related to medicines' influence on people's choice of prescription drugs. In the present study we were especially interested in the differences between people who had refused GS and those who had allowed GS.

The aim of this present study was to explore what factors related to medicines influence people's choice of prescription drugs five years after generic substitution was introduced in Finland.

Methods

This population survey was carried out during the autumn of 2008. A random sample was drawn from five mainland counties: Southern Finland, Eastern Finland,

Western Finland, Oulu, and Lapland. The sixth county, Åland, was excluded from the sample because of its divergent drug use culture compared with the other counties [19]. We wanted to include in the sample individuals who had substituted their medicines, individuals who had refused substitution, and also those who had no experience with GS. According to the register of The Social Insurance Institution of Finland, in 2008 only 10% of Finnish pharmacy customers refused GS. Because the proportion was so small, we wanted to make sure we included enough individuals who had refused GS in the sample. Therefore, we obtained statistics, by hospital district, about people who had refused GS during 2007 from The Social Insurance Institution of Finland. The hospital districts were located in the counties. In 2007 altogether 778,902 individuals (excluding Åland) refused generic substitution in Finland. Of these, 38% lived in Southern Finland, 11% in Eastern Finland, 40% in Western Finland, 7% in Oulu, and 4.5% in Lapland. The random sample (n = 3000) was formulated on the grounds of these percentage values. So, the sample included 1140 persons from Southern Finland, 340 persons from Eastern Finland, 1190 persons from Western Finland, 220 persons from Oulu, and 110 persons from Lapland. A flow chart of the postal survey process is presented in Figure 1.

A questionnaire was mailed to a random sample of 3000 people at least 18 years old and living in Finland. The sampling was conducted by the Finnish Population Register Centre from their database. Two reminders were sent after the first mailing round. The first page of the questionnaire was meant for all respondents. The second page was meant for respondents who had substituted their medicines at least once and the third page was meant for respondents who had refused substitution at least once. The last page was reserved for free comments. The questionnaire consisted of both structured and open-ended questions. The questionnaire was developed on the basis of our previous study of pharmacy customers in 2003 [17], when GS was introduced in Finland. The questionnaire was piloted the first time in 2003 and again in 2008 after editing. Factors that influenced the subjects' choice of medicines were asked with a following question "Which of the following are important when you are choosing a medication." The question contained 11 propositions that were price, availability, familiarity, domestic product, excipients, shape of the tablet/capsule, color of the tablet/capsule, appearance of the package, manufacturer, splittability, and brand name. The respondents could choose (circle) more than one proposition. The propositions were almost the same as in the earlier study. However, we added three propositions (splittability, manufacturer, brand name) that emerged in the earlier study. Background information

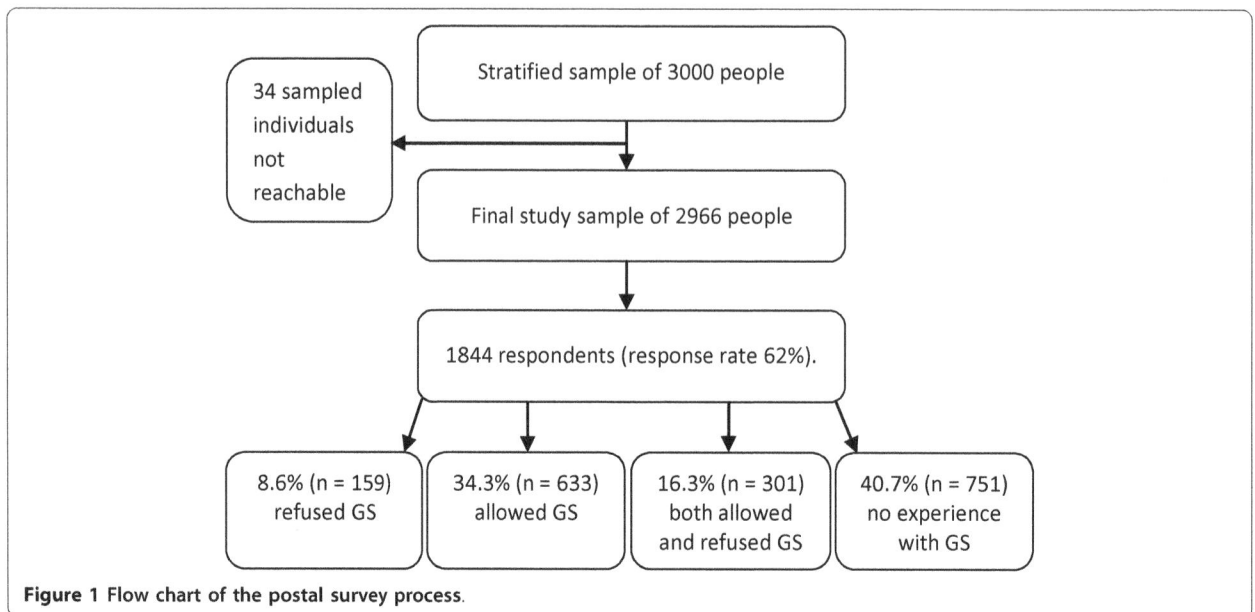

Figure 1 Flow chart of the postal survey process.

(sex, year of birth, county) were asked with structured questions. Use of prescription drugs was asked with the question "Do you use one or more prescription drugs regularly?"

The study setting and the complete anonymity of the respondents were in accordance with the local ethical instructions for researchers. In Finland, questionnaire studies are not required to be approved by the ethics committee. The ethics committee states that respondents give their approval when they answer the questionnaire.

The data were analyzed with SPSS 17.0.1 statistical software (SPSS Inc. Chicago, IL) using frequencies and cross-tabulations for descriptive analysis.

Results

Thirty-four questionnaires did not reach the recipients for various reasons (e.g. addresses were wrong; the intended recipient had moved abroad; death) or because the recipients were excluded due to poor health or institutional care. A total of 1844 of the remaining 2966 questionnaires were returned (response rate, 62%). The percentage of female respondents was 55%. The mean age of the respondents was 54 years and their median age was 55 years. The detailed characteristics of the study population are presented in Table 1.

Price (72%), familiarity (56%), and availability (42%) were the three most important factors that influenced the choice of medicines (Table 2). Other characteristics

Table 1 Summary of study population

	Total		Patients who refused GS		Patients who allowed GS		Patients who had refused and allowed GS		Patients who had no experience with GS	
	No.	(%)	No.	(%)	No.	(%)	No.	(%)	No.	(%)
All	1844	(100)	159	(9)	633	(34)	301	(16)	751	(41)
Sex										
Male	826	(45)	54	(34)	254	(40)	130	(43)	388	(52)
Female	1018	(55)	105	(66)	379	(60)	171	(57)	363	(48)
Age, yr										
18-59	1118	(61)	70	(45)	404	(64)	154	(52)	490	(66)
60-94	706	(39)	87	(55)	227	(36)	145	(48)	247	(34)
Not reported	20		2		2		2		14	
Mean (SD)	54	(17)	61	(18)	53	(16)	57	(19)	52	(17)
Median	55		62		53		59		52	
Regularly uses prescription drugs										
Yes	1085	(59)	140	(88)	440	(70)	239	(80)	266	(36)
No	748	(41)	19	(12)	190	(30)	60	(20)	479	(64)
Not reported	11		0		3		2		6	

Table 2 Three most important factors that influence the choice of prescription medicines

			Price		Familiarity		Availability	
		No.	No.	%	No.	%	No.	%
All respondents		1551	1112	(72)	874	(56)	643	(42)
Gender	Men	688	492	(72)	366	(53)	298	(43)
	Women	863	620	(72)	508	(59)	345	(40)
Prescription medicines in	Yes	919	633	(69)	474	(52)	403	(44)
regular use	No	624	472	(76)	396	(64)	237	(38)
Age, years	< 60	952	742	(78)	554	(58)	402	(42)
	≥ 60	585	363	(62)	314	(54)	230	(39)
Patients who had refused GS								
All		134	60	(45)	95	(71)	50	(37)
Gender	Men	45	21	(47)	32	(71)	15	(33)
	Women	89	39	(44)	63	(71)	35	(39)
Prescription medicines in	Yes	117	52	(44)	85	(73)	44	(38)
regular use	No	17	8	(47)	10	(59)	6	(35)
Age, years	< 60	63	36	(57)	45	(71)	23	(37)
	≥ 60	70	24	(34)	49	(70)	26	(37)
Patients who had allowed GS								
All		538	448	(83)	242	(45)	203	(38)
Gender	Men	212	170	(80)	87	(41)	84	(40)
	Women	326	278	(85)	155	(48)	119	(37)
Prescription medicines in	Yes	380	308	(81)	159	(42)	151	(40)
regular use	No	155	137	(88)	82	(53)	50	(32)
Age, years	< 60	340	297	(87)	159	(47)	133	(39)
	≥ 60	196	150	(77)	83	(42)	69	(35)
Patients who had refused and allowed GS								
All		251	178	(71)	137	(55)	119	(47)
Gender	Men	108	81	(75)	46	(43)	52	(48)
	Women	143	97	(68)	91	(64)	67	(47)
Prescription medicines in	Yes	200	137	(69)	103	(52)	103	(52)
regular use	No	49	39	(80)	32	(65)	16	(33)
Age, years	< 60	124	101	(82)	76	(61)	58	(47)
	≥ 60	125	76	(61)	60	(48)	60	(48)
No experience								
All		628	426	(68)	400	(64)	271	(43)
Gender	Men	323	220	(68)	201	(62)	147	(46)
	Women	305	206	(68)	199	(65)	124	(41)
Prescription medicines in	Yes	222	136	(61)	127	(57)	105	(47)
regular use	No	403	288	(72)	272	(68)	165	(41)
Age, years	< 60	425	308	(73)	274	(65)	188	(44)
	≥ 60	194	113	(58)	122	(63)	75	(39)

Respondents could choose several options.

of the medicines, such as domestic product (25%), splittability (24%), excipients (16%), manufacturer (10%), brand name (8%), shape of the tablet/capsule (6%), color of the tablet/capsule (1%), and appearance of the package (1%), were not as important factors to the respondents.

For the people who had refused GS, the familiarity of the medicine was the most important factor that influenced their choice of medicine (Table 2). People who used prescription medicines regularly valued that characteristic more often than patients who did not use prescription medicines regularly.

People who had allowed GS considered price the most important characteristic in their choice of medicine, in contrast to people who had refused GS (Table 2). Price was a very important characteristic especially for women, for people who did not use any prescription medicine regularly, and for people under 60 years of age.

People who had both refused and allowed GS also appreciated price as the most important characteristic (Table 2). People who did not use any prescription medicines regularly considered price more important than people who used prescription medicines regularly. Also, people under 60 years of age considered price a very important characteristic.

For the respondents who had no experience with GS, price and familiarity were the most important characteristics in their choice of medicines.

Discussion

According to our study, price, familiarity, and availability were the three most important factors that influenced the choice of prescription medicines. People who allowed GS or who had both refused and allowed GS considered price the most important factor. People who had refused GS considered familiarity much more important than price. People who had no experience at all with GS appreciated both of these factors. The fact that price was the most important factor for people is in line with our earlier study, where savings were the main reason for accepting GS [17,18]. Finnish people also have confidence in the effect of cheaper medicines [18]. They also held the opinion that GS does not cause any risk to drug safety.

The people who had refused GS were a little older than the people in the other groups. It is obvious that especially older people appreciated the familiarity and price of medicines. Many old people often have someone else buy their medicines for them. If the possibility of GS had not been discussed before, it is probable that the representative would refuse GS. However, if the representative allows GS, it is possible that he/she cannot take into account the familiarity of the medicine to the old person being represented. Before GS was introduced it was thought it would confuse patients when the names, colors, packages, etc., of drug products changed [1,2]. Although people did not usually choose prescription medicines on the grounds of these external characteristics of medicines, confusions could be possible. The Finnish Medicines Agency, Fimea, publishes an interchangeable drug list quarterly. For example, in 2008 (list July 2008-September 2008) the list included 23 simvastatin products (20 mg), 39 mirtazapine products (15 mg), and 23 amlodipine products (10 mg). While pharmacies cannot stock all these interchangeable products, there still are many drug products to choose from.

The response rate of 62% was quite good, since the present study was based on a population survey and the sample also included individuals who did not know

what GS is. The response rate was 67% for women and 56% for men. The difference between sexes, in proportion and response rate, was similar in a previous Finnish population survey [20-22]. The age distribution of the respondents was quite similar to the age distribution of the sample and background population. Young age groups were somewhat under-represented among the respondents. Young people usually use less medicine than older age groups, and maybe for that reason they were not motivated to answer our questionnaire. Also, the proportion of men (45%) and women (55%) respondents was quite well in line with the sample (men 49%, women 51%) and the population (men 49%, women 51%).

Conclusions

Price, familiarity, and availability were important factors in the choice of prescription medicines. The external characteristics of medicines, for instance the color and shape of the tablet/capsule or the appearance of the package, were not significant characteristics for people.

Acknowledgements and funding
None

Author details
[1]University of Eastern Finland, Faculty of Health Sciences, School of Pharmacy, Social Pharmacy, P.O.Box 1627, FI-70211 Kuopio, Finland. [2]University of Eastern Finland, Faculty of Health Sciences, School of Medicine, Department of Primary Health Care, P.O.Box 1627, FI-70211 Kuopio, Finland. [3]Kuopio University Hospital, Unit of Primary Health Care, P.O.Box 1777, FI-70211 Kuopio, Finland.

Authors' contributions
RH designed and carried out the postal survey and drafted the manuscript. PM participated in the design of the postal survey and helped draft the manuscript. RA participated in the design of the postal survey and helped draft the manuscript. All the authors read and approved the final manuscript.

Competing interests
The authors declare that they have no competing interests.

References
1. Finnish Medical Association: *Lausunto luonnoksesta hallituksen esitykseksi eduskunnalle lääkelain ja sairausvakuutuslain muuttamiseksi. Statement for the Ministry of Social Affairs and Health* 2002, [in Finnish].
2. Pharma Industry Finland: *Lausunto luonnoksesta lakiehdotukseksi geneerisen substituution toteuttamiseksi Suomessa. Statement for the Ministry of Social Affairs and Health* 2002, [in Finnish].
3. Gore P, Madhavan S, McClung G, Riley D: **Consumer involvement in nonprescription medicine purchase decisions.** *J Health Care Mark* 1994, **14**:16-23.
4. Hanna LA, Hughes CM: **Public's views on making decisions about over-the-counter medication and their attitudes towards evidence of effectiveness: A cross-sectional questionnaire study.** *Patient Educ Couns* 2011, **83**:345-351.
5. Wazaify M, Shields E, Hughes CM, McElnay JC: **Societal perspectives on over-the-counter (OTC) medicines.** *Fam Pract* 2005, **22**:170-176.

6. The Proprietary Association of Great Britain: *A Summary Profile of the OTC Consumer* London; 2005.

7. Andersen ML, Laursen K, Schaumann M, Rubak SL, Olesgaard P, Mainz J, Lauritzen T: **How do patients evaluate the newly introduced system of substituting prescriptions?** *Ugeskr Laeger* 2000, **162**:6066-6069, [in Danish].

8. Rubak SL, Andersen ML, Mainz J, Olesgaard P, Lauritzen T: **How do practitioners evaluate the newly introduced system of substituting prescriptions?** *Ugeskr Laeger* 2000, **162**:6070-6073, [in Danish].

9. Rubak SL, Andersen ML, Mainz J, Olesgaard P, Laursen K, Schaumann M, Lauritzen T: **How do pharmacists evaluate the newly introduced system of substituting prescriptions?** *Ugeskr Laeger* 2000, **162**:6074-6077, [in Danish].

10. Socialstyrelsen: *Patientsäkerhet vid utbyte av läkemedel på apotek* Stockholm; 2004, [in Swedish].

11. Frisk P, Rydberg T, Carlsten A, Ekedahl A: **Patients' experiences with generic substitution: a Swedish pharmacy survey.** *Journal of Pharmaceutical Health Services Research* 2011, **2**:9-15.

12. Gill L, Helkkula A, Cobelli N, White L: **How do customers and pharmacists experience generic substitution?** *International journal of pharmaceutical and healthcare marketing* 2010, **4**:375-395.

13. Håkonsen H, Toverud EL: **Special challenges for drug adherence following generic substitution in Pakistani immigrants living in Norway.** *Eur J Clin Pharmacol* 2011, **67**:193-201.

14. Toverud EL, Roise AK, Hogstad G, Wabo I: **Norwegian patients on generic antihypertensive drugs: a qualitative study of their own experiences.** *Eur J Clin Pharmacol* 2011, **67**:33-38.

15. Sorensen L, Stokes JA, Purdie DM, Woodward M, Roberts MS: **Medication management at home: medication risk factor prevalence and inter-relationships.** *J Clin Pharm Ther* 2006, **31**:485-491.

16. Van Wijk BL, Klungel OH, Heerdink ER, de Boer A: **Generic substitution of antihypertensive drugs: does it affect adherence?** *Ann Pharmacother* 2006, **40**:15-20.

17. Heikkilä R, Mäntyselkä P, Hartikainen-Herranen K, Ahonen R: **Customers' and physicians' opinions of and experiences with generic substitution during the first year in Finland.** *Health Policy* 2007, **82**:366-374.

18. Heikkilä R, Mäntyselkä P, Ahonen R: **Do people regard cheaper medicines effective? Population survey on public opinion of generic substitution in Finland.** *Pharmacoepidemiol Drug Saf* 2011, **20**:185-191.

19. Lahnajärvi L, Klaukka T, Enlund H: **Ahvenanmaa - itsehallittua lääkekulutusta.** Helsinki: Kansaneläkelaitos; 1997.

20. Ylinen S, Hameen-Anttila K, Sepponen K, Lindblad AK, Ahonen R: **The use of prescription medicines and self-medication among children-a population-based study in Finland.** *Pharmacoepidemiol Drug Saf* 2010, **19**:1000-1008.

21. Turunen JH, Mäntyselkä PT, Kumpusalo EA, Ahonen RS: **Frequent analgesic use at population level: prevalence and patterns of use.** *Pain* 2005, **115**:374-381.

22. Pohjanoksa-Mäntylä M, Bell JS, Helakorpi S, Närhi U, Pelkonen A, Airaksinen MS: **Is the Internet replacing health professionals? A population survey on sources of medicines information among people with mental disorders.** *Soc Psychiatry Psychiatr Epidemiol* 2011, **46**:373-379.

11

Exploring the relationship between safety culture and reported dispensing errors in a large sample of Swedish community pharmacies

Annika Nordén-Hägg[*], Sofia Kälvemark-Sporrong and Åsa Kettis Lindblad

Abstract

Background: The potential for unsafe acts to result in harm to patients is constant risks to be managed in any health care delivery system including pharmacies. The number of reported errors is influenced by a various elements including safety culture. The aim of this study is to investigate a possible relationship between reported dispensing errors and safety culture, taking into account demographic and pharmacy variables, in Swedish community pharmacies.

Methods: A cross-sectional study was performed, encompassing 546 (62.8%) of the 870 Swedish community pharmacies. All staff in the pharmacies on December 1st, 2007 were included in the study. To assess safety culture domains in the pharmacies, the Safety Attitudes Questionnaire (SAQ) was used. Numbers of dispensed prescription items as well as dispensing errors for each pharmacy across the first half year of 2008 were summarised. Intercorrelations among a number of variables including SAQ survey domains, general properties of the pharmacy, demographic characteristics, and dispensing errors were calculated. A negative binomial regression model was used to further examine the relationship between the variables and dispensing errors.

Results: The first analysis demonstrated a number of significant correlations between reported dispensing errors and the variables examined. Negative correlations were found with SAQ domains Teamwork Climate, Safety Climate, Job Satisfaction as well as mean age and response rates. Positive relationships were demonstrated with Stress Recognition (SAQ), number of employees, educational diversity, birth country diversity, education country diversity and number of dispensed prescription items. Variables displaying a significant relationship to errors in this analysis were included in the regression analysis. When controlling for demographic variables, only Stress Recognition, mean age, educational diversity and number of dispensed prescription items and employees, were still associated with dispensing errors.

Conclusion: This study replicated previous work linking safety to errors, but went one step further and controlled for a variety of variables. Controlling rendered the relationship between Safety Climate and dispensing insignificant, while the relationship to Stress Recognition remained significant. Variables such as age and education country diversity were found also to correlate with reporting behaviour. Further studies on the demographic variables might generate interesting results.

Background

The potential for unsafe acts to result in harm to patients is a constant risk to be managed in any health care delivery system. In pharmacies these unsafe acts might consist of dispensing errors that can result in patients receiving the wrong medicine. In community pharmacies, these errors are present in a frequency varying between 0.01% [1,2] and 22% [3], depending on the definition of dispensing errors and the method used to assess these errors. Types of errors include selection errors such as improper choice of medicines, dosage forms, strengths or quantities, as well as erroneous dosage instructions [1,2,4-7]. The causes of dispensing errors vary but commonly noted causes are look-alike packages and similar brand names [1,8]. The context in

* Correspondence: annikanordn.h@telia.com
Department of Pharmacy, Uppsala University, Box 570, Uppsala S-751 23, Sweden

which these errors occur also have a strong impact and includes such variables as fatigue, high workload, overwork and interruptions [2,5,9].

A variety of measures are used to prevent and manage errors [2,7,9]. One of the main measures is the use of reporting systems, providing possibilities to analyse and subsequently prevent errors. However, research findings show that such structured attempts to collect reports on errors are not always successful and the relationship between actual numbers of errors and the reported number of errors is not clear-cut, since reporting is influenced by a number of elements resulting in lack of reports [10,11]. The reasons include inadequate and unsatisfactory safety procedures, resulting in a lack of common definitions and classification of errors [12], staff ignorance of the purpose of reporting, [13] or shortcomings in staff abilities to follow existing guidelines. [14] They also include the impact of inter- and intra-professional values and interactions. [14] Other reasons can be attributed to the safety culture in the workplace, including employees' shared perceptions of policies, practices, and procedures that are rewarded, supported and expected [15].

The safety culture is thus an important part of the context, regarding error handling and patient safety issues in health care, including pharmacies., In search for valid yet feasible methods for conducting annual assessments of safety culture, healthcare organisations have used survey questionnaires that measure frontline caregiver perceptions. These provide a snapshot of the larger culture through multiple dimensions such as safety climate, teamwork climate, and stress recognition [16,17].

Studies on the relationship between safety culture and dispensing errors are scarce. In an American study, the overall safety climate of a hospital unit was found to predict medication errors, and a more positive safety culture was associated with fewer incidents [18,19]. A strong safety culture might reinforce adherence to medication administration practices and encourage an open and constructive response to errors [18]. In a strong safety culture, employees tend to perceive procedures as suitable and safety information as available. The norm is to openly confer about safety issues and the willingness to report treatment errors is high [19].

There might be other factors contributing to incidence and reporting of errors. These include demographic variables. Seniority has been found to bring about experience [20], which might reduce the risk for error making. Cultural differences and language difficulties between health care personnel increase the risk for medical misunderstandings [21], which may potentially increase the risk for errors. The term diversity is used to describe the variance of demographic characteristics such as for instance age, education and role at worksite [22]. This aspect, although complex, might add important information about the impact of staff composition on reporting of errors. Pharmacy characteristics may also be related to reported dispensing errors.

The relationship between errors and culture has, to our knowledge, not been systematically studied in community pharmacies. Thus, the aim of this study is to investigate the possible relationship between reported dispensing errors and safety culture, taking into account demographic and pharmacy variables, in Swedish community pharmacies. It has to be pointed out that this is an explorative study only and further analyses on variables might be a next step, given that co-variation is found.

Methods

A cross-sectional study was performed, using routinely collected pharmacy data and a separately conducted survey distributed to staff at Swedish community pharmacies.

Setting

Until June 2009 Swedish community pharmacies were owned by the National Corporation of Pharmacies. The corporation was responsible for all of the approximately 870 community pharmacies in Sweden at the time of this study. (Since 2009, a deregulation of the pharmacies in Sweden is in effect, and the pharmacy market has been opened to all interested parties.) There were approximately 7,000 staff members in these pharmacies; the largest professional category was made up of pharmacists (61%) [23].

Measures
Reported dispensing errors

Reporting dispensing errors in Swedish pharmacies is mandatory by law [24]. These reports were, at the time of the study, submitted through a national, web-based error reporting system and kept at the headquarters of the National Corporation of Pharmacies. In December 2007, 14.99 dispensing errors per 100,000 dispensed prescription items were reported in the Swedish community pharmacies [25].

A dispensing error, is a deviation that includes incorrect dispensing, counseling of service to a patient (by the National Corporation of Pharmacies, 2008). This comprises

- Wrong medicine, wrong strength or wrong dispensing form
- Wrong quantity
- Wrong dosage
- Passed expiry date
- Wrong written or verbal information
- Wrong patient or unit
- Missing medicine

- Missing or delayed delivery
- Not noted interaction or double prescribing

Monthly compilations on numbers of reported dispensing errors for each pharmacy from January 2008 until June 2008 were included.

The safety attitudes questionnaire

Information on safety culture in Swedish pharmacies was collected using the Safety Attitudes Questionnaire [23]. It is a validated survey instrument that provides a snapshot of staff perceptions, attitudes, and beliefs about quality of safety and teamwork in a particular work setting. The SAQ has six dimensions including Teamwork Climate, Safety Climate, Perceptions of Management, Job Satisfaction, Working Conditions and Stress Recognition [16]. Together these scales provide a multidimensional profile of the safety-related norms in a given work setting. Higher scores on each of these scales, represent more safety awareness and readiness to manage risk by the staff.

All the people listed as employed in all Swedish community pharmacies on December 1st, 2007 were asked to participate in the survey on safety climate; SAQ. The survey was translated and adapted for use and distributed to staff in Swedish community pharmacies in 2008 [23].

Demographic variables

Respondent demographic items included age, country of birth, educational level as well as in which country the education was provided, and role in pharmacy (e.g. pharmacy manager) [23].

Dispensed prescription items

Numbers of dispensed prescription items; DPIs, were available from the National Corporation of Pharmacies. These data were compiled for each pharmacy from January through June of 2008. Inclusion criteria for pharmacies, based on volume, included only pharmacies with at least 1,000 dispensed prescription items during this period. Only one pharmacy had less than 1,000 DPIs[a] and was hence excluded in this study.

Response rate

Response rate was studied as an extra control variable in order to investigate if general responsiveness among the staff had an impact on the possible relationship between safety climate and dispensing errors.

Study group

Pharmacies with at least three respondents were included. Out of the total number of pharmacies 546 (62.8%), including 3,654 (54.7%) respondents, met the inclusion criteria of at least three respondents and 1,000 dispensed prescription items during the first half year of 2008.

The SAQ is originally validated for units with at least five respondents [16]. The rationale behind this threshold was to protect the confidentiality of respondents and to target a minimum number of individuals to assess a culture [26]. However, a considerable number, approximately 27%, of Swedish pharmacies have three or less employees. Allowing the use of lower threshold of respondents per pharmacy would meaningfully increase the usability of this survey tool. Consequently, the validity of a lower threshold of respondents in pharmacies was tested, under the assumption that a unit with at least three individuals may also have a joint culture. The psychometric validation of this group of respondents is included in Additional file 1: Appendix A.

Statistics

Level of analysis

The analysis was conducted at the pharmacy level. Individual questionnaire responses were aggregated by calculating, for each pharmacy, the mean scores of each variable. The SAQ uses consensus assessments whereby group-level perceptions are garnered to see what views the pharmacy personnel have in common [27-29]. To justify the aggregation of scores from the individual to the pharmacy level of analysis, homogeneity of scores or a within-unit agreement and between-unit variance should be demonstrated. James, Demaree, and Wolf's $r_{wg(j)}$ index [30] was computed; this is a measure of intra-group agreement of homogeneity. The $r_{wg(j)}$ agreement index represents the interchangeability of respondents and is used to determine the appropriateness of aggregating data to higher levels of analysis. It attempts to determine whether one group member's response is basically identical to another group member's response. The $r_{wg(j)}$ is a group-specific index; that is, it is an index that is calculated for each of the groups in the sample. Any $r_{wg(j)}$ values greater than 0.70 are viewed as providing acceptable support for aggregating data to a unit level of analysis [31].

ICC(1) (Intraclass Correlation Coefficient) values represent the amount of variance in individual perceptions that can be explained by unit or team membership; i.e. being a staff member in a specific pharmacy. ICC(2) is an index that represents the reliability of the group mean within a sample and varies as a function of group size and the ICC(1) value. ICC(1) was computed from a one-way ANOVA. In this ANOVA the SAQ dimensions comprise the variable of interest (dependent variable) and pharmacy membership is the independent variable [31]. ICC(2) was computed from ICC(1) via the Spearman-Brown formula [31]. Many researchers simply evaluate the statistical significance of the ICC(1) value to assess whether there is meaningful non-independence among survey responses [32,33] which is also done in this study. Together, this package of indices gives insight into how much the members of a pharmacy agree with one another and how different teams are from one another, both of which are important for understanding the impact of combining individual team member perceptions into team-level metrics. The analyses were carried out using functions provided in the multilevel package for R; version 2.10.0, 2010.

The result of the $r_{wg(j)}$ analyses is included in Additional file 1. The $r_{wg(j)}$ agreement index presented for the SAQ domains shows moderate (Stress Recognition, Perceptions of Management), but mainly strong agreement within pharmacies (Table 1). ICC(1) values were all statistically significant, demonstrating between-unit significance for all survey domains. However some variation was present, and while 19% of the variability in any one respondent's rating of Teamwork Climate is a function of the pharmacy group to which the individual belongs, only 4% of Stress Recognition is a function of this group belonging. The ICC(2) values for Job Satisfaction and Perceptions of Management are reasonable. Acceptable within-unit homogeneity was however present across survey domains, with the exception of the Stress Recognition domain. In the case of Stress Recognition, there is significant variability between pharmacies, but relative to the other scales, the source of variation coming from within the pharmacy as a *collective view* was lower. This suggests that Stress Recognition is less of a consensus perception than the other domains, which is consistent with previously published studies [16,34]. Thus Stress Recognition might be considered as an additive construct [29].

Data analysis

In a descriptive analysis, intercorrelations for all the variables in the questionnaire, as well as number of employees per pharmacy, dispensed prescription items per pharmacy, response rate and errors were calculated using R.

Based on these intercorrelations, a negative binomial regression model was used to further examine the relationship between pharmacy characteristics and domains of the SAQ and the outcome dispensing errors. This model is appropriate when modelling a non-zero, count-based outcome in which there is overdispersion [35]. Functions in the MASS package of R were used to estimate the negative binomial models. The results are to be interpreted as follows: For a one unit change in the predictor variable, i.e. the difference in the logs of expected counts of the response variable is expected to change by the respective regression coefficient, holding all other variables constant.

Approval of ethics committee

No approval was required from the ethics committee according to the Swedish law[b] at the time of the data collection. Ethical considerations were met however; responding to the questionnaire was voluntary and all answers were de-identified to maintain confidentiality.

Results

In the descriptive analysis the means, standard deviations, and correlations among the variables at the pharmacy were calculated (Tables 2 and 3). A number of significant correlations between dispensing errors and SAQ dimensions were found. A significant negative correlation was found between dispensing errors and Teamwork Climate (−0.09), Safety Climate, (−0.12) and Job Satisfaction (−0.12) respectively; high levels in these SAQ dimensions were associated with low levels of errors. A significant positive relationship was demonstrated between the Stress Recognition dimension (0.10) and dispensing errors, i.e., respondents that acknowledged the impact of stress on their performance, were more likely to report dispensing errors.

Reported errors were significantly positively correlated to number of employees, educational diversity (i.e. a higher value indicates greater variety across pharmacy members in their education background), birth country diversity, education country diversity, and number of dispensed prescription items. Thus pharmacies with higher numbers of reported dispensing errors were also likely to have a high number of staff, a diverse staff (education level/country of education/country of birth) and also, a high number of dispensed prescription items. A significant, but negative, correlation was found between reported dispensing errors and mean age, i.e. the older the staff the lesser the numbers of dispensing errors. A negative correlation was also demonstrated between response rates and reported dispensing errors; pharmacies with high response rates on our survey demonstrated fewer dispensing errors.

A second analysis was carried out; i.e. those variables displaying a significant relationship to reported dispensing errors in the descriptive analysis, were included in a

Table 1 Aggregation metrics for team-level consensus composition constructs[ab]

	ICC(1)	ICC(2)	X̄ $r_{wg(j)}$	SD $r_{wg(j)}$
Teamwork Climate	0.19**	0.58	0.82	0.26
Safety Climate	0.15**	0.50	0.88	0.18
Job Satisfaction	0.22**	0.68	0.83	0.25
Stress Recognition	0.04**	0.21	0.68	0.32
Perceptions of Management	0.23**	0.65	0.70	0.27
Working conditions	0.16**	0.47	0.74	0.25

[a] Individual N = 3,654; Pharmacy N = 546.

[b] *p < .05, **p < .01 two-tailed.

Table 2 Pharmacy-Level means, standard deviations and intercorrelations of SAQ dimensions and dispensing errors[abc]

	M	SD	Teamwork Climate	Safety Climate	Job Satisfaction	Perceptions of management	Working Conditions	Stress Recognition
Teamwork Climate	4.42	0.46	(0.90)					
Safety Climate	4.28	0.38	0.79**	(0.87)				
Job Satisfaction	4.32	0.50	0.75**	0.74**	(0.92)			
Perceptions of Management	3.81	0.55	0.59**	0.61**	0.63**	(0.85)		
Working Conditions	3.88	0.52	0.58**	0.62**	0.57**	0.63**	(0.78)	
Stress Recognition	3.88	0.45	−0.09*	−0.12**	−0.16**	−0.26**	−0.18**	(0.74)
Dispensing errors	6.35	5.82	−0.09*	−0.12**	−0.12**	−0.06	−0.07	0.10*

[a] Pharmacy-level N = 546.
[b] For correlations |0.09|, p < .05; |0.11|, p < .01.
[c] Pharmacy-level inter-item reliability (i.e., Cronbach's α) for multi-item scales is in parentheses along the diagonal.

negative binomial regression analysis, displayed in Table 4. The number of dispensed prescription items and number of employees were both significantly and positively related to reported dispensing errors. Mean age was significantly and negatively related to these errors. Pharmacies that were more diverse with respect to whether staff members had received their education outside Sweden tended to report more errors. When controlling for respondent demographics, the only SAQ survey domain significantly related to dispensing errors was Stress Recognition; pharmacies in which respondents reported higher levels of stress recognition had higher frequencies of reports on dispensing errors.

Discussion

This study explores the relationship between safety climate and the reporting of dispensing errors in a national sample of community pharmacies in Sweden. An association between safety climate and errors has been established in other parts of health care [18,19]. No significant relationship between reported dispensing errors in Swedish community pharmacies and Safety Culture, after controlling for variability in respondent and pharmacy demographics, was found. The presence of an unusually strong safety culture in these community pharmacies, as compared to other health care settings in the USA [23], has been previously reported. An explanation for this strong culture might be the fact that the National Corporation of Pharmacies for a long time put great effort into quality management and worked intensively on initiating measures for continuous improvements [37]. This included elements like definite guidelines; i.e. standard operation procedures for the dispensing process and other processes. Various indicators were used to assess quality in pharmacies and for instance all staff went through quality education around 2000. Thus it could be assumed that good quality awareness, with a

Table 3 Pharmacy-level means, standard deviations, and intercorrelations of pharmacy characteristics and dispensing errors[ab]

	M	SD	1	2	3	4	5	6	7	8	9	10
1 Number of employees	6.69	3.77	-									
2 Mean age	49.85	5.66	−0.05	-								
3 Mean education	2.20	0.26	0.13**	0.06	-							
4 Age diversity[1]	10.25	3.69	0.14**	−0.45**	−0.06	-						
5 Education diversity[1]	0.43	0.19	0.37**	−0.12**	0.26**	0.10*	-					
6 Birth country diversity[2]	0.15	0.21	0.12**	−0.23**	−0.13**	0.09*	0.24**	-				
7 Education country diversity[2]	0.08	0.15	0.12**	−0.17**	−0.16**	0.05	0.28**	0.71**	-			
8 Role diversity[2]	0.53	0.13	0.06	0.03	0.38**	−0.04	0.50**	0.02	0.06	-		
9 Response rate	66.68	21.56	0.06	0.04	0.08*	0.02	−0.03	−0.06	−0.04	0.15**	-	
10 DPI[3]	50276.59	26562.48	0.79**	−0.08	0.03	0.10*	0.32**	0.16**	0.14**	−0.03	−0.39**	-
11 Dispensing errors	6.35	5.82	0.53**	−0.11*	−0.01	0.07	0.25**	0.19**	0.20**	−0.02	−0.26**	0.64**

[a] Pharmacy-level N = 546.
[b] For correlations |0.09|, p < .05; |0.11|, p < .01.
[1] Age diversity and Education diversity is an assessment of Standard Deviation.
[2] Birth Country Diversity, Education Country Diversity and Role Diversity is calculated using Blau's index; an index to measure variety across categories. It ranges from 0 to 1, with 1 indicative of more variety in a given grouping [36].
[3] Dispensed Prescription Items.

Table 4 Results of negative binomial regressions predicting number of dispensing errors[abc]

	1	2	3	4
Intercept	1.71	1.71	1.70	1.70
Number of DPI[1]	0.01**	0.01**	0.01**	0.01**
Number of employees	0.05**	0.06**	0.05**	0.05**
Response rate	−0.01**	−0.01**	−0.01**	−0.01**
Mean education		−0.10	−0.12	−0.07
Mean age		−0.01	−0.01*	−0.01*
Education diversity			0.34	0.31
Education country diversity			0.47*	0.47*
Age diversity			−0.01	−0.01
Teamwork climate				0.09
Safety climate				0.12
Job satisfaction				−0.15
Perceptions of management				0.12
Working conditions				−0.15
Stress recognition				0.19*
AIC	2916.90	2913.7	2906.2	2836.20

[a] Pharmacy N = 546.
[b] *p < .05, **p < .01 two-tailed.
[c] All predictor variables are mean- centred.
[1] Dispensed prescription items.

ruling influence on safety issues in pharmacies, was present and impacted the outcome of this survey.

Thus one possible explanation for the lack of association is that a ceiling effect may have reduced the possibility to discriminate between pharmacies. Anecdotally, recent work at Johns Hopkins Hospital suggests that the more mature a reporting system is, the more the relationship between SAQ dimensions and error reporting declines [38]. Perhaps it is the case that, as staff build confidence and trust around safety standards and reporting procedures, the predictive power of safety culture as a proxy for "safety-related trust" is diminished. The system becomes a natural part of the work place and therefore only an increasingly weak relationship with reported dispensing errors would be found, which could be one explanation to the pattern of results found in the current study. The differences between settings in this study compared to those in the other studies; i.e. hospital units vs. pharmacies, as well as difference in instruments used for assessing safety climate and error-reporting systems used, also make direct comparisons difficult. As our study is larger than the other studies, lack of power is however not likely to explain the lack of association, if there is one.

The SAQ dimension Teamwork Climate has also been demonstrated to be strong in Swedish community pharmacies, [23] and presumed to reveal prevalence of good

co-operation and respect among staff [39,40]. As already noted, no relationship was found with dispensing errors in this study, after controlling for demographic variables. Again, a ceiling effect might partially explain this.

The only Safety Attitudes Questionnaire domain that was significantly, positively, correlated with dispensing errors, after controlling for demographics, was Stress Recognition. In SAQ this dimension is an indicator of individual attitudes rather than of group attitude, since the dimension, unlike all other dimensions, is dominated by items referring to "I" rather than "we" (see Additional file 1). It might be questioned whether there is a place for a dimension primarily assessing individual's self-awareness within the framework of the presumed collective safety climate area. The within-unit and between-unit analysis has however ensured that this variable performs satisfactorily at group level, although considerably poorer than the other dimensions. When staff members in a pharmacy experience dispensing errors, the awareness of the risk of errors may increase, with increased stress recognition among staff as one possible outcome. This may explain the counterintuitive relationship between stress recognition and dispensing errors, where more self aware staff members, with regard to how they behave under pressure, is associated with more reported dispensing errors. This seems to be contrary to prior research linking higher stress recognition to better performance in commercial aviation pilots [41], but further investigation is warranted. In an American study, safety climate was negatively related to incident reporting volume, while stress recognition was independently positively related to incident reporting volume, which correlates with our findings [42] The difference between that study, and the current study, is that this national sample of community pharmacies included far more demographic variables, which were not controlled for in the American study. If controlling for demographic variables diminishes the predictive power of safety culture over incident reporting, then the current study has identified the importance of controlling for respondent and site demographic variables. It is possible that the size of this nation-wide study was so large, and the number of demographic variables was so comprehensive, that few other studies (to date) into incident reporting have the ability to attempt such an analysis.

Relationships were found between high levels of dispensing errors and high numbers of dispensed prescription items and employees, respectively. This might be an indication of the fact that the bigger the pharmacy, in terms of number of employees and prescription volumes the busier the surroundings are. It might become difficult to convey information on safety issues and prescriptions and have informative communication between colleagues; misunderstandings might be more common. It will also become harder to get to know your colleagues [43].

A relationship was also found between age and dispensing errors; the higher the mean age in a pharmacy is, the lower the number of dispensing errors is. Seniority has been found to bring about experience [20]. The senior staff might make fewer errors, as they are more experienced, know the pitfalls and can avoid them. Who makes most errors – the experienced staff or the more junior staff? This question has been evaluated by O'Shea [44] in a literature review, but the answer was inconclusive.

In the first correlation analysis a number of relationships regarding demographic diversity were found and significant relations were found between reported errors and education, birth country as well as education country. The only remaining relationships, after having controlled for covariates in the regression analysis were education background diversity and an association between having a heterogeneous staff with regard to educational background (non-Swedish/Swedish) and dispensing errors. The more multifaceted the educational background is, the more errors are reported. Misunderstandings between different cultural groups of health care personnel have been reported in Sweden [21]. Cultural differences and language barriers in pharmacies might lead to misunderstandings and misinterpretations, resulting in more errors. A non-native health-care staff might also experience a more difficult working situation in relation to patients, due to cultural differences [45] and communication problems [46] which might increase the risk for errors. It is important, however, to remember that these problems are balanced by the advantages of having multicultural competence at the working site and the degree of advantages depends largely on leadership [47]. This exploration suggests a possible relationship between demographic diversity variables and reported errors. The theory behind demographic diversity is complex [22] and an in-depth analysis might be worthwhile.

A negative association was found between the numbers of dispensing errors and response rate. A high response rate on a questionnaire about safety attitudes might be a measure of the staff's attentiveness to these issues. If so, a high response rate might be an indicator of responsible behaviour, which in turn might be associated with deliberate and careful dispensing behaviour.

A high agreement between reported errors and actual errors is assumed, based on the fact that the reporting system is relatively mature [23]. The Swedish reporting system is now over 10 years old and administrative procedures are in place. There is a clear-cut definition of a dispensing error and specific guidelines regarding handling of errors. Such clarity is considered to positively incentivize reporting behaviour [12,14. Several

measurements have been made over the years, which has put a focus on dispensing errors in the National Corporation of Pharmacies, e.g. the introduction of an intervention, targeted to reduce specific errors [22]. Feed-back has been provided to the users on a regular basis over the years. Other studies have demonstrated that when safety climate is very positive (i.e. safety "trust" is high), the reported number of errors is closer to the actual number of errors [48]. Experiences of previous handling of errors influence the way staff behave, i.e. a mature and non-punitive approach to errors will result in a higher degree of detecting and reporting of errors.

Conclusion

This study replicated previous work linking safety climate to reporting behaviour, but went one step further and controlled for a variety of demographic variables. After controlling these variables, the relationship between safety climate and dispensing errors was rendered insignificant, while the relationship to stress recognition remained significant. A few demographic variables; i.e. age and education country diversity also were found to impact reporting behaviour. Further studies on the demographic variables might generate interesting results.

Endnotes

[a]This pharmacy was judged either to have very limited opening hours or to be in the process of closing.

[b]http://www.riksdagen.se/sv/Dokument-Lagar/Lagar/Svenskforfattningssamling/Lag-2003460-om-etikprovning_sfs-2003-460/ [Swedish only]. The law state that ethical approval is needed if: 1. the research involves storing sensitive personal data 2. The research involves storage of data on crime and sentences 3. If there is an intended physical or psychological impact from the research (e.g. clinical trials of medicine, testing new therapies) and 4. The research involves tissue from humans. None of this is applicable on this research. No data was stored that could link an answer to a specific individual.

Additional file

Additional file 1: Appendix A.

Competing interests
Annika Nordén-Hägg and Sofia Kälvemark Sporrong were, at the time of planning and data collection, employed by the National Corporation of Swedish Pharmacies.
Åsa Kettis has no competing interests.

Acknowledgements
We gratefully acknowledge the contribution of J Bryan Sexton, who provided valuable input and discussion in performing the study and the compilation of the manuscript. We also gratefully acknowledge the contribution of Andrew Knight, who performed the statistical calculations and provided statistic input to the manuscript.

Authors' contributions

ANH - Initiating project, planning project, acquisition of data, analysis and interpretation of data, drafting of manuscript, revising manuscript, final approval. SKS - Planning project, analysis and Interpretation of data, revising manuscript, final approval. AKL - Planning project, analysis and interpretation of data, revising manuscript, final approval. All authors read and approved the final manuscript.

References

1. Knudsen P, Herborg H, Mortensen A, Knudsen M, Hellebek A: **Preventing medication errors in community pharmacy: frequency and seriousness of medication errors.** *Qual Saf Health Care* 2007, **16:**291–296.
2. Thorsted C: **Kun få fejl på apotekerne [Danish].** *Farmaci* 2005, **6:**12–14.
3. Flynn EA, Barker KN, Berger BA, Lloyd KB, Brackett PD: **Dispensing errors and counseling quality in 100 pharmacies.** *J Am Pharm Assoc* 2009, **49:**151–152.
4. Lynskey D, Haigh S, Patel N, Macadam A: **Medication errors in community pharmacy: an investigation into the types and potential causes.** *Int J Pharm Pract* 2007, **15:**105–112.
5. Aschcroft D, Quinlan P, Blenkinsopp A: **Prospective study of the incidence, nature and causes of dispensing errors in community pharmacies.** *Pharmacoepidemiology and drug safety* 2005, **14:**327–332.
6. Flynn E, Barker K, Camahan B: **National observational study of prescription dispensing accuracy and safety in 50 pharmacies.** *J Am Pharm Assoc* 2003, **43:**191–200.
7. Chua S, Wong ICK, Edmondson H, Allen C, Chow J, Peacham J, Hill G, Grantham J: **A feasibility study for recording of dispensing errors and 'near misses' in four UK primary care pharmacies.** *Drug Safety* 2003, **26:**803–813.
8. *National Health Service. Building a safer NHS for patients. Implementing an organisation with a memory.* London: Department of Health; 2001.
9. Peterson G, Wu M, Bergin J: **Pharmacists' attitudes towards dispensing errors: their causes and prevention.** *J Clin Pharm Ther* 1999, **24:**57–71.
10. Flynn E, Barker K, Pepper G, Bates D, Mikeal R: **Comparison of methods for detecting medication errors in 36 hospitals and skilled nursing facilities.** *Am J Health Syst Pharm* 2002, **59:**436–446.
11. Taylor J, Brownstein D, Christakis D, Blackburn S, Strandjord T, Klein E, Shafii J: **Use of incident reports by physicians and nurses to document medical errors in pediatric patients.** *Pediatrics* 2004, **114:**729–735.
12. Tamuz M, Thomas E, Franchois K: **Defining and classifying medical error: lessons for patient safety reporting systems.** *Qual Saf Health Care* 2004, **13:**13–20.
13. *Socialstyrelsen [National Board of Health and Welfare]. [Swedish]:* Tillsynsavdelningens verksamhetsberättelse 2006; 2007. http://www. socialstyrelsen.se/Publicerat/2007/9696/2007-118-10.htm.
14. Kingston M, Evans S, Smith B, Berry J: **Attitudes of doctors and nurses towards incident reporting: a qualitative analysis.** *Medical J Australia* 2004, **181:**36–39.
15. Schneider B: **Organizational climate: An essay.** *Personnel Psychology* 1975, **28:**447–479.
16. Sexton J, Helmreich RL, Neilands T, Rowan K, Vella K, Boyden J, Roberts PR, Thomas EJ: **The safety attitudes Questionnaire: psychometric properties, benchmarking data, and emerging research.** *BMC Heal Serv Res* 2006, **6:**44.
17. Colla J, Bracken A, Kinney L, Weeks W: **Measuring patient safety comate: a review of surveys.** *Qual Saf Health Care* 2005, **14:**364–366.
18. Hofmann D, Mark B: **An investigation of the relationship between safety climate and medication errors as well as other nurse and patient outcomes.** *Pers Psychol* 2006, **59:**847–869.
19. Naveh E, Katz-Navon T, Stern Z: **Readiness to report medical treatment errors. The effects of safety procedures, safety information and priority of safety.** *Med Care* 2006, **44:**117–123.
20. Sorlie V, Lindseth A, Udén G, Norberg A: **Women physicians' narratives about being in ethically difficult care situations in paediatrics.** *Nursing Ethics* 2000, **7:**47–62.
21. Berbyuk N, Allwood J, Edebäck C: *Being a non-Swedish physician in Sweden: A comparison of the views on work related communication of*

non-Swedish physicians and Swedish health care personnel. Communication: Journal of Intercultural; 2005:8.
22. Lau D, Murnighan J: **Demographic Diversity and Faultlines: The Compositional Dynamics of Organizational Groups.** *Acad Manag Rev* 1998, **23:**325–340.
23. Norden-Hägg A, Sexton J, Kälvemark-Sporrong S, Ring L, Kettis-Lindblad Å: **Assessing Safety Culture in Pharmacies: The psychometric validation of the Safety Attitudes Questionnaire (SAQ) in a national sample of community pharmacies in Sweden.** *BMC Clin Pharmacol* 2010, **10:**8. http://www.biomedcentral.com/1472-6904/10/8.
24. *Socialstyrelsen [National Board of Health and Welfare].:* Ledningssystem för kvalitet och patientsäkerhet i hälso- och sjukvården [Swedish] SOSFS; 2005:12. http://www.socialstyrelsen.se/sosfs/2005-12
25. Norden-Hägg A, Andersson K, Kälvemark-Sporrong S, Ring L, Kettis-Lindblad Å: **Reducing dispensing errors in Swedish pharmacies: the impact of a barrier in the computer system.** *Qual Saf Health Care* 2010, **19:**1–5.
26. Pronovost P, Berenholtz S, Goeschel C, Needham D, Sexton J, Thompson D, Lumbomski LH, Marseller JA, Makary MA, Hunt E: **Creating high reliability in health care organizations.** *Heal Serv Res* 2006, **41:**1599–1617.
27. Sexton JB, Holzmueller CG, Pronovost P, Thomas EJ, Mcferran S, Nunes J, Thopson DA, Knight AP, Penning DH, Fox HE: **Variation in caregiver perceptions of teamwork climate in labor and delivery units.** *J Perinatol* 2006, **26:**463–470.
28. Kozlowski SJ, Klein K, Kozlowski SJ, Klein K: **A multilevel approach to theory and research in organizations: Contextual, temporal, and emergent processes.** In *Multilevel theory, research, and methods in organizations: Foundations, extensions, and new directions.* Edited by Klein K, Kozlowski SJ, Klein K, Kozlowski SJ. San Francisco, CA, US: Jossey-Bass; 2000:3–90.
29. Chan D: **Functional relations among constructs in the same content domain at different levels of analysis: A typology of composition models.** *J Appl Psychol* 1998, **83:**234–246.
30. James L, Demaree R, Wolf G: **rwg: An Assessment of Within-Group Interrater Agreement.** *J Appl Psychol* 1993, **78:**306–309.
31. Bliese P: **Within-group agreement, non-independence, and reliability: Implications for data aggregation and analysis.** In *Multilevel theory, research, and methods in organizations: Foundations, extensions, and new directions.* Edited by Klein K, Kozlowksi S. San Francisco, CA, US: Jossey-Bass; 2000.
32. Kenny D, Lavoie L: **Separating individual and group effects.** *J Personal Soc Psychol* 1985, **48:**339–348.
33. Gelman A, Hill J: *Data Analysis Using Regression and Multilevel/Hierarchical Models.* New York: Cambridge University Press; 2007.
34. Deilkås E, Hofoss D: **Psychometric properties of the Norwegian version of the Safety Attitudes Questionnaire (SAQ), Generic version (Short Form 2006).** *BMC Heal Serv Res* 2008, **8:**191.
35. Long J: *Regression models for categorical and limited dependent variables.:* Sage Publications; 1997.
36. Harrison D, Klein K: **What's the difference? Diversity constructs as separation, variety, or disparity in organizations.** *Acad Manag Rev* 2007, **32:**1199–1228.
37. Arrhenius K: *Personal communication.* Stockholm: National Corporation of Pharmacies; 2010.
38. Paine L: *Personal communication.* Hospital: Johns Hopkins; 2009.
39. Hedlund G: **Managing International Business: A Swedish Model.** In *Sweden at the Edge: Lessons for American and Swedish Mangers.* Edited by Maccoby M. Philadelphia: University of Pennsylvania Press; 1991:201–220.
40. World value survey; 2009. http://margaux.grandvinum.se/SebTest/wvs/articles/folder_published/article_base_111.
41. Helmreich R: **Cockpit management attitudes.** *Human Factors: The journal of the human Factors and Ergonomics Society* 1984, **26:**583–589.
42. Taylor J: *Utility of patient safety case finding methods and correlations among organizational safety climate, nurse injuries, and errors.* Johns Hopkins University: Dissertation; 2007.
43. Westerlund T, Almarsdóttir A, Melander A: **Factors influencing the detection rate of drug-related problems in community pharmacy.** *Pharmacy World & Science* 1999, **21:**245–250.
44. O'Shea E: **Factors contributing to medication errors: a literature review.** *J Clin Nurs* 1999, **8:**496–504.
45. Tindall W, Bearsley R, Kimberlin C: *Communication Skills in Pharmacy Practice. A practical guide for students and practitioners.* Philadelphia: Lipincott Williams & Wilkins; 2003.

46. Berbyuk Lindström N: *Intercultural communications in the health care. Non-Swedish physicians in Sweden.* University of Gothenburg, Sweden: Dissertation; 2008.

47. Halbur K: *DA H.* Essentials of cultural competence in pharmacy practice. Washington: American Pharmacists Association; 2008.

48. Edmondson AC: **Learning from failure in health care: Frequent opportunities, pervasive barriers.** *Qual Saf Health Care* 2004, **13**:3–9.

12

Data for drugs available through low-cost prescription drug programs are available through pharmacy benefit manager and claims data

Vivienne J Zhu[1,2*], Anne Belsito[1], Wanzhu Tu[1,2] and J Marc Overhage[2,3]

Abstract

Background: Observational data are increasingly being used for pharmacoepidemiological, health services and clinical effectiveness research. Since pharmacies first introduced low-cost prescription programs (LCPP), researchers have worried that data about the medications provided through these programs might not be available in observational data derived from administrative sources, such as payer claims or pharmacy benefit management (PBM) company transactions.

Method: We used data from the Indiana Network for Patient Care to estimate the proportion of patients with type 2 diabetes to whom an oral hypoglycemic agent was dispensed. Based on these estimates, we compared the proportions of patients who received medications from chains that do and do not offer an LCPP, the proportion trend over time based on claims data from a single payer, and to proportions estimated from the Medical Expenditure Panel Survey (MEPS).

Results: We found that the proportion of patients with type 2 diabetes who received oral hypoglycemic medications did not vary based on whether the chain that dispensed the drug offered an LCPP or over time. Additionally, the rates were comparable to those estimated from MEPS.

Conclusion: Researchers can be reassured that data for medications available through LCPPs continue to be available through administrative data sources.

Keywords: Low-cost prescription program, Oral antihyperglycemic agents, Pharmacy benefit manager, Claims data

Background

When pharmacies dispense a medication for a patient who has a drug benefit, they typically submit an electronic transaction to a pharmacy benefit management (PBM) adjudication system as a method to confirm eligibility and to request payment. The PBM returns a transaction which contains status data about the adjudication and later transfers the transaction data to the payer who contracted with them for services.

In 2006, pharmacies introduced low-cost prescription programs (LCPP) offering selected generic medications that included those for common diseases, such as diabetes, hypertension, and asthma, for $5 or less for a 30-day supply (they sometimes offer a 90-day supply for $10 to $15) [1]. Researchers and others who rely on claims data became concerned that, since the dispensing pharmacy would be unlikely to receive additional reimbursement from the payer and there may be direct and indirect costs associated with submitting the claim, the pharmacy might often not submit a claim when the patient purchased one of these low cost prescriptions using cash. [2,3] Failing to submit claims for these drugs, many of which are commonly used, would diminish the value of administrative data sources for research [4]. Even if the drug in question was not the primary focus of a study, important confounding or comorbidity data could be lost.

In order to determine whether LCPPs have an effect on the availability of low-cost medication dispensing data through claims, we analyzed data from a large

* Correspondence: jiazhu@iupui.edu
[1]Regenstrief Institute, Inc, IndianapolisIndiana, USA
[2]Indiana University School of Medicine, Indianapolis, IN, USA
Full list of author information is available at the end of the article

health information exchange and compared the proportion of patients receiving each oral hypoglycemic medication available through LCPPs at pharmacy chains with and without LCPPs. We also compared the proportion of patients who had at least one prescription for an oral hypoglycemic medication before and after pharmacies implemented LCPPs. Our hypothesis was that, if patients pay cash for medications available through LCPPs, the proportion of patients appearing to use these medications would appear lower for chains with LCPP compared to chains without these programs. Similarly, we would expect the proportion of patients receiving each of these medications to appear to fall after the pharmacy chains implemented LCPPs.

Methods

This study was approved by the Institutional Review Board of Indiana University. We chose to base our evaluation on patients with type 2 diabetes, a common disease that requires treatment with medications chronically. We chose to study patients with a specific condition in order to allow us to estimate usage rates (proportion of patients who received a prescription for a drug) which we could compare across chains with and without LCPPs from 2008 to 2010, before and after the LCPP implementation from 2002 to 2010, as well as with estimates based on the most recent Medical Expenditure Panel Survey, a nationally representative survey of medical care use and expenditures.

Indiana network for patient care

The Indiana Network for Patient Care (INPC) is an operational regional health information exchange, which collects and transfers healthcare information electronically across organizations within a region, community or hospital system [5]. The INPC services more than 75 participating hospitals as well as laboratories, radiology centers, public health departments, long-term care facilities, payers, some pharmacies, and PBMs, and the INPC has served Indianapolis for more than 15 years [1,6]. In particular the INPC includes pharmacy claims data from the largest public and private payors as well as medication history data from PBMs obtained *via* the Surescripts network. Surescripts is the country's largest electronic prescribing network providing electronic access to prescription information. It connects all of the nation's major chain pharmacies, many of the nation's leading payers, and over 10,000 independent pharmacies nationwide. The medication data usually include patient identifying data, such as name, gender, ethnicity, and address; drug data, including a coded identifier, whether the drug dispensed was branded, and the number of days' supply dispensed; and dispensing pharmacy information, including the National Council for Prescription

Drug Programs (NCPDP) pharmacy code. We map the coded drug identifiers (almost always National Drug Codes but sometimes pharmacy specific codes) indirectly to the RxNORM codes (a standardized nomenclature for clinical drugs and drug delivery devices developed and maintained in the National Library of Medicine), which allowed us to aggregate drugs at the level of active ingredients. We selected commonly used antidiabetic medications (First DataBank Standard Therapeutic Class Code: 71), including selected oral hypoglycemic agents (OHA) therapeutic classes: sulfonylurea, biguanides, thiazolidinediones, α-glucosidase inhibitors, meglitinides, dipeptidyl-peptidase-4 inhibitors, and antidiabetic combinations.

Pharmacy data

Using the NCPCP pharmacy database, we aggregated dispensing locations into chains by store name. We defined an LCPP as a program that offered 30-day supplies of medications for $5 or less and which did not have obvious barriers to participation, such as annual membership fees or difficult enrollment processes. In addition to reviewing the grey and published literature [4,7], we reviewed both the current and past versions of the websites for each of the 14 chains in our database to determine which offered an LCPP and which antidiabetic medications were currently included in the program. [7,8] Using these data, we identified five major chains which implement LCPP and provide generic antidiabetic medication (glimepiride, glipizide, glyburide,and metformin). While the chains implemented their LCPPs at slightly different times, they essentially started in the 4th quarter of 2006, and most were implemented by the 4th quarter of 2007.

Measurements

In order to construct a measure of the rate of medication use for each category, we identified all patients in the Indianapolis Metropolitan Statistical Area (MSA) who had at least one clinical encounter with type 2 diabetes (ICD-9-CM codes 250.X0 or 250.X2 as the primary diagnosis) from 2008 to 2010. We then assigned each patient who had at least 3 medication dispensing records (assuming that patients with a chronic disease on chronic medications would have a minimum of 4 dispensing events over the course of 1 year, even if they received 90-day supplies and were only being treated with 1 drug) to the pharmacy chain through which they received their prescriptions. We excluded patients who received prescriptions from more than 1 chain during the study period from the cohort in order to eliminate any cross-over effects. Next, we computed the rate at which each drug was used in each pharmacy chain cohort of patients. If a patient had at least 1 dispensing

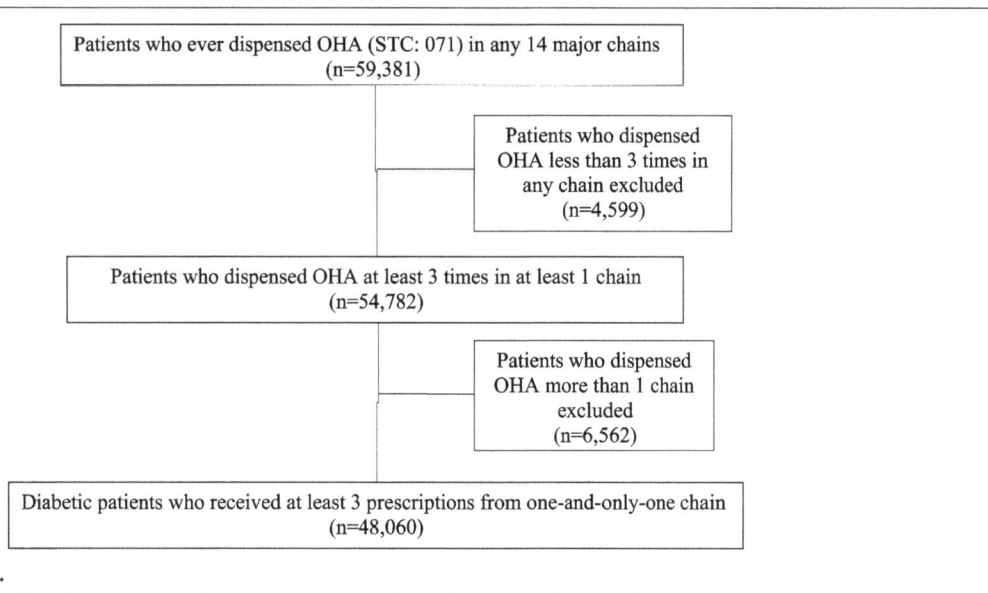

Figure 1 Patient selection.

event for the drug, we included them in the numerator, while the total number of diabetic patients attributed to the pharmacy chain was used as the denominator. Using the same approach, we measured the proportion of patients using individual OHA longitudinally (2002 to 2010) for a single payer.

In order to obtain comparable independent estimates of rates of use of these drugs nationally, we extracted data from the Medical Expenditure Panel Survey (MEPS) 2008 Prescribed Medicines dataset (file: HC-118A). [9] The MEPS study is a large-scale survey of families and individuals, their medical providers, and employers across the United States by the Agency for Healthcare Research and Quality (http://www.meps.ahrq.gov/meps-web/). The estimated proportion of diabetes patients using each OHA drug in the year 2008 was used as a reference measure. We selected patients who had at least 1 diagnosis code for diabetes and used the MEPS weightings to project the proportion of diabetic patients receiving each active ingredient to the U.S. population.

Analysis

Primarily, we compared the rates at which a specific medication was dispensed to diabetic patients between chains offering and not offering an LCPP. In the generalized linear mixed models (GLMM), the dispensing event of low-cost medications was the dependent variable, and the low-cost program was used as the independent variable. Odds ratios (OR) were used to quantify the magnitude of associations between these 2 variables. Both adjusted and unadjusted associations were estimated. Patient age, gender, race, and pharmacy chain were used as covariates (fixed effects) for the adjusted analysis.

Patients were included in the model as the random effect.

In order to take account into secular trends, we secondarily evaluated longitudinal trends of the proportion of patients using low-cost medication in major chains with and without LCPP. The interrupted time series analyses with control group were performed to assess the immediate changes of proportion of low-cost OHA use after LCPP implementation and to analyze if any detectable change was caused by the LCPP. For this analysis,

Table 1 Patient characteristics

Chains	Number of Patients	Age of dispensing (Mean±SD)		Female	White
Chain1†	424	63.9	± 12.0	50.70%	83.20%
Chain2	489	61.2	± 13.0	43.90%	87.50%
Chain3	693	66.4	± 10.4	51.50%	81.70%
Chain4†	727	60.7	± 13.1	45.20%	91.20%
Chain5†	810	53.5	± 12.3	52.30%	84.20%
Chain6‡	966	57.3	± 12.6	45.60%	83.60%
Chain7	1,708	60.8	± 11.0	40.10%	89.60%
Chain8	2,892	60.8	± 10.2	40.80%	91.80%
Chain9	3,461	64.0	± 11.0	43.10%	87.80%
Chain10†	3,932	59.1	± 12.8	51.00%	87.70%
Chain11†	5,623	57.6	± 12.3	50.80%	82.40%
Chain12	7,971	58.2	± 12.8	51.70%	75.10%
Chain13	9,882	66.6	± 10.6	43.10%	85.10%
Chain14†	16,788	59.1	± 12.9	49.00%	79.00%
MEPS	13.7million	60.7	± 12.8	44.2%	66.8%

† Chain with a LCPP.
‡ Chain with LCPP for Chlorpropamide only.

the proportion of low-cost OHA use was measured quarterly. Changes of proportion of low-cost OHA use and changes of the slopes between pre-intervention period (2002, quarter 1 to 2006, quarter 4) and post-intervention period (2007, quarter 1 to 2010, quarter 4) were estimated and compared for chains with LCPP (intervention) and without LCPP (control).

Results

We identified 48,060 diabetic patients who received at least 3 prescriptions from one-and-only-one of 14 pharmacy chains (4,129 individual pharmacies) which cover more than 95% of INPC patients who had OHA dispensing records (Figure 1). The demographic characteristics of the patient cohorts were similar across chains (Table 1). Among a total of 620,648 OHA dispensing events, 268,473 were dispensed from chains without an LCPP and 352,175 were dispensed from chains with an LCPP. Overall, the percentage of dispensing events of low-cost medications was higher in pharmacy chains which have low-cost programs: 71.7% vs. 66.1%. After

controlling for patient gender, race, and chain, chains with an LCPP are more likely to dispense an OHA which is available as a low-cost medication (OR: 1.21,95% CI [1.19,1.22], p < 0.0001). Proportions of patients for which each OHA was dispensed are similar for drugs across chains whether they offer an LCPP or not (Figure 2). In addition, the proportions of diabetic patients receiving each medication based on projections from the MEPS data were similar to those in our Indianapolis cohorts (Table 2).

From the longitudinal (2002–2010) dataset, a total of 18,775 patients were identified (14,220 for LCPP with 154,525 low-cost OHA dispensing events, and 4,555 for non-LCPP with 74,738 low-cost OHA dispensing events). Figure 3 demonstrates the results of segmentation regression for 36-quarter intervals. In the LCPP group post-LCPP implementation and controlling for baseline trends, no sudden changes of the proportion of low-cost medication use were found (p = 0.14), and a slight decline of slope was observed (–0.01, p < 0.0001). Similarly, in the non-LCPP group, there was also no

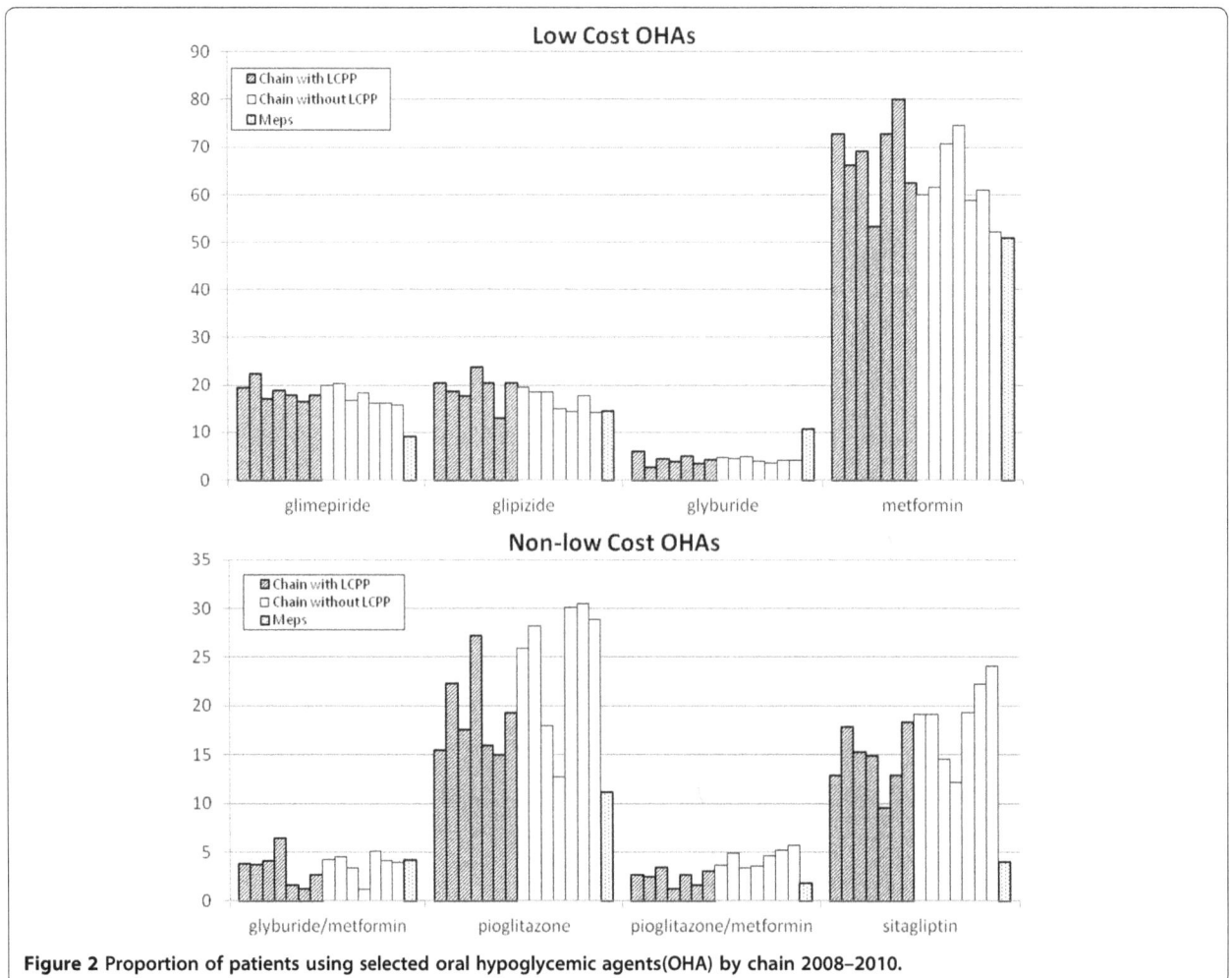

Figure 2 Proportion of patients using selected oral hypoglycemic agents(OHA) by chain 2008–2010.

Table 2 Proportion of patients using selected oral hypoglycemic agent (OHA) by chain

Ingredient	MEPS	Chain14	Chain11	Chain1	Chain10	Chain4	Chain2	Chain5	Chain13
Chlorpropamide *	0.2	0.04	0.01	0	0.02	0	0	0	0.03
Glimepiride *	9.1	17.1	19.4	18.8	18.0	17.8	22.4	16.5	19.9
Glipizide *	14.5	17.6	20.3	23.8	20.4	20.3	18.6	12.9	19.6
Glyburide *	10.7	4.3	5.9	3.7	4.9	4.2	2.6	3.4	4.6
Metformin *	51.0	69.1	72.8	53.3	72.8	62.4	66.2	80.0	59.9
Acarbose	0.1	0.4	0.3	0.9	0.4	0.2	0.2	0.2	0.4
Glimepiride/Pioglitazone	0.3	0.2	0.26	1.1	0.2	0.1	0.8	0.1	0.2
Glimepiride/Rosiglitazone	0.5	0.4	0.17	0.4	0.4	0.6	0.4	0.2	0.5
Glipizide/Metformin	0.1	0.6	0.56	0.9	0.5	0.8	0.6	0.2	0.7
Glyburide/Metformin	4.1	4.0	3.8	6.3	1.5	2.6	3.6	1.2	4.1
Pioglitazone	11.1	17.5	15.4	27.1	15.9	19.2	22.2	14.9	25.8
Pioglitazone/Metformin	1.8	3.3	2.5	1.1	2.6	3.0	2.4	1.6	3.6
Repaglinde	0.8	0.8	0.5	0.9	0.6	0.9	0.8	0.1	1.0
Rosiglitazone	0.5	3.0	2.3	6.8	3.1	3.0	3.4	2.3	5.6
Rosiglitazone/Metformin	0.6	1.4	1.1	2.3	1.6	1.5	1.8	1.2	2.0
Sitagliptin	4.0	10.8	9.0	12.2	9.4	12.7	12.2	8.8	14.3
Sitagliptin/Metformin	1.1	4.9	4.3	2.8	4.5	6.7	6.1	4.5	5.3
Low-cost OHA		85.3	89.0	78.5	89.0	83.2	83.4	90.0	79.0
Non-low-cost OHA		55.3	33.8	52.1	34.4	43.4	43.7	29.3	52.2

*low-cost oral antidiabetic medication.

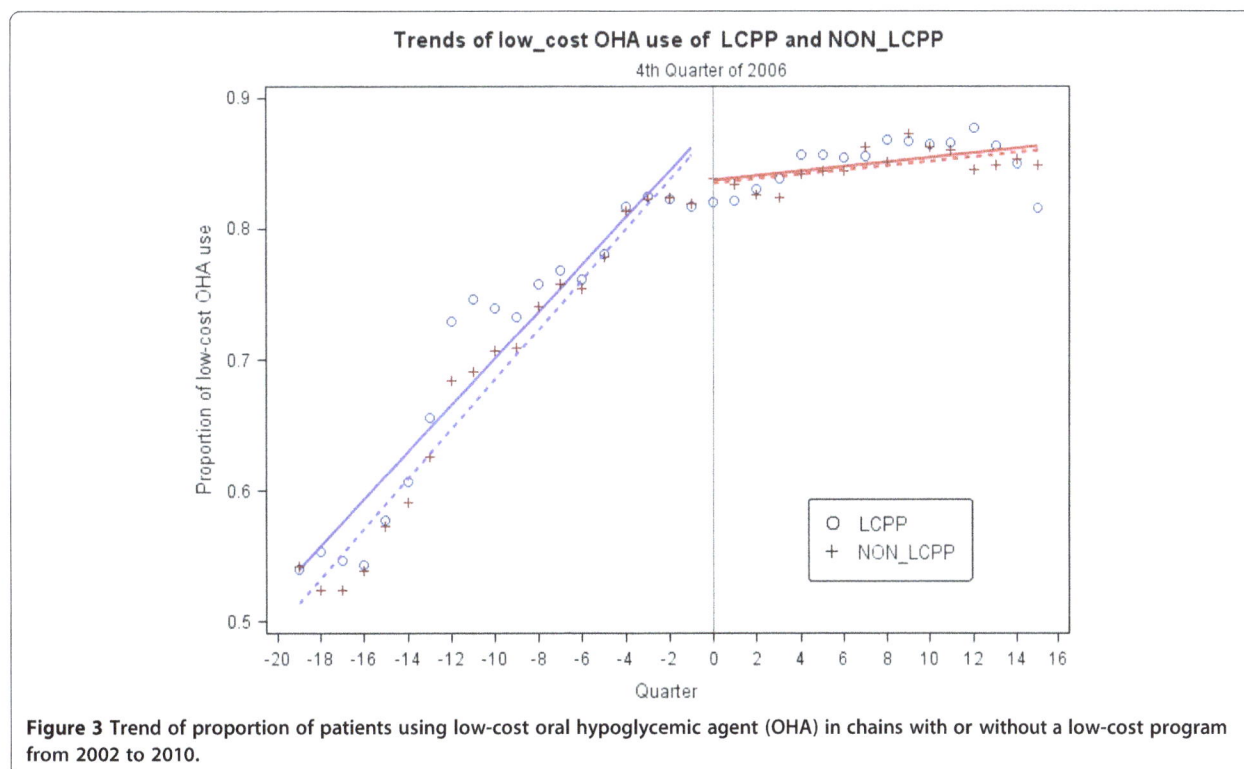

Figure 3 Trend of proportion of patients using low-cost oral hypoglycemic agent (OHA) in chains with or without a low-cost program from 2002 to 2010.

significant drop of low-cost medication use (p = 0.06); however, there was a change in slope (−0.01, p < 0.0001) over time. In the segmentation regression with two groups, there was no difference between the groups in prior trend (p = 0.35). After LCPP implementation, the immediate change was not significantly different for the LCPP and non-LCPP groups (p = 0.88), and there was no significant difference between the LCPP and non-LCPP groups in the change in slope (p = 0.57).

Discussion

To our knowledge, this is the first study that investigated whether LCPPs decrease data availability of low-cost medication dispensing events. We did not find any evidence to support the concern voiced by some researchers that pharmacies may not be sending claims for low-cost generic medications to PBMs. The estimated proportion of patients receiving each anti-diabetic medication was comparable not only across chains, regardless of whether they offered an LCPP, but also before and after the time frame in which chains implemented LCPPs. In addition, from the longitudinal data, we further observed no significant difference in changes in the level and slope of the proportion of low-cost medication use after LCPP implementation between chains with and without LCPP.

In the longitudinal data set, low-cost OHA use has been rapidly increasing from 2002 to 2006. A slower growing of the proportion of low-cost medication use has been observed in chains with and without LCPP in the beginning of 2007. Possible explanation could be an amount of patients dispensed preferred branded antidiabetic medications even the insurance program has encouraged using generic OHAs. In addition, some patients in this population might be eligible for Medicare Part D program when it was implemented in 2006, which we might not capture complete medication dispensing information for these patients.

The proportions for anti-diabetic drugs which are not included in the LCPPs were similar between chains offering LCPPs and those that do not, which increases our confidence in our estimation process. In addition, the similarities of the proportion of patients using each OHA between our estimates based on pharmacy claims and estimates from the MEPS data increase support our belief that our claims-based estimates are reasonable.

From these experiences, we did not find evidence to support the concern that the PBMs do not capture dispensing events of low-cost medications in chains with LCPP. We speculate that because of the level of automation of the submission process in most pharmacies and the minimal cost of transmitting these transactions that, unless a patient pays cash and specifically requests that the pharmacy not share the data with the patient's payor, the pharmacy will send the claim to the patient's PBM. To not send in the claim, the technician or the pharmacist would have to change the patient's payer to "cash", which would require more work than submitting a claim to the third-party when the patient has active prescription drug coverage in their profile.

Limitation

It is possible that the central Indiana population may not be representative of other populations but the demographics are similar to the overall US population. We only studied OHAs in diabetic patients who have active insurance coverage. Findings may not apply to other medications in the LCPP or to patients without active insurance coverage. In addition, we were not able to directly measure the proportion of patients receiving OHAs to compare with the estimate based on claims transactions, but we believe that our approach of comparing the proportions for patients receiving medications from chains with and without LCPPs are a good proxy. Note that provider orders would not provide a good gold standard since so many prescriptions go unfilled. We might not have identified all diabetic patients and may have included some Type 1 diabetics, but this should not introduce any systematic bias. Further, assignment of patients to pharmacy chains was reasonable based on at least 3 OHA dispensing events during the study period, which might exclude information from patients who had less than three OHA dispensing records in the INPC. However, this assignment may provide information for a more stable study population for each chain.

Conclusion

Our findings should reassure researchers that dispensing data for medication available through LCPPs are not selectively excluded from PBM or claims datasets.

Competing interest
The authors declare that they have no competing interests.

Ackowledgements
We would like to thank Roberta Ambuehl (senior data analyst) at the Regenstrief Institute, Inc.

Author details
[1]Regenstrief Institute, Inc, IndianapolisIndiana, USA. [2]Indiana University School of Medicine, Indianapolis, IN, USA. [3]Siemens Healthcare, Malvern, PA, USA.

Authors' contributions
VZ participated in literature research, study design, data analysis/ interpretation, and manuscript preparation. AB participated in study design and data acquisition. WZ participated in study design and data analysis. JMO led manuscript definition of intellectual content, study design, data analysis/ interpretation, and manuscript preparation. All authors read and approved the final manuscript.

References

1. Overhage JM, Tierney WM, McDonald CJ: **Design and implementation of the Indianapolis Network for Patient Care and Research.** *Bull Med Libr Assoc* 1995, **83**(1):48–56.

2. Choudhry NK, Shrank WH: **Four-Dollar Generics — Increased Accessibility, Impaired Quality Assurance.** *N Engl J Med* 2010, **363**(20):1885–1887. Available at http://www.nejm.org/doi/pdf/10.1056/NEJMp1006189. Accessed September 5, 2011.

3. Kaiser Family Foundation and Health Research and Education Trust: **Employer health Benefits: 2009 annual survey.** 2011, Available at: http://ehbskfforg/pdf/2009/7936pdf. Accessed June 17.

4. Czechowski JL, Tjia J, Triller DM: **Deeply discounted medications: Implications of generic prescription drug wars.** *J Am Pharm Assoc (2003)* 2010, **50**(6):752–757. Available at: http://japha.metapress.com/media/f6pnujmwlrnfd7nwdrwq/contributions/h/6/1/2/h6122644558q197h.pdf. Acessed September 5, 2011.

5. AHRQ: **Health Information Exchange.** 2009, Available at: http://www.healthit.ahrq.gov/hie (accessed May 2012).

6. McDonald CJ, Overhage JM, Barnes M, *et al*: **INPC Management Committee. The Indiana network for patient care: a working local health information infrastructure: An example of a working infrastructure collaboration that links data from five health systems and hundreds of millions of entries.** *Health Aff (Millwood)* 2005, **24**(5):1214–1220. Available at: http://content.healthaffairs.org/cgi/pmidlookup?view=long&pmid=16162565. Accessed September 5, 2011.

7. : **Generic Retail Drug Pricing and States: $4 and free drug promotions by large chains affected by state laws.**, . Avaliable at: http://wwwncslorg/defaultaspx?tabid=14440. Accessed in June, 2011.

8. Keivn Lu CJ, Ronald Tamler: *"Wal-Mart Effect" Is a Mixed Blessing for Diabetes Drug Prices.* San Diego: American Diabetes Association. 71th Scientific Session. A1177-P; 2011.

9. Agency of Health Research and Quality: **Trends in the pharmaceutical treatment of diabetes, 1997 to 2007.** 2010, Available at: http://www.meps.ahrq.gov/mepsweb/data_files/publications/rf30/rf30.shtml, Accessed September 5, 2011.

13

Electrophysiological and pharmacological evaluation of the nicotinic cholinergic system in chagasic rats

Rafael Bonfante-Cabarcas[1,3]*, Erlymar López Hincapié[1,3], Eliezer Jiménez Hernández[1,3], Ruth Fonseca Zambrano[1,3], Lady Ferrer Mancini[1,3], Marcos Durand Mena[1,3] and Claudina Rodríguez-Bonfante[2,3]

Abstract

Background: Two theories attempt to explain the changes observed in the nicotinic acetylcholine receptors (nAChRs) in chagasic cardiomyopathy. The neurogenic theory proposes that receptor changes are due to loss of intracardiac ganglia parasympathetic neurons. The immunogenic theory proposes that the nAChRs changes are the result of autoantibodies against these receptors. Both theories agreed that nAChRs functional expression could be impaired in Chagas disease.

Methods: We evaluated nAChRs functional integrity in 54 Sprague Dawley rats, divided in two groups: healthy and chronic chagasic rats. Rats were subjected to electrocardiographic studies in the whole animal under pentobarbital anesthesia, by isolation and stimulation of vagus nerves and in isolated beating hearts (Langendorff's preparation).

Results: Nicotine, 10 μM, induced a significant bradycardia in both groups. However, rats that had previously received reserpine did not respond to nicotine stimulation. β-adrenergic stimulation, followed by nicotine treatment, induced tachycardia in chagasic rats; while inducing bradycardia in healthy rats. Bilateral vagus nerve stimulation induced a significantly higher level of bradycardia in healthy rats, compared to chagasic rats; physostigmine potentiated the bradycardic response to vagal stimulation in both experimental groups. Electric stimulation (e.g., ≥ 2 Hz), in the presence of physostigmine, produced a comparable vagal response in both groups. In isolated beating-heart preparations 1 μM nicotine induced sustained bradycardia in healthy hearts while inducing tachycardia in chagasic hearts. Higher nicotine doses (e.g.,10 – 100 uM) promoted the characteristic biphasic response (i.e., bradycardia followed by tachycardia) in both groups. 10 nM DHβE antagonized the effect of 10 μM nicotine, unmasking the cholinergic bradycardic effect in healthy rats only. 1 nM α-BGT alone induced bradycardia in healthy hearts but antagonized the 10 μM nicotine-induced tachycardia in chagasic rats. In healthy but not in chagasic hearts, 10 μM nicotine shortened PQ and PR interval, an effect counteracted by MA, DHβE and αBGT

Conclusion: Our results suggest that cholinergic function is impaired in chronic Chagas disease in rats, a phenomena that could be related to alteration on the nAChR expression.

Keywords: Vagal stimulation, Isolated beating hearts, Nicotine, Chagas disease, Mecamylamine, DHβE, α-BGT

* Correspondence: rcabarca@ucla.edu.ve
[1]Biochemistry Research Units, Health Sciences School, Universidad Centro Occidental Lisandro Alvarado, Barquisimeto, Lara, Venezuela
[3]Libertador Av. con Andrés Bello, Unidad de Bioquímica, Decanato de Ciencias de la Salud, Universidad Centro-Occidental "Lisandro Alvarado", Barquisimeto, Estado Lara Código Postal: 3001, Venezuela
Full list of author information is available at the end of the article

Background

Chagas disease, caused by *Trypanosome cruzi* (*T cruzi*), is considered a serious public health problem in Central and South America countries [1]. In Venezuela, approximately 4 million people are at risk to develop Chagas disease [2]. The chagasic chronic cardiomyopathy (CCC) is the most common complication of this disease; approximately 25-30% of infected patients developed CCC [1].

Although the CCC pathogenesis is not completely understood, two theories attempt to explain it: the neurogenic theory postulates that CCC is the result of myocardial denervation. During the acute phase of the disease, *T cruzi's* invasion of the myocardium results in a selective, mechanical destruction of the intracardiac post-ganglionic parasympathetic neurons. The destruction of the parasympathetic neurons allows for a sustained non-counteracted sympathetic tone; this unbalanced sympathetic stimulation initiates trophic changes that result in the myocardial remodeling that culminates in arrhythmias and heart failure [3].

The immunogenic theory explains the CCC pathogenesis as the result of an aberrant immune response that includes loss of self-tolerance and the development of cross-reacting antibodies. Due to molecular mimicry, cross-reacting antibodies bind and neutralize surface receptors such as nAChRs. These cross-reacting antibodies (i.e., autoantibodies) affect the activity and number of those receptors population [4-7].

Nicotinic acetylcholine receptors (nAChRs) are pentameric, ligand-gated ion channels, formed by α and β subunits. Eight α subunits (α_2- α_7, α_9, α_{10}) and three β subunits (β_2-β_4) have been described; the combination of these subunits produces a wide variety of functional receptors [8]. Intracardiac ganglion neurons can express α_2 to α_9 and β_2 to β_4 subunits, assembled predominantly as α_3/β_2, α_3/β_4, $\alpha_3/\beta_2/\beta_4$, $\alpha_3/\beta_2/\alpha_5$, $\alpha_3/\beta_4/\alpha_5$, and monomeric α_7. For example, the canine intracardiac ganglion expresses predominately α_3/β_2 nAChRs, with a smaller levels of $\alpha7$ nAChRs [9-12].

Both neurogenic and immunogenic theories propose alterations in the function of the cholinergic system. Recently, our group demonstrated the existence of trophic and functional disturbances of the muscarinic cholinergic receptor system on *in vivo* and *in vitro* rats' models of Chagas disease [13,14]. In the present study, we analyzed the functionality of the nAChRs in the whole animal and in isolated beating-heart preparations, of healthy and chagasic Sprague Dawley rats.

Methods

All drugs and chemicals were purchased from Sigma-Aldrich Co (St. Louis, MO, USA) and prepared as mg/ml or M stocks solution by dissolving the drugs in purified deionized water. Stocks solutions were alliquoted and stored at 5°C until use.

Animal model

All experiments were carried out on 54 Sprague Dawley rats, randomly distributed according to the experiment: 16 (8 healthy and 8 chagasic rats) for the whole animal experiments, 15 (8 healthy and 7 chagasic) were treated with reserpine, and 23 (11 healthy and 12 chagasic) were used in vagal stimulation and isolated beating heart experiments. The MHOM/VE/92/2-92-YBM trypomastigotes strain was used to induce infection. Experimental animal (i.e., rats) were inoculated with 1.000 trypomastigotes per gram of body weight (chagasic group). Chagasic animals develop an acute disease with a parasitemia peak of $67.27 \pm 25.05 \times 10^6$ parasites/ml at the third week of infection. At the time of performing the experiments, the animals had 7.84 ± 0.45 months-old, weighted 504.9 ± 10.74 and 418.5 ± 15.10 grs for healthy and chagasic rats, respectively; and only two chagasic animals displayed parasites in a blood sample, giving a parasitemia of 114.9 ± 84.43 parasites/ml. Animals were individually housed in a temperature-controlled environment with a 12:12 light/dark cycle and free access to food and water. Experimental protocols were approved by the ethical committee of the School of Health Sciences following the American Physiological Society guidelines.

Vagus nerve stimulation (VNS)

The animals were anesthetized using a pentobarbital (20-40 mg/Kg) and ketamine (50 mg/Kg) cocktail administered intraperitoneally. The animals' respiration was mechanically aided through a tracheal cannula connected to a volume-controlled rodent respirator at a frequency of 70 strokes/min to facilitate ventilation in spontaneously breathing rat. The cervical vagus nerve was exposed bilaterally and severed at the caudal terminus. Platinum bipolar electrodes were attached to the nerves ending leading toward the heart. The electrodes were connected to a PowerLab/8sp system to generate frequency of heart pacing . During the experiments performance, the electric pulses were modified according to the protocol. Impulses were delivered either at a fixed frequency (1.5 Hz) but different potency ranges (0.25 to 3 V) or in a range of frequencies (1-4 Hz) but fixed potency (2 V). All experiments were performed in the absence and presence of 0.3 mg/Kg physostigmine.

Isolated beating-heart system

The animals were anesthetized as described above and the hearts removed under aseptic conditions. The isolated hearts were connected to a Langendorff's perfusion system by cannulation of the aorta. The hearts were perfused with a tepid (37°C) modified physiological solution (pH 7.40 ± 0.05), aerated with a 95% O_2 and 5% CO_2 mixture. Perfusion was conducted at a rate of 7-10 mL/min maintaining a pressure range of 50 to 100 mmHg. The perfusion solution composition included 10 mM glucose, 1 mM $MgSO_4$, 116 mM NaCl, 18 mM $NaHCO_3$, 2.5 mM $CaCl_2$, 5 mM KCl, and 1 mM malate.

To evaluate the effect of nicotine stimulation on the chagasic and control hearts' rate, the isolated hearts were perfused, for 5 minutes, with 1, 10 or 100 μM of nicotine. The heart preparations were allowed a 10 min rest period between doses – maintaining perfusion with modified physiological solution. The effect of the following nAChRs' antagonists, on the isolated hearts' rate, was evaluated: 1 μM mecamylamine (MA, α_3/β_4 nAChR antagonist), 10 nM dihydro-β-erythroidine (DHβE; α_4/β_2 nAChR antagonist), and 1 nM α-bungarotoxin (α-BGT; α_7 nAChR antagonist) [15]. The antagonists were administered in the perfusion solution for 10 minutes, in the absence of nicotine, and for additionally 5 minutes in the presence of 10 μM nicotine. The preparations were allowed a 10 minutes resting period – perfusion with modified physiological solution – between antagonists administration.

EKG recording

In the VNS experiments, the hearts' electric activity was monitored using needle electrodes placed subcutaneously on the sternum xiphoid process and on both shoulders – the left shoulder electrode served as reference electrode. In the isolated heart preparations, the positive electrode was inserted into the heart's apex and the negative electrode into the right atrium. Analogical EKG signals were amplified using BioAmp, transformed in digital signals by Power Lab 8 data acquisition unit, recorded and analyzed using Lab Chart software (ADInstruments).

Data analysis

Data are expressed either as mean of absolute values ± SEM or normalized to be expresed as percentages ± SEM. Paired and non-paired Student's t-test were used to analyze the effect of a drug on a particular group in matched observations or when a variable for the control group was compared with the same variable of the *T cruzi* infected group, respectively. Repeated measure analysis of variance (rANOVA) followed by a Dunnet's post-test were peformed to determine the statistical significance of drug concentration and time effect per group. In all analyses, a p value < 0.05 was considered statistically significant. Statistical analysis were performed using the GraphPad Prism 4 for Windows software (GraphPad Software Inc, La Jolla, CA).

Results

EKG study in intact animals

The significant bradycardia induced by 10 μM nicotine, in healthy and chagasic rats, was reverted by 0.1 μM d-tubocurarine (Figures 1A and 1C). Lower concentrations of nicotine appear to have no effect on the heart rate of the animals.

In order to determine whether the catecholaminergic neurons were involved in the bradycardic response, the synaptic amine content was depleted with reserpine (1 mg/Kg/day for three days) in both control and chagasic animals. It was observed that reserpine-treated animals (both groups) had a lower basal heart rate and nicotine was unable to induce bradycardia (Figure 1B and 1D).

When adrenergic tone was enhanced (0.01 mg/Kg of isoproterenol), a similar tachycardic response (p = 0.14) was induced in both animals groups (i.e., 117.2% ± 1.54 in the healthy group and 120.6% ± 1.68 in the chagasic rats). After administration of 10 uM of nicotine, we observed that nicotine induced bradycardia in the healthy group while, surprisingly, inducing a significant tachycardia in the chagasic animals (Figure 2).

NVS study in intact animals

Stimulation of both vagus nerves induced a proportional bradycardia to the frequency of the stimulus. However, the bradycardic response was significantly higher in healthy rats, compared with chagasic rats (Figure 3A). Physostigmine potentiated the bradycardic response, in both experimental groups; at low frequencies (1 and 1.5 Hz) the bradycardic response was significantly higher in healthy rats but, a higher frequencies (2 to 4 Hz) bradycardia was similar in both groups (Figure 3B).

Likewise, at low frequency stimulation (1.5 Hz), a significant bradycardic response was elicited as the voltage intensity increased above 0.5 V. A significant difference between the groups was observed at 3 V when the vagus nerves' data were analyzed together (Figure 3C). Physostigmine potentiated the bradycardic response, with the resulting response significantly higher, at 2 and 2.5 V, for healthy rats compared with chagasic rats (Figure 3D).

Isolated beating-hearts study
Heart rate

Figure 4 illustrates the effect of nicotine on the heart rate of healthy and chagasic hearts. Nicotine (1 μM) slow-down the heart rate for 150 sec in healthy hearts (-4.9 ± 2.1%; p < 0.05), while in the chagasic hearts induced a transient but non-significant, decrease on the hearts rate (20 s), followed by a significant tachycardia (+2.6 ± 1%, p <0.05) (see Figure 4A). The response of healthy and chagasic hearts to 10 μM nicotine stimulation (Figure 4B) was comparable to that induced by 1 μM nicotine in the chagasic hearts. Initially, 10 μM nicotine induced a non-significant bradycardia

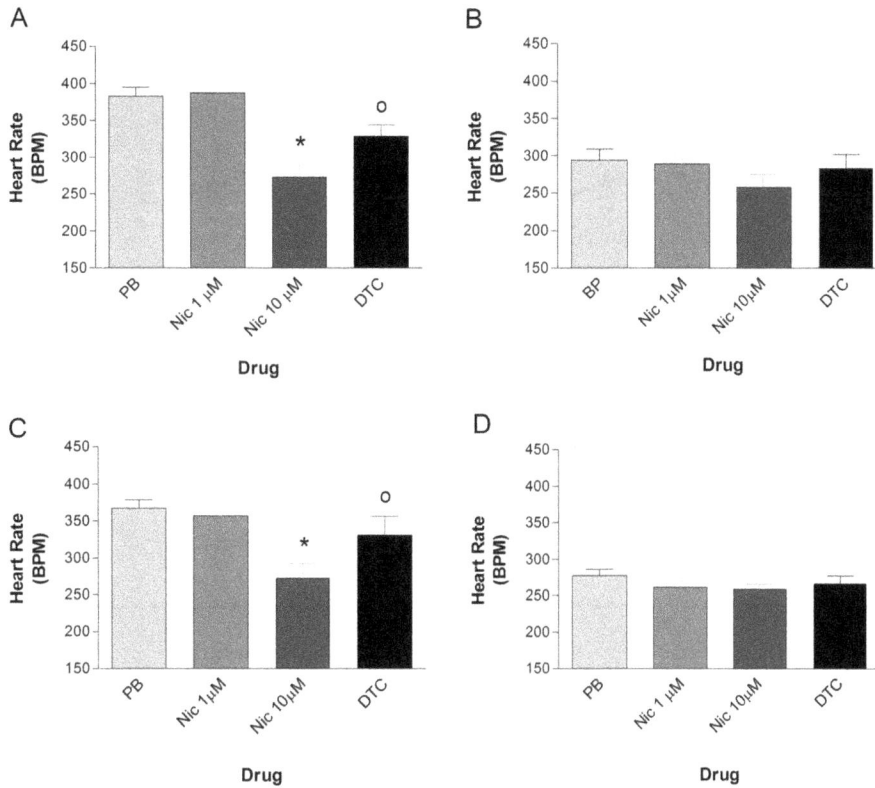

Figure 1 Nicotine affects the heart rate of anesthetized whole-animals. 10 µM Nicotine (Nic) induced a significant bradycardic response, while 1 µM D-tubocurarine reversed it, in both healthy (**A**) and chagasic (**C**) rats. Lower doses of Nic (i.e., 1 µM) have no effect on the heart rate of these animals. EKG results from healthy (**B**) and chagasic (**D**) rats, treated daily with 1 mg/Kg of reserpine for 3 days, showed a significant decrease of heart rate compared to untreated animals; however, 10 µM of nicotine has no bradycardic effect on reserpine-treated healthy (**B**) or chagasic (**C**) animals.

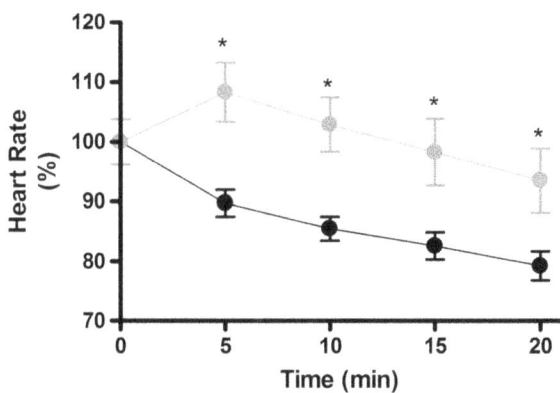

Figure 2 Nicotine effect on sympathetic-stimulated whole-animals. Anesthetized rats (n=10 per group) were treated successively with isoproterenol (0.01 mg/Kg) followed by nicotine (10 µM) at 20 min intervals. Nicotine induced bradycardia in healthy rats (black circles), while inducing tachycardia in chagasic rats (gray squares). *means $p < 0.05$ when both groups are compared at the indicated time.

(-2 ± 1.5%, $p > 0.05$) that was followed by a significant tachycardia (+5.8 ± 3.5% in healthy group; +4 ± 1.9% in chagasic group. $p < 0.05$). The effect of 100 µM nicotine was similar to that induced by 10 µM nicotine in both groups.

In the absence of nicotine stimulation, healthy hearts response to MA was a slight but significant ($p < 0.05$) bradycardia (2.24 to 2.92%). Chagasic hearts response to MA was non-significant. However, 1 µM MA abrogated the tachycardia elicited by 10 µM nicotine, in both, healthy and chagasic hearts.

Figure 5A shows that on healthy hearts α-BGT (full circles) induced a significant bradycardia (-6.8 ± 3.1%; $p < 0.05$); however, in the presence of 10 µM nicotine (open squares) α-BGT blocked the nicotine-induced tachycardia. Figure 5B shows that the α-BGT, by itself, had no effect on chagasic hearts' heart rate (full circles), but effectively blocked the nicotine-induced tachycardia (open squares).

In healthy hearts 10 nM DHβE, by itself, failed to induce a significant tachycardia ($p > 0.05$); however, in the presence of nicotine (10 µM), DHβE induced a significant ($p < 0.05$) bradycardia (Figure 5C). The chagasic hearts

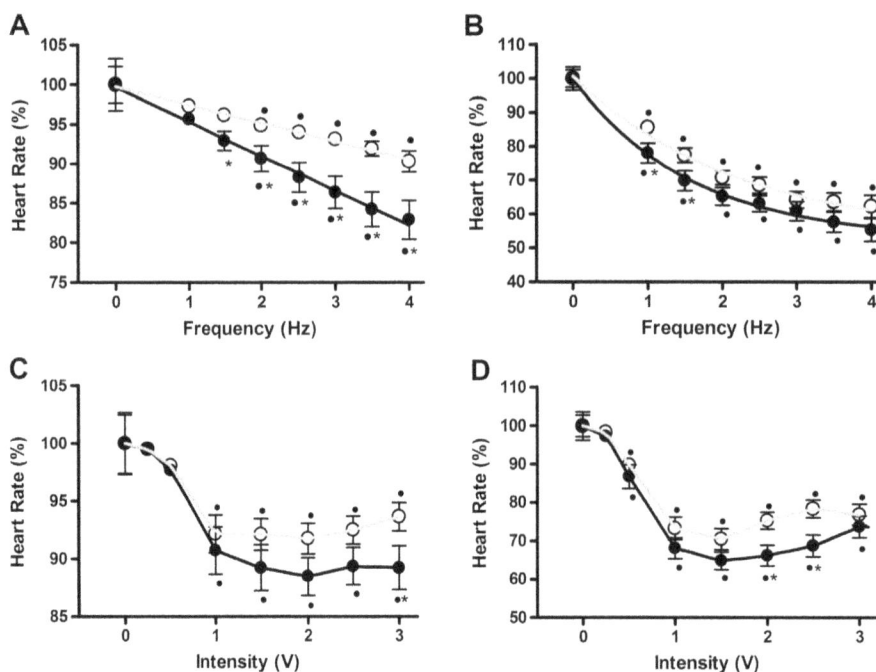

Figure 3 Vagal nerve stimulation in whole-animals. A 2 ms electric stimulation was delivered to the vagal nerve – at increasing frequency but fixed voltage (2 V) or increasing voltage at a fixed frequency (1.5 Hz) – in the absence (**A** and **C**) or presence of 0.3 mg/Kg physostigmine (**B** and **D**). In absence of physostigmine chagasic rats (open circles) the heart rate decreased proportionally to stimulus frequency (panel **A**) or intensity (panel **C**). Physostigmine increased the vagal response in both groups; however, when higher stimulation frequencies were applied (i.e., ≥ 3 Hz), the vagal response of chagasic animals became similar as compared with healthy rats. $p < 0.05$ indicated statistical significant differences between groups (*) or to the basal rate (˙).

response to DHβE stimulation alone was a delayed brady-cardia (i.e., 10 min after stimulation). In the presence of nicotine, the delayed was abrogated (Figure 5D) and the response was comparable to that observed in the healthy hearts group.

PQ and PR intervals
Chagasic hearts had significantly prolonged PQ and PR intervals when compared to healthy hearts (healthy Rats:

PQ = 46.82 ± 2.49 and PR: 53.70 ± 2.37 ms; chagasic rats: PQ = 54.17 ± 2.55 and PR = 61.92 ± 2.48 ms; p = 0.049 and 0.041, respectively). The PQ interval in healthy hearts was significantly decreased by nicotine 10 μM, during the desensitized period (5 min), an effect that was antagonized by MA, DHβE and α-BGT. No significant effect in chaga-sic hearts in the PQ interval was observed. Similar effects were observed for the PR intervals. When healthy and chagasic hearts were compared in a particular protocol

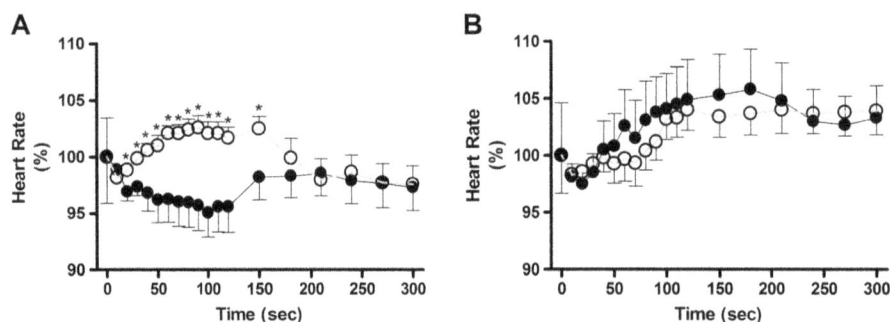

Figure 4 Nicotine induces a biphasic response in isolated beating-heart preparations. Nicotine at concentrations of 1 μM (left panel) and 10 μM (right panel) was perfused during 5 min. The bipolar 400 Hz acquisition rate EKG records indicated that 1 μM nicotine increased the heart rate of chagasic hearts (open circles), while decreasing it in healthy hearts (filled circles). 10 μM nicotine induced a biphasic effect (i.e., transiently bradychardia followed by sustained tachycardia) on both healthy and chagasic animals' heart rate. * $p < 0.05$ indicated statistically significant difference compared to pre-drug basal rate.

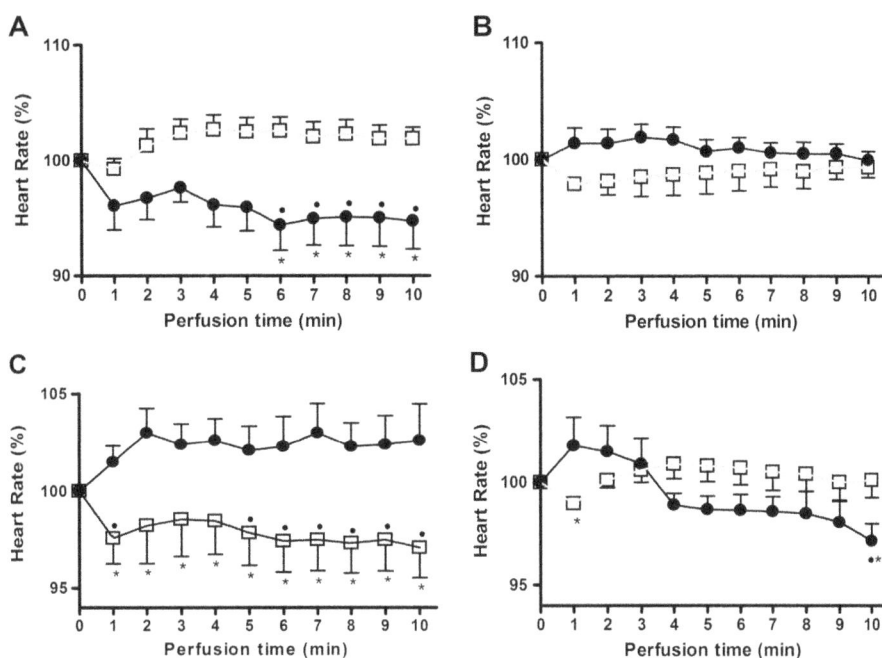

Figure 5 α-BGT and DHβE pharmacological effects on isolated beating-heart preparations. The nicotinic antagonists α-BGT (panels **A** and **B**) and DHβE (panels **C** and **D**) were perfused in the absence (black circles) or presence (open squares) of 10 μM nicotine in healthy (panels **A** and **C**) and chagasic (panel **B** and **D**) hearts. Observe that α-BGT or DHβE, in healthy hearts, induced a significant bradycardia that counteracted the nicotine effect. $p < 0.05$ indicates statistically significant difference between drug's group (*) or to the basal heart rate (•).

variable, we observed significant differences with 10 μM nicotine during the desensitizing period, 100 μM nicotine during the activation period, DHβE and αBGT (Table 1).

QT and QTc intervals

No significant effects on either of the intervals were observed when healthy and chagasic hearts were compared. Furthermore, we did not observe any significant effect of nicotine on both intervals; however, in chagasic hearts with the addition of 10 μM nicotine (activation period), DHβE and α-BGT significantly increased the QTc interval when compared to nicotine only. When healthy and chagasic hearts were compared in a particular protocol variable we observed significant differences with 10 μM nicotine during the desensitizing period and DHβE.

T and QRS amplitude

QRS amplitude was higher in healthy hearts when compared with chagasic hearts (HR: 709 ± 103.8 μV; CH: 462.1 ± 62.53 μV; p = 0.05). In healthy hearts, 10 μM nicotine in the presence of MA and DHβE only, induced a significantly decrease of the QRS amplitude; while in chagasic hearts 1 μM nicotine and 10 μM nicotine in the presence of DHβE induced a significant decrease of QRS amplitude. When healthy and chagasic hearts were compared in a particular protocol variable we observed significant differences

with 100 μM nicotine during the desensitizing period and DHβE.

No differences for the T wave amplitude were observed between healthy and chagasic hearts. In healthy and chagasic hearts nicotine 10 μM in addition to DHβE induced a significant decrease of the T amplitude during the desensitizing period. When healthy and chagasic hearts were compared in a particular protocol variable we observed significant differences with 10 μM nicotine in addition to MA during the desensitizing period.

Perfusion pressure

In healthy and chagasic hearts 10 μM nicotine induced a significant increases of the pressure wave amplitude during the activation period, an effect that was blocked by MA and DHβE in healthy hearts and by MA, DHβE and αBGT in chagasic hearts. The use of 100 μM nicotine also induced an increase of the pressure wave amplitude during the activation period in healthy hearts but not in chagasic ones. When healthy and chagasic hearts were compared in a particular protocol variable we observed significant differences with 10 μM nicotine in addition to αBGT during activation and desensitizing periods (Table 1).

Discussion

This work represents the first study that evaluates the functional integrity of the nicotinic cholinergic system in

Table 1 Effect of nicotine and a selective nicotinic antagonist on electrocardiographic parameters in isolated beating heart

Protocol Sequence	PQ interval				Aorta Pressure Wave			
	Healthy Hearts		Chagasic Hearts		Healthy Hearts		Chagasic Hearts	
	AV (msec)	%	AV (msec)	%	AV (mmHg)	%	AV (mmHg)	%
Basal	46.8±2.5	100	54.2±2.6[@]	100	14.1±2.3	100	14.4±1.4	100
Nic 1 µM A	44.9±1.7	97.2±3.0	53.0±2.5	96.2±0.3	15.8±2.6	141.0±29.72	15.6±2.2	110.7±11.2
Nic 1 µM D	47.1±2.4	101.7±4.3	53.3±3.0	95.7±1.3	13.6±1.9	124.7±28.72	13.3±1.5	96.0±10.0
Wash 1	49.9±1.9	100	53.7±2.2	100	11.6±1.6	100	12.9±1.5	100
Nic 10 µM A	48.9±2.0	98.1±2.2	53.8±2.3	100.3±1.7	16.7±1.9*	180.9±37.74	16.9±1.9*	134.8±9.8
Nic 10 µM D	45.4±2.2*	90.7±2.2	54.2±2.5	104.6±2.0[@]	14.6±1.6	159.5±31.96	13.6±1.3	112.8±8.7
Wash 2	47.9±1.9	100	55.8±2.6	100	11.8±1.2	100	12.6±1.5	100
Nic 100 µM A	48.3±2.0	101.0±2.4	57.1±2.5	109.0±1.5[@]	16.5±1.7*	150.4±17.21	14.5±1.5	120.1±9.7
Nic 100 µM D	48.7±2.0	101.4±2.9	54.5±2.6	100.5±1.2	12.8±1.6	107.1±5.75	13.4±1.5	112.7±12.6
Wash 3	48.1±2.1	100	51.2±2.6	100	12.9±1.4	100	13.1±1.2	100
MA	47.4±2.0	99.6±3.8	53.0±2.4	103.4±1.7	11.7±1.5	90.5±8.13	12.3±1.3	95.3±6.4
MA+Nic 10 µM A	48.2±2.3	100.3±2.1	52.7±2.05	104.3±1.1	12.5±2.3	92.7±9.64	11.4±1.3	88.7±6.0°
MA+Nic 10 µM D	48.6±2.9	101.2±2.8°	53.6±2.4	102.8±0.4	12.4±1.6	94.4±7.88	11.4±1.4	87.7±6.6°
Wash 4	46.6±2.4	100	53.9±2.1	100	10.3±1.5	100	11.5±1.3	100
DHβE	47.4±2.4	101.7±1.7	55.4±2.5	107.8±0.5[@]	12.4±2.1	121.9±15.10	10.7±1.2	95.4±3.7
DHβE+Nic 10 µM A	49.0±2.6	105.5±1.8°	55.8±2.5	104.7±0.6	11.2±1.8	110.0±12.80°	11.0±1.2	98.5±4.5°
DHβE+Nic 10 µM D	48.8±1.9	105.6±2.2°	55.6±2.3	106.8±0.7	10.4±1.7	99.8±8.64°	10.8±1.2	96.3±4.4
Wash 5	48.4±2.1	100	55.8±2.6	100	10.0±1.9	100	10.1±0.9	100
αBGT	50.6±2.1	104.9±2.9	55.3±2.5	97.2±0.9[@]	7.7±1.4	84.3±7.33	10.6±1.0	104.2±3.8
αBGT+Nic 10 µM A	50.3±1.9	104.4±1.9°	56.0±2.9	81.3±3.6	9.4±1.7*	96.5±5.52°	8.9±1.2	99.0±5.2°[@]
αBGT+Nic 10 µM D	49.4±1.8	102.6±2.4	57.4±2.6	106.6±1.7	10.3±2.1	105.2±12.35	9.7±1.2	95.4±3.8[@]
Wash 6	50.3±2.1	-	57.8±2.7	-	10.4±1.0	-	9.3±1.7	-

A: agonist activation period at 30 sec of perfusion; D: agonist desensitization period at 5 min of perfusion; AV: absolute values; Nic: nicotine; MA: mecamylamine; DHβE: dihydro-beta-erythroidine; αBGT: alfa-bungarotoxin; * means p < 0.05 when absolute values are compared against basal or wash periods by repeated measure ANOVA followed by Dunnet post-test; ° means p < 0.05 when % values are compared in the presence and absence of the antagonist by Wilconxon matched pairs test; [@] means p < 0.05 when % values are compared between healthy and chagasic groups by Mann-Whitney test.

rats with chronic chagasic disease, using electrophysiological tools. We were able to determine that rats with Chagas disease have a dysfunction of nicotinic cholinergic system when compared with healthy rats.

In our whole-animal model, nicotine induced bradycardia, an effect that could be mediated by the simultaneous activation of the post-synaptic autonomic neurons and inhibition of adrenergic pre-synaptic terminals innervating the heart. The inhibition of the adrenergic response most likely is mediated by M2 muscarinic AChRs. M2-mediated inhibitory effect has been demonstrated in guinea pig, where muscarinic agonists reduced norepinephrine overflow, in a concentration-dependent manner, and such effect was selectively antagonized by the M2-specific antagonist AF-DX-116 [16].

The tachycardia induced by nicotine, in the presence of isoproterenol, indicates an impairment in the vasovagal reflex in chagasic rats. Isoproterenol increases the systolic pressure, due to the increment on heart rate and ejection fraction. The damaged cholinergic parasympathetic efferents favored a post-synaptic β-adrenergic dominance over

the heart rate. This observation was consistent with reports that, in rats, phenylephrine-induced bradycardia was diminished in the indeterminate phase of Chagas disease as well as in chronic chagasic cardiomyopathy [14].

Direct stimulation of the vagus nerve, in rats with chronic Chagas disease, decreased the bradycardic response as a function of stimuli frequency and intensity, indicating a reduced vagal function in chagasic rats. The importance of the vagus nerve's functional integrity has been documented in rats with acute chagasic myocarditis using direct vagal stimulation [17]. In these studies, the chronotropic response to stimulation, with low frequencies pulses, was significantly different between chagasic rats and healthy rats. These groups have comparable chronotropic response to higher frequency stimuli suggesting decrease in the fibers' excitability and change in their response threshold in chagasic rats, due to acute nerve inflammation.

In Chagas disease, the diminished cholinergic function has been explained as a direct consequence of the presence of autoantibodies against both types of AChRs (i.e., nicotinic and muscarinic receptors). The chronic binding of these autoantibodies to the nAChR could induce a decrease in the population of functional nAChRs and consequently contribute to the alterations described in the course of chronic Chagas' disease [6,7]. In our experiments, we observed that when physostigmine, a well known acetyl cholinesterase inhibitor, was administered at the same time of high frequencies stimuli, the vagal response was restored. By mass-action law, a high level of synaptic acetylcholine would competitively displace the autoantibodies from the receptor sites.

In our isolated beating-heart model, nicotine stimulation induced the classic biphasic heart rate, which has been described for both nicotine and other non-selective AChR agonists [18-21]. However, our study demonstrated the nicotine-induced effect was dose-dependent. While 1 μM nicotine induced a bradycardia only, 100 μM of nicotine induced a biphasic effect in control rats. These differential responses were blocked by 1 μM mecamylamine, indicating that the action of nicotine used the ganglionic α3β4 nicotine acetylcholine receptor (nAChR) signaling.

The need of an intact ganglionic transmission has been demonstrated on elegant studies using hexamethonium. This ganglionic nAChR antagonist blocked the nicotine-induced biphasic heart rate [10,19-21]. However, the exact nAChR population involved in the nicotine-induced bradycardia has not been identified. Successful blockade of nicotine-induced bradycardia by α-BGT suggest that α7 nAChR subtype could be involved in the biphasic heart-rate response to nicotine stimulation [19]. Involvement of other nAChR subtypes or even the contribution of specific subunits cannot be ignored. nAChR with high affinity for nicotine are preferentially formed by α2, α4 and β2 subunits [22-24]. α2β2 and α4β2 receptors have been described to be expressed on intracardiac neurons [9]. DHβE, an α4β2 nAChR selective antagonist, prevented nicotine-induced bradycardia, while a selective agonist (RJR2403) reproduced the nicotine effect [20,21]. Cytisine, a selective β4 subunit agonist, and metillycaconitine (selective α7 antagonist) have opposites effect on the heart rate [19-21].

Our results indicated that pre-synaptic α7 nAChRs are involved in the nicotine-induced tachycardic phase as it was blocked by α-BGT. The bradycardic response to α-BGT perfused alone suggested that α7 subunit is also present in nAChR intrinsic adrenergic neurons. Recent studies have found that autonomic dysfunction; especially a decrease of vagal activity, is related to worsening of cardiovascular diseases. Autonomic imbalance with increased adrenergic and reduced parasympathetic activity is involved in the development and progress of heart failure (HF) [25]. M2-AChR knockout mice exhibit impaired ventricular function and increased susceptibility to cardiac stress, suggesting a protective role of the parasympathetic nervous system in the heart [26]. Furthermore, vagal stimulation has been shown to be beneficial in cases of heart failure, because it inhibited cardiac remodeling associated with heart dysfunction [27,28].

Our results suggest that nicotinic receptors are involved in the regulation of electrical transmission between sinusal and AV nodes, however chagasic hearts have lost this capability because nicotine was unable to shorten PQ and PR intervals in them, indicating a disregulation of nicotinic receptors in these structures. Indeed a lost of nicotinic receptors could explain a prolongued PQ and PR intervals observed in chagasic hearts in basal conditions.

The increase of perfusion pressure wave induced by nicotine in both groups reflects a positive inotropic effect of the agonist acting on nicotinic receptors. It has been already reported that nicotine produced a concentration-dependent positive inotropic effect on electrical evoked contraction of isolated toad ventricle [29].

Conclusions

Our results support the hypothesis that cholinergic dysfunction in Chagas disease is the result of a combined disruption of the vagal transmission and trophic remodeling of intracardiac neurons and receptors. The importance of our findings is to demonstrated that alterations in cardiac nicotinic cholinergic transmission is present in Chagas disease in an early phase of cardiomyopathy evolution, before a dilated cardiomyopathy with congestive heart failure will be installed. Therefore cardiac nicotinic cholinergic functionality could be useful as prognostic marker of the disease.

Competing interest
The authors declare that they have not competing interests.

Authors' contribution
RBC and CRB: made substantial contributions to conception and design, carried out whole-animal studies including data acquisition, analysis and interpretation, and wrote the draft and final version of the manuscript. ELH, RFZ and LFM: contributed to conception, design and performance of isolated beating-heart studies including data acquisition and analysis, involved in drafting the manuscript. MDM and EJM: contributed to conception, design and performance of vagal nerve stimulation studies, including data acquisition and analysis and were involved in drafting the manuscript. All authors read and approved the final version of the manuscript.

Acknowledgements
This study was funded by the "Consejo de Desarrollo Científico, Humanístico y Tecnológico" (CDCHT) grants N° 002-ME-2004 and 006-ME-2008, Universidad Centro Occidental "Lisandro Alvarado", Barquisimeto, Lara, Venezuela. The authors would like to thank Dr. Carla R. Lankford (US FDA, Silver Spring, Maryland, USA) for poof-reading this manuscript.

Author details
[1]Biochemistry Research Units, Health Sciences School, Universidad Centro Occidental Lisandro Alvarado, Barquisimeto, Lara, Venezuela. [2]Medical Parasitology Research Units, Health Sciences School, Universidad Centro Occidental Lisandro Alvarado, Barquisimeto, Lara, Venezuela. [3]Libertador Av. con Andrés Bello, Unidad de Bioquímica, Decanato de Ciencias de la Salud, Universidad Centro-Occidental "Lisandro Alvarado", Barquisimeto, Estado Lara Código Postal: 3001, Venezuela.

References

1. Rassi A Jr, Rassi A, Marin-Neto JA: Chagas disease. *Lancet* 2010, 375(9723):1388–1402.
2. Aché A, Matos AJ: Interrupting Chagas disease transmission in Venezuela. *Rev Inst Med Trop Sao Paulo* 2001, 43:37–43.
3. Dávila DF, Santiago JJ, Odreman WA: Vagal dysfunction and the pathogenesis of chronic Chagas disease. *Int J Cardiol* 2005, 100:337–339.
4. Kierszenbaum F: Where do we stand on the autoimmunity hypothesis of Chagas disease? *Trends Parasitol* 2005, 21:513–516.
5. Sterin-Borda L, Borda E: Role of neurotransmitter autoantibodies in the pathogenesis of chagasic peripheral dysautonomia. *Ann N Y Acad Sci* 2000, 917:273–280.
6. Goin JC, Venera G, Biscoglio de Jimenez Bonino M, Sterin-Borda L: Circulating antibodies against nicotinic acetylcholine receptors in chagasic patients. *Clin Exp Immunol* 1997, 110:219–225.
7. Hernández CC, Barcellos LC, Giménez LE, Cabarcas RA, Garcia S, Pedrosa RC, Nascimento JH, Kurtenbach E, Masuda MO, Campos de Carvalho AC: Human chagasic IgGs bind to cardiac muscarinic receptors and impair L-type Ca2+ currents. *Cardiovasc Res* 2003, 58:55–65.
8. Fischer H, Liu DM, Lee A, Harries JC, Adams DJ: Selective modulation of neuronal nicotinic acetylcholine receptor channel subunits by Go-protein subunits. *J Neurosci* 2005, 25:3571–3577.
9. Poth K, Nutter T, Cuevas J, Parker M, Adams D, y Luetje C: Heterogeneity of nicotinic receptor class and subunit mRNA expression among individual parasympathetic neurons from rat intracardiac ganglia. *J Neurosci* 1997, 2:586–596.
10. Bibevski S, Zhou Y, McIntosh M, Zigmond R, y Dunlap M: Functional nicotinic acetylcholine receptors that mediate ganglionic transmission in cardiac parasympathetic neurons. *J Neurosci* 2000, 13:5076–5082.
11. Cuevas J, Berg D: Mammalian nicotinic receptor with alpha 7 subunits that slowly desensitize and rapidly recover from alpha-bungarotoxin blockade. *J Neurosci* 1998, 18:10335–10344.
12. Purnyn HE, Rikhalsky OV, Skok MV, Skok VI: Functional nicotinic acetylcholine receptors in the neurons of rat intracardiac ganglia. *Fiziol Zh* 2004, 50:79–84.
13. Peraza-Cruces K, Gutiérrez-Guédez L, Castañeda Perozo D, Lankford CR, Rodríguez-Bonfante C, Bonfante-Cabarcas R: Trypanosoma cruzi infection induces up-regulation of cardiac muscarinic acetylcholine receptors in vivo and in vitro. *Braz J Med Biol Res* 2008, 41:796–803.
14. Labrador-Hernández M, Suárez-Graterol O, Romero-Contreras U, Rumenoff L, Rodríguez-Bonfante C, Bonfante-Cabarcas R: The cholinergic system in cyclophosphamide-induced Chagas dilated myocardiopathy in Trypanosoma-cruzi-infected rats: an electrocardiographic study. *Invest Clin* 2008, 49:207–224.
15. Alkondon M, Albuquerque EX: Diversity of nicotinic acetylcholine receptors in rat hippocampal neurons. I. Pharmacological and functional evidence for distinct structural subtypes. *J Pharmacol Exp Ther* 1993, 265:1455–1473.
16. Haunstetter A, Haass M, Yi X, Krüger C, Kübler W: Muscarinic inhibition of cardiac norepinephrine and neuropeptide Y release during ischemia and reperfusion. *Am J Physiol* 1994, 267:R1552–R1558.
17. Dávila DF, Gottberg CF, Donis JH, Torres A, Fuenmayor AJ, Rossell O: Vagal stimulation and heart rate slowing in acute experimental chagasic myocarditis. *J Auton Nerv Syst* 1988, 25:233–234.
18. Cardinal R, Pagé P: Neuronal modulation of atrial and ventricular electrical properties. In *Basic and Clinical Neurocardiology*. Edited by Armour JA, Ardell JL. NY: Oxford University Press; 2004:315–399.
19. Ji S, Tosaka T, Whitfield BH, Katchman AN, Kandil A, Knollmann BC, Ebert SN: Differential rate responses to nicotine in rat heart: evidence for two classes of nicotinic receptors. *J Pharmacol Exp Ther* 2002, 301:893–899.
20. Li YF, Lacroix C, Freeling J: Cytisine induces autonomic cardiovascular responses via activations of different nicotinic receptors. *Auton Neurosci* 2010, 154:14–19.
21. Li YF, LaCroix C, Freeling J: Specific subtypes of nicotinic cholinergic receptors involved in sympathetic and parasympathetic cardiovascular responses. *Neurosci Lett* 2009, 462:20–23.
22. Chavez-Noriega LE, Crona JH, Washburn MS, Urrutia A, Elliott KJ, Johnson EC: Pharmacological characterization of recombinant human neuronal nicotinic acetylcholine receptors h alpha 2 beta 2, h alpha 2 beta 4, h alpha 3 beta 2, h alpha 3 beta 4, h alpha 4 beta 2, h alpha 4 beta 4 and h alpha 7 expressed in Xenopus oocytes. *J Pharmacol Exp Ther* 1997, 280:346–356.
23. Xiao Y, Kellar KJ: The comparative pharmacology and up-regulation of rat neuronal nicotinic receptor subtype binding sites stably expressed in transfected mammalian cells. *J Pharmacol Exp Ther* 2004, 310:98–107.
24. Parker MJ, Beck A, Luetje CW: Neuronal nicotinic receptor beta2 and beta4 subunits confer large differences in agonist binding affinity. *Mol Pharmacol* 1998, 54:1132–1139.
25. Klein HU, Ferrari GM: Vagus nerve stimulation: A new approach to reduce heart failure. *Cardiol J* 2010, 17:638–644.
26. LaCroix C, Freeling J, Giles A, Wess J, Li YF: Deficiency of M2 muscarinic acetylcholine receptors increases susceptibility of ventricular function to chronic adrenergic stress. *Am J Physiol Heart Circ Physiol* 2008, 294:H810–H820.
27. Castro RR, Porphirio G, Serra SM, Nóbrega AC: Cholinergic stimulation with pyridostigmine protects against exercise induced myocardial ischaemia. *Heart* 2004, 90:1119–1123.
28. Lara A, Damasceno DD, Pires R, Gros R, Gomes ER, Gavioli M, Lima RF, Guimarães D, Lima P, Bueno CR Jr, Vasconcelos A, Roman-Campos D, Menezes CA, Sirvente RA, Salemi VM, Mady C, Caron MG, Ferreira AJ, Brum PC, Resende RR, Cruz JS, Gomez MV, Prado VF, de Almeida AP, Prado MA, Guatimosim S: Dysautonomia due to reduced cholinergic neurotransmission causes cardiac remodeling and heart failure. *Mol Cell Biol* 2010, 30:1746–1756.
29. Koley J, Saha JK, Koley BN: Positive inotropic effect of nicotine on electrically evoked contraction of isolated toad ventricle. *Arch Int Pharmacodyn Ther* 1984, 267:269–278.

14

Allosteric transition: a comparison of two models

Niels Bindslev

Abstract

Introduction: Two recent models are in use for analysis of allosteric drug action at receptor sites remote from orthosteric binding sites. One is an allosteric two-state mechanical model derived in 2000 by David Hall. The other is an extended operational model developed in 2007 by Arthur Christopoulos's group. The models are valid in pharmacology, enzymology, transportology as well as several other fields of biology involving allosteric concentration effects.

Results: I show here that Hall's model for interactions between an orthoster, an alloster, and a receptive unit is the best choice of model both for simulation and analysis of allosteric concentration-responses at equilibrium or steady-state.

Conclusions: As detailed knowledge of receptors systems becomes available, systems with several pathways and states and/ or more than two binding sites should be analysed by extended forms of the Hall model rather than for instance a Hill type exponentiation of terms as introduced in non-mechanistic (operational) model approaches; yielding semi-quantitative estimates of actual system parameters based on Hill's unlikely simultaneity model for G protein-coupled receptors.

Background

A sizeable decline in development of classical agonists and antagonist for medication [1-3] has elicited a drug-hunt to construct and develop allosters in laboratories of academia [4-8] and industry (e.g., Novasite Pharmaceuticals Inc; Addex Pharmaceuticals), including positive and negative allosters as well as ortho-allosters for therapeutic purposes. In doing so, it has become important to simulate and analyse concentration-response data for allosters by models that are as close to the systems mechanistic function as possible.

Optimal allosteric models are in great demand, since mechanistic simulations may be combined with structural analysis of alloster binding, receptor multi-merization and association of molecules as G proteins, arrestins, and RAMPs into synthesis of QSARs for ligand binding and receptor activation [9-16].

Data from equilibrium concentration-response experiments involving allosteric modulators are presently interpreted by unlike choices of model. Therefore, with such schism in selection of model, especially true for data from cell-systems expressing subtype 7TMRs [17], it seems worth a discussion about which direction analysis of synagics data for allosters should take. For possible outcomes of including allosters consult Figure 1. For definitions of terms related to allostery see Table 1.

Two actual allosteric models - ATSM and EXOM. One model is the allosteric two-state model, ATSM, introduced by Hall in 2000, implemented and further discussed by others [5,17-25]. Another model we could call the "extended operational model", EXOM for short [26], is based on combining the original operational model, BLM [27], with the ternary-complex model, TCM [28], as later further detailed [29-31]. EXOM is implemented and presently advocated by several lead-modellers [7,8,32-38]. There are other approaches taken to model the behaviour of allosters in the field of 7TMRs [20,33,39-42].

ATSM is a mechanistic model. ATSM-analysis with extracted numbers for model parameters supposes direct information about mechanical interactions between allosters, receptors and orthosters at a molecular scale. Thus, one might gain a quantitative and dynamic handle on molecular processes *per se* within receptors. The other model, EXOM, a non-mechanistic model, is a close relative of ATSM and has the same number of independent parameters to be determined. EXOM is used assuming that individual physical parameters of multi-step processes as such cannot be extracted, as they are composite. EXOM may give quantified estimates on

Correspondence: bindslev@sund.ku.dk
Synagics Lab, Endocrinology Section, Department of Biomedical Sciences, The Medical Faculty, Panum Building, University of Copenhagen, Blegdamsvej 3, DK-2200, Copenhagen N, Denmark

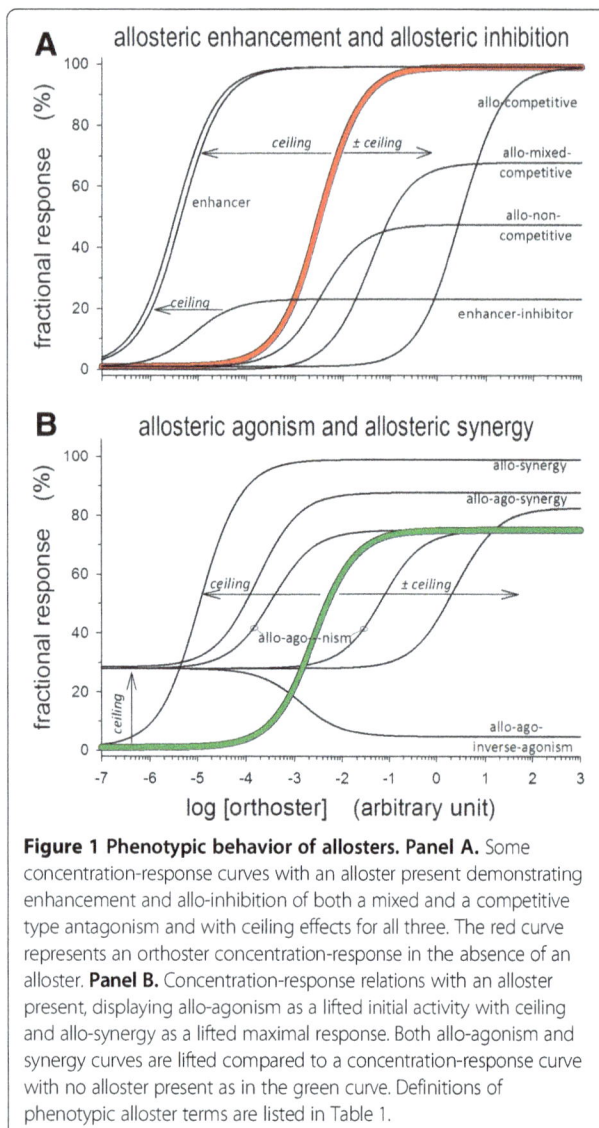

Figure 1 Phenotypic behavior of allosters. Panel A. Some concentration-response curves with an alloster present demonstrating enhancement and allo-inhibition of both a mixed and a competitive type antagonism and with ceiling effects for all three. The red curve represents an orthoster concentration-response in the absence of an alloster. **Panel B.** Concentration-response relations with an alloster present, displaying allo-agonism as a lifted initial activity with ceiling and allo-synergy as a lifted maximal response. Both allo-agonism and synergy curves are lifted compared to a concentration-response curve with no alloster present as in the green curve. Definitions of phenotypic alloster terms are listed in Table 1.

Table 1 Terms and definitions for allosteric synagics (see Figure 1)

Term	Definition
orthoster	primary ligand, binds at orthosteric (primary) receptor binding site and covers ligands as agonists, inverse agonists and (neutral) antagonists
alloster or allosteric modulator	secondary ligand, binds to a non-overlapping (secondary or allosteric) binding site distinct from an orthosteric binding site
ago-alloster	an alloster which can activate the receptor even in the absence of an orthoster, but with ceiling for the increased activity
allo-agonism	the effect of an ago-alloster
syn-alloster	alloster, at high orthoster concentrations it can still lift the response further with ceiling;
allo-synergy or synergy	the effect of syn-allosters, different from super-agonism
ago-syn-alloster	alloster, both activates receptors in absence of orthoster and increases activity even at high orthoster concentration. Both increases in activity have ceiling
allo-ago-synergy	the effect of ago-syn-allosters, different from super-agonism
enhancer	alloster, moves orthoster d-r curves to the left with ceiling
allo-competitor	alloster, moves orthoster d-r curves right with or without ceiling
allo-mixed-competitor	alloster, decreases activity and changes apparent affinity constants for orthosters. Orthoster d-r curves with allo-mixed-competitor are right-shifted but may have increased affinity
enhancer-inhibitor	alloster that both increases apparent affinity constants and decreases activity for orthosters. With enhancer-inhibitor, orthoster d-r curves move left with ceiling
ago-inverse-alloster	alloster, stimulates activity from an allosteric site in its own right, but with an activity which is reduced with increasing orthoster concentrations
ortho-alloster or bitopic ligand	compound with moieties for simultaneous binding and activation at both orthosteric and allosteric receptor binding sites
synagics	the study of equilibrium and steady-state concentration-responses of ligand interactions with receptive units such as protein macromolecules
positive and negative allosteric modulators	(PAMs* and NAMs**) - ligands that increase or decrease receptor activity directly or indirectly from an allosteric binding site.

*PAMs cover both ago-allosters, syn-allosters, and ago-syn-allosters. Enhancers may be included here. ** NAMs cover both allo-mixed-competitors, enhancer-inhibitors, and ago-inverse-allosters. Allo-competitors may be included here.

elicited cooperative binding and efficacy for orthosters and allosters interacting at receptors [26,34]. By selecting similar assumptions for ATSM as for EXOM, ATSM may cover the EXOM-scenario and yield estimates of parameters for lumped multi-steps rather than single steps, and thus become a black-box model as the EXOM.

In both ATSM and EXOM, allosters may behave as enhancers with ceiling and as competitive antagonists without ceiling. Furthermore, they are also efficient in simulating allo-agonism and allo-synergy both with ceiling effects; observed as lifts of concentration-response curves by allosters at low and high orthoster concentrations [17,26,37]. However, EXOM lacks ATSM's advantage of being a mechanistic model and for describing spontaneous activity of receptive units. Additionally, from a theoretical point of view, a parameter in EXOM to describe cooperative activity is amputated, yielding

illogic results. For this latter conclusion, see details in the next to last sections of Methods and Results and Discussion.

Here I focus on ATSM and EXOM and compare them for simulation and analysis of experimental data. It is demonstrated that there are no arguments as posited [8,17] for employing EXOM instead of ATSM, quite the other way about. Therefore, my goal is to convince future modellers to use ATSM and possible extended forms for analysis and simulation of allosteric concentration-response relations rather than EXOM.

Methods

One basic model - cTSM

In simulation of synagics for orthosters and allosters, the basis of most models is often two simple reaction schemes; the cyclic-two-state model, cTSM, and the ternary-complex model, TCM. Since this paper is about modelling as opposed to general statements about ligand-receptor interactions it is paramount with precise definitions including aspects of cTSM and TCM. This has been discussed before [22] and may seem superfluous. However, in order to validate and compare newly derived ATSM and EXOM in a coherent fashion, concepts related to cTSM and TCM must be brought together and systematized. cTSM is dealt with first.

The gist of the cTSM, Figure 2A, is its explicit description of a conformational switch between an inactive and active state of a non-bound receptor. It specifically includes spontaneous activity in form of non-liganded receptor R*. The behaviour of cTSM has been scrutinized [43,44]. cTSM has two interesting parameters. L describes the distribution between unliganded inactive and active receptor states, R $\rightleftharpoons$ R*, such that $L = $ R*/R, Figure 2A. Deriving cTSM's distribution equation for activity, the free non-active receptor state R is equated with "1". Thus, the unliganded, active receptor state R* is equal to L. The second parameter, a, is a concomitant

constant for activation of receptor forms bound with ligand S, RS $\rightleftharpoons$ R*S. This step has $a \cdot L$ as its efficacy constant. By assuming multi-steps, $a \cdot L$ is identical to Stephenson's efficacy constant [45] and Black & Leff's transducer ratio τ [27]. A_s is the equilibrium affinity constant for S binding to non-active forms of R, Figure 2A. Therefore, a is also a concomitant constant for binding of S to already activated receptors. The affinity constant for S+R* $\rightleftharpoons$ R*S is thus $a \cdot A_s$.

Arguments still appear on how to understand activation of protein molecules when ligands are applied - is it by *induction* after ligands bind or is it rather by ligand *selection* and stabilization of already activated molecules? Jacques Monod early on favoured a selection process [46] and this understanding crystallized in the famous MWC-model [47]. The MWC explicitly introduces an unliganded switch R$\rightleftharpoons$R* as the "allosteric transition" [48]. Contrary, Koshland argued for induction after binding [49]. "Selection" follows one leg of cTSM while "induction" follows another [50], Figure 2A. They are two views on a single process [18] chapter 5. Below, when either "induction" or "selection" is used on activation of receptive units as ligands bind, it covers both pathways in cTSM.

Another basic model - TCM

The TCM, Figure 2B, looks fairly simple, but possesses surprising allosteric regimes. Depending on which of the liganded complexes are included for activity, TCM can simulate enhancement with ceiling and competitive ("surmountable") inhibition, besides allo-agonism without ceiling and "mixed competitive inhibition". TCM

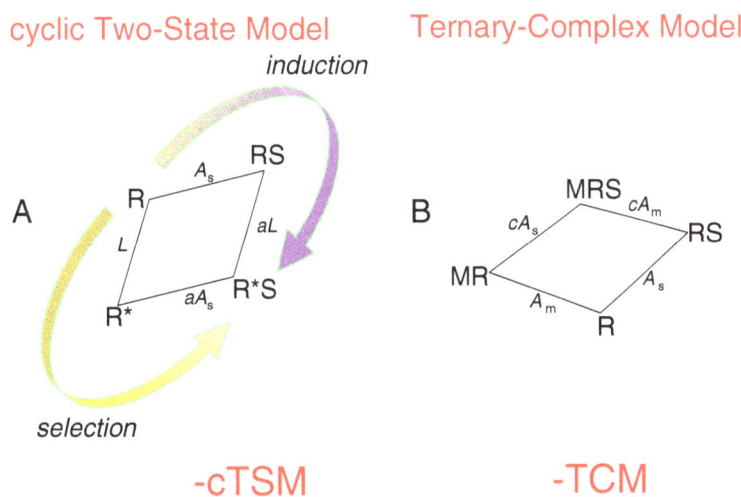

Figure 2 Two simple reaction schemes. **Panel A.** The cyclic two-state model, cTSM, with selection and induction arrows indicating two separate but simultaneous pathways from an inactive and non-liganded receptor conformation R to an active and agonist S liganded receptor conformation R*S. A_s is an equilibrium association constant for S, L is a conformational efficacy constant for non-bound receptors, and parameter a is an efficacy constant for ligand bound receptor conformations from RS to R*S. **Panel B.** The ternary-complex model, TCM, in which symbol M represents the term and concentration for an additional alloster ligand. A_m is an equilibrium association constant for M, and parameter c is a cooperativity coefficient for two-ligand binding.

with tacit active conformations has no allo-synergy or spontaneous activity. Ten sub-models derived from TCM are characterized in Table 2. Three of these sub-models are further described in the Results section and some simulations by these three models are shown in a figure in the Results section.

Operational models

To understand the present use of "stimulus", "efficacy" and "intrinsic efficacy" in operational models as EXOM, it is necessary to go back to their definitions [45,51,52]. Stephenson's stimulus concept seems obsolete today by accepting two-step receptor schemes with straightforward derived distribution equations [18] chapter 2; [50] and when needed, apt assumptions of more than two steps. Two-step schemes yield equations identical to initially derived operational models based on the stimulus-response idea [27,51,53]. Concepts as "stimulus", "transducer ratio" and "fitting parameter" are of course justified in selecting operational model approaches rather than mechanistic ones. Spontaneous activity often seen in studies with 7TMRs is not included in the realm of operational models, although recently serious attempts have appeared [54,55].

Meanwhile, users of operational models should recognize that their assumptions for derivation put a veil over underlying physical systems and that any involved "operational" assumption may just as well be applied to the ATSM. For instance, as mentioned, $a \cdot L$ can be conceived as equal to transducer ratio τ.

Distribution equation for ATSM and EXOM

Reaction schemes of ATSM and EXOM are depicted in Figure 3A and 3B. The intention with EXOM was to derive a stimulus-equation for activating receptors, including alloster-activated units, while explicitly excluding non-liganded active conformations [26]. Thus, three bound species RS, MR, and MRS in EXOM can switch to active forms R*S, MR*, and MR*S. But, in order to exclude constitutive activity, non-liganded R is not allowed a switch to active R*, Figure 3B. Thus, EXOM is a pure "induction" reaction scheme in Koshland-sense, as free forms of receptor R must be bound before activation. The three bound and active forms of the receptor are equated as "stimulus" and transformed through a hyperbolic expression for activity, as for the BLM. The result is a distribution equation with three active conformations to a total of seven conformation, as even a possible inactive R*-conformation is considered non-existent [26].

To simplify a comparison of EXOM with ATSM, distribution equations for both are expressed parallel to earlier expressions for ATSM [18] chapter 7.

Table 2 Phenotypic concentration-responses for allosters in 10 sub-models from TCM

Type of TCM model	#	Enhancement ←	w/ ceiling ←	Allo-agonism ↑	w/ ceiling ↑	Strict allo-synergy ↑	Allo-modification w/ ceiling → ↓
(S)/4	1	no	na	no	na	no	modifier - EC_{50} ↓
(S+MS)/4	2	yes	yes	no	na	no	competitive
(S+M+MS)/4	3	yes	yes	yes	no	no	na
(S+M)/4	4	no	na	inverse	yes	no	yes
(MS)/4	5	(yes)	yes	no	na	(yes)	na
(S)/3	6	no	na	no	na	no	modifier - EC_{50} ↓
(S+MS)/3	7	yes	→	no	na	no	no
(MS)/3	8	(yes)	no	no	na	(yes)	no
(S)/3*	9	no	na	no	na	no	competitive**
(S+M)/3*	10	no	na	yes	no	no	no

For model types in the left column, terms S, M, and MS in parenthesis indicate active forms of the liganded receptor as either R*S, M*R or MR*S, and with the total number of receptor conformations after the slash. In models 6–8, complex MR is not formed. Model 7 is the classical uncompetitive reaction scheme. * In models 9–10, complex MRS is not formed. **Model 9 is classical type II reaction scheme for competitive inhibition with no ceiling, the same as assuming parameter $c = 0$. Arrows indicate direction of affinity change and direction of ceiling effects.

na = not applicable, (yes) indicates that there is an effect in form of co-agonism, i.e., no response for ligand S alone.

Simulations of concentration-response relations for tabulated sub-models 1–4, in column 2, are shown in Figure 4 panels A-I. S stands for orthoster and M for alloster. Ceiling effects for enhancement (= parameter $c > 1$) in sub-model 2 starts at $A_m \cdot M > 1$, panel D in Figure 4. Allo-competitive antagonism (= parameter $c < 1$) in sub-model 2 requires $c \cdot A_m \cdot M > 10$ for a ceiling effect to appear. Thus, sub-model 2 simulates genuine competitive antagonism as long as the product $c \cdot A_m \cdot M$ is below 10, Figure 4 panel F. This dependence on product $A_m \cdot M > 1$ for ceiling effects of enhancement and on product $c \cdot A_m \cdot M > 10$ for ceiling effects in allo-competitive inhibition are also characteristics of both ATSM, Figure 5 panels A and C, and EXOM, Figure 5 panels D and F.

Tabulated ternary-complex sub-model 1 and 6 with parameter $c < 1$ are characterized as (mixed) modifier mechanisms in enzymology. Their mixed allo-modification includes a possible simulation of classical non-competitive antagonism with a fixed EC_{50}, when $c = 1$, Figure 4 panel B. Furthermore, both sub-models 1 and 6 have increasing affinity for increasing modifier concentration, indicated by EC_{50} ↓ in column 8. Sub-type model 4, excluding the ternary complex MRS as active, may show inverse agonism with decreasing ceiling values for the apparent affinity EC_{50} when parameter $c > 1$ and increasing ceiling levels for EC_{50} when parameter $c < 1$, Figure 4 panels J-L.

Sub-models 5 and 8 demonstrate co-agonism, which means that both ligand S and ligand M have to be present for an activity to show up, simulations not shown. Sub-model 7 is identical to the classical un-competitive reaction scheme. Sub-models 9 and 10 are based on the classical type II competitive reaction scheme, excluding the double-liganded MRS conformation ([18] chapter 2), and therefore do not qualify as true TCMs.

Two characteristics for ATSM and EXOM are not covered by any of the listed TCM reaction schemes in Table 2, viz. a strict allo-synergy, Figure 5 panels M and N, and ceiling effects for allo-agonism, compare Figure 4 panels G-I with Figure 5 panels G-H, J-K, M-N, Q-R, and T-U.

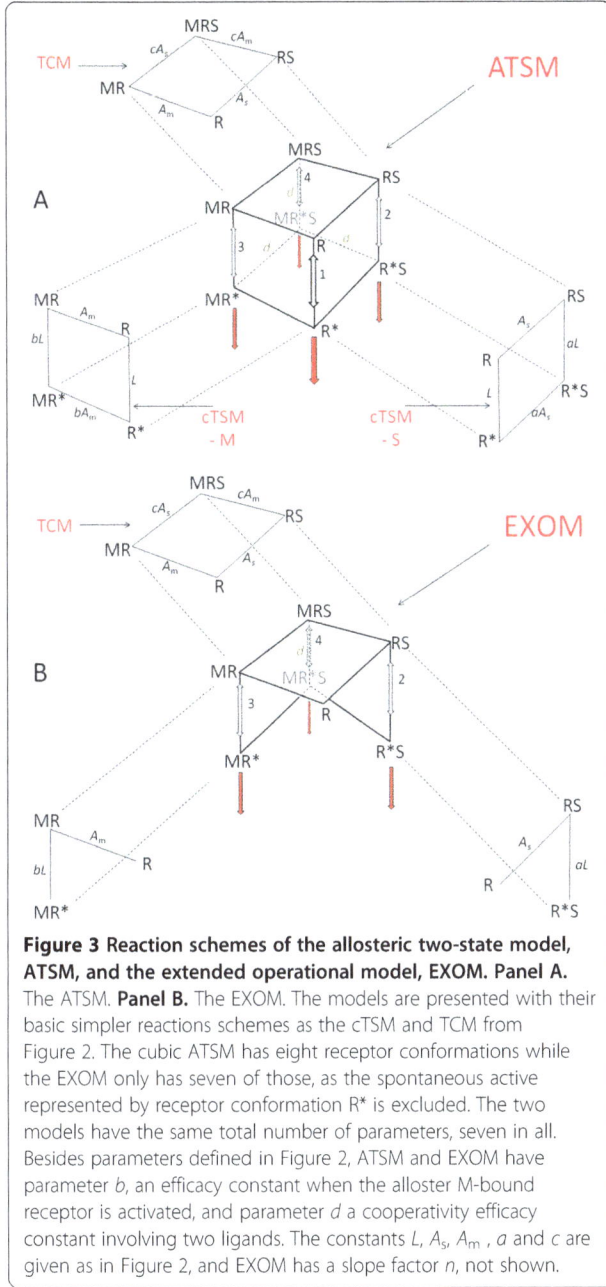

Figure 3 Reaction schemes of the allosteric two-state model, ATSM, and the extended operational model, EXOM. **Panel A.** The ATSM. **Panel B.** The EXOM. The models are presented with their basic simpler reactions schemes as the cTSM and TCM from Figure 2. The cubic ATSM has eight receptor conformations while the EXOM only has seven of those, as the spontaneous active represented by receptor conformation R* is excluded. The two models have the same total number of parameters, seven in all. Besides parameters defined in Figure 2, ATSM and EXOM have parameter b, an efficacy constant when the alloster M-bound receptor is activated, and parameter d a cooperativity efficacy constant involving two ligands. The constants L, A_s, A_m, a and c are given as in Figure 2, and EXOM has a slope factor n, not shown.

and for activity in ATSM:

Deviations between the two models are marked by bracketed and bolded symbols. Definitions of symbols listed below are followed by symbols in parenthesis from Leach [26] and Hall [22]: E = actual response; E_m = maximal activity; S = orthoster (A; A); M = alloster (B; B); A_s = equilibrium association constant for ligand S ($1/K_A$, K); A_m = equilibrium association constant for ligand M ($1/K_B$, M); a = efficacy constant for S (τ_A; α); b = efficacy constant for M (τ_B; β); c = binding cooperativity constant (α; γ); and d = activation cooperativity constant (β; δ). Parameter β for EXOM is only defined for cooperativity of an alloster on orthoster activation, but not reciprocally as in ATSM. Further, unlike ATSM, EXOM has a Hill type exponentiation parameter, n, for terms of summed activity and inactivity. The benefits of including such a Hill exponentiation may be questioned as discussed earlier [18] chapter 10. Indeed, Hill-type exponentiation may also be applied to ATSM. However, as ATSM is a mechanistic approach, it seems more logical to derive equations based on formulation for an extended ATSM with more than two binding sites [18,25].

In absence of an orthoster the initial efficacy, IntEff, for ATSM is given by: $L/[L+(1+ A_m \cdot M)/ (1+b \cdot A_m \cdot M)]$, and for EXOM, assuming $n = 1$, by: $1/[1+(1+A_m \cdot M)/ (1+b \cdot A_m \cdot M)]$.

For high values of the orthoster, $S \Rightarrow \infty$, maximum activity, MaxEff, as a function of alloster concentration for ATSM is given by: $L/[L + (1 + c \cdot A_m \cdot M)/(a \cdot (1 + \boldsymbol{b} \cdot c \cdot d \cdot A_m \cdot M))]$, and for EXOM, assuming $n = 1$, by: $1/[1 + (1 + c \cdot A_m \cdot M)/ (a \cdot (1 + c \cdot d \cdot A_m \cdot M))]$. Differences between ATSM and EXOM expressions are indicated with bolded types.

Best-fit analyses to experimental data for ATSM and EXOM
The analyses were performed in the following manner. Selected allosteric effects were obtained from data-figures in the literature, data-figure 1 ([38], Figure 2B), data-figure 2 ([37], Figure 2B), and data-figure 3 ([56], Figure 3). Model parameters a and A_s were first evaluated by fitting the distribution equations for ATSM and

$$E = \frac{E_m \cdot [a \cdot A_s \cdot S + b \cdot A_m \cdot M + a \cdot c \cdot d \cdot A_s \cdot S \cdot A_m \cdot M]^{(n)}}{[1 + A_s \cdot S + A_m \cdot M + c \cdot A_s \cdot S \cdot A_m \cdot M]^{(n)} + [a \cdot A_s \cdot S + b \cdot A_m \cdot M + a \cdot c \cdot d \cdot A_s \cdot S \cdot A_m \cdot M]^{(n)}}$$

This yields for activity in EXOM:

$$E = \frac{E_m \cdot (\boldsymbol{L} \cdot)[(1+)a \cdot A_s \cdot S + b \cdot A_m \cdot M + a \cdot (\boldsymbol{b} \cdot)c \cdot d \cdot A_s \cdot S \cdot A_m \cdot M]}{1 + A_s \cdot S + A_m \cdot M + c \cdot A_s \cdot S \cdot A_m \cdot M + (\boldsymbol{L} \cdot)[(1+)a \cdot A_s \cdot S + b \cdot A_m \cdot M + a \cdot (\boldsymbol{b} \cdot)c \cdot d \cdot A_s \cdot S \cdot A_m \cdot M]}$$

EXOM to response data at zero alloster concentration. The obtained values for a and A_s were then inserted into the distribution functions for the two models and used for an ensuing fitting of the remaining parameters listed in the last Table, parameters b, c, d, and A_m. By varying the initial values for each parameter in three steps, at least 12 fits were performed on each curve for every alloster concentration in all three data-figures. Only fitted parameter values with convergence to a tolerance of 10^{-10} in SigmaPlot software were accepted.

Thus, concentration-response curves at three different alloster concentrations yields three best-fit values for each of the four parameters. Obtained results for the single parameter in the last Table represent a ratio between the two best-fit values with the largest mutual difference of the three determinations for each parameter at different alloster concentrations. A global fit to data sets for all four parameters [57] was not possible.

A fourth data set, data-figure 4 ([36], Figure 1C), was also analysed but neither ATSM nor EXOM fitted well to these data with a 44% spontaneous activity and a 56% alloster/ orthoster response. The failure of fitting was mostly due to a lack in obtaining a reasonable determination of maximal response for several of the concentration-response curves.

Results and discussion
TCM - three and ten variants
Three functional variants of TCM are briefly described below and examples of their simulations shown in Figure 4, while characteristics of ten different forms derived from TCM are listed in annotated Table 2.

In a first form, complex RS tacitly moves to R*S as the sole source of activity. Simulation of this allo-scheme can resemble classical non-competitive antagonism for orthosters in functional assays, where only the maximal effect attenuates as the concentration of an alloster increases while the dissociation constant for the agonist stays constant. This happens for activity when constant c is unity. An example is shown in Figure 4B. Note, that in TCM occupancy, alloster effects can never be non-competitive-like, i.e., with reduced activity and fixed EC_{50}.

In a second form, S-liganded conformations, RS and MRS, move tacitly to R*S and MR*S as source of activity. This reaction scheme gives us models of activity and occupancy that behave in an identical manner as their distribution equations are identical. This reaction scheme includes enhancement for constant $c > 1$ and with ceiling when $A_m \cdot M > 1$ and competitive inhibition when $c < 1$, but with a ceiling effects for both binding and activation by an alloster when $c \cdot A_m \cdot M > 10$, Figure 4D and 4F. This model is identical to the uncompetitive reaction scheme.

In a third form, all liganded conformations, i.e., RS, MR, and MRS, are sources of activity, Figure 2B. In

EXOM, this is the basic TCM. TCM sub-type 3 may simulate allo-agonism for activity, but without ceiling effects as indicated by black circles for limiting EC_{50} values as M → ∞, Figure 4G-I.

Since the term "competitive inhibition", according to an informative review [48], meant inhibition through an overlap or steric hindrance at binding sites [58], the term "allosteric inhibition" was used from the start of the 1960s merely to indicate negative feedback different from competitive inhibition. Nothing more. TCM with its two remote binding sites has no mutual exclusion by steric hindrance or by overlap. Meanwhile, TCM may still simulate "competitive inhibition", either by its un-competitive form as shown in Figure 3F, or by mutual exclusion of triple complex MRS through remote or inter-molecular conformational changes, not shown. Thus, TCM has allosteric inhibition in the MWC-sense. "Competitive inhibition" by mutual exclusion in TCM requires that the cooperative binding constant c goes to insignificantly small values, thus preventing detectable levels of MRS and of its tacitly active form, MR*S. Such allosteric mutual exclusion, as one type II competitive inhibition ([18], chapter 2) has been cartooned ([58], Figure III-1, panel 5). Thus, as "allosteric" solely refer to ligand binding at remote, non-overlapping binding sites and without steric hindrance, "allosteric" becomes a pleonasm in "allosteric ternary complex model", ATCM, as TCM is defined by having two, non-overlapping binding sites without steric hindrance. As both acronyms cover the exact same model, it remains a matter of taste using either ATCM or TCM. Contrary, the signifier "allosteric" in "allosteric transition" [48] becomes indicative for two-state models as MWC and ATSM, involving cTSM.

Comparison of simulations from ATSM and EXOM
A comparison is made between ATSM and EXOM simulations of concentration-responses of activity with orthoster concentration as independent variable and with varying alloster concentration M. Thus, the following are principal statements about parameter influences on initial and maximal efficacies, on ceiling effects for enhancement, competitive and mixed inhibition, on allo-agonism and -synergy, as well as on apparent dissociation constant EC_{50}. To simplify the comparison, EXOM slope factor n is assumed unity. The results reveal a few crucial differences between the two models even based on homologous parameters as A_s, A_m, a, c, and d.

As indicated above, IntEff for EXOM is dependent on parameter b, while for ATSM it is dependent on both b and L. For ATSM, MaxEff is dependent on $L \cdot a$, whilst EXOM-MaxEff is only dependent on a. Thus, when comparing ATSM and EXOM, choice of values for a and b in EXOM should match with values for $L \cdot a$ and $L \cdot b$ in ATSM. Accordingly, in selection of parameter

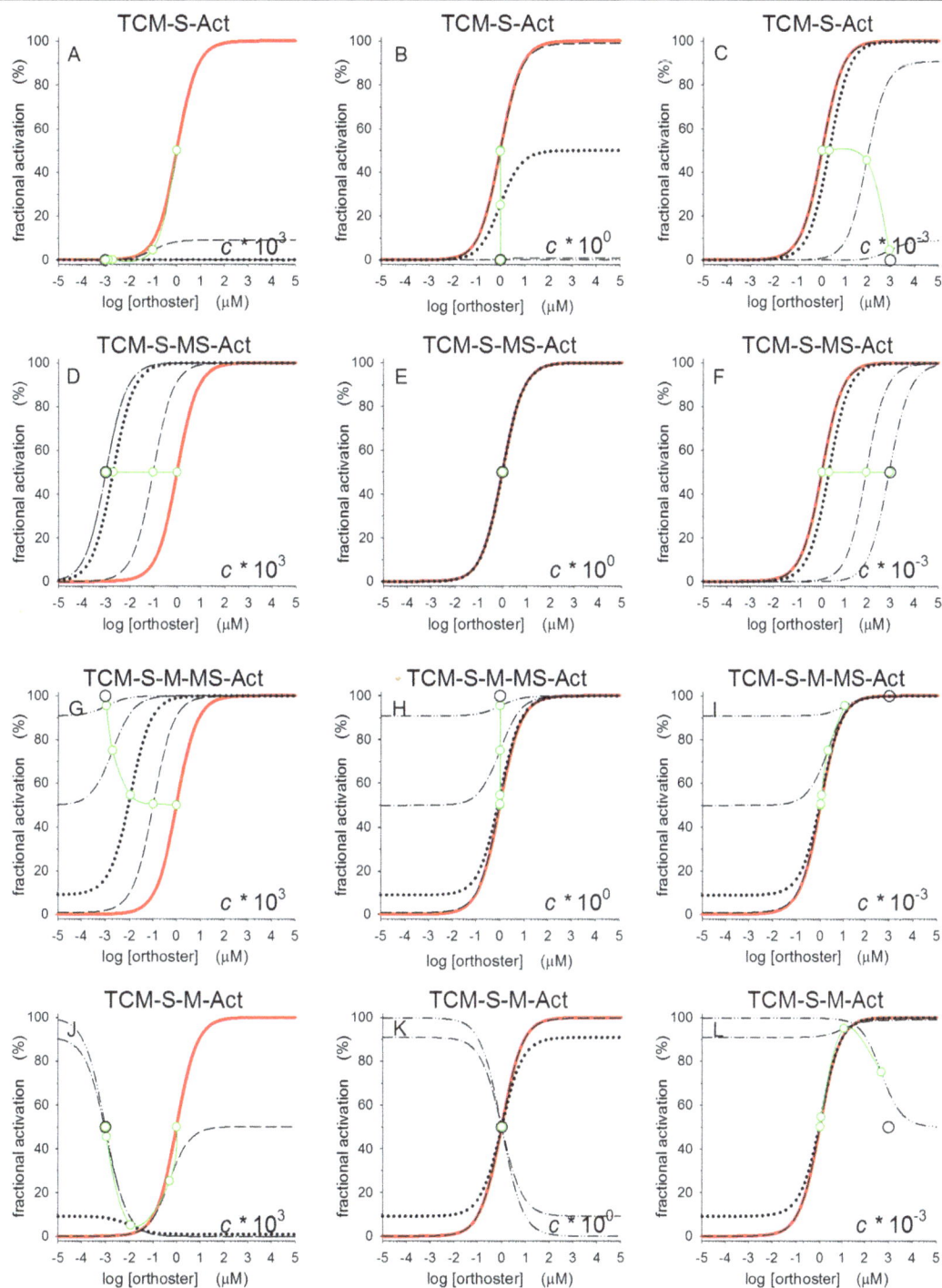

Figure 4 Simulations from four sub-models of the ternary-complex model, TCM. For sub-model definitions see Table 2. Parameters A_s and A_m, equilibrium association constants for ligands S and M, are kept at unity. Parameter c, the cooperativity constant for binding, is varied by a factor 10^3 in three steps for each sub-model as indicated in the panels. Red curves indicate orthoster concentration-response curves in the absence of an alloster. In all panels the alloster M concentration is varied in four steps: in panels A-I by a factor 10^2 from 1×10^{-2} to 1×10^4; in panels G-K by a factor 10 from 1×10^{-2} to 1×10^1 and in panel L by a factor 10^2 from 1×10^{-3} to 1×10^3. Green curves with circles show the actual EC_{50} and the black circle represents the position of a limiting EC_{50} for M $\rightarrow \infty$.

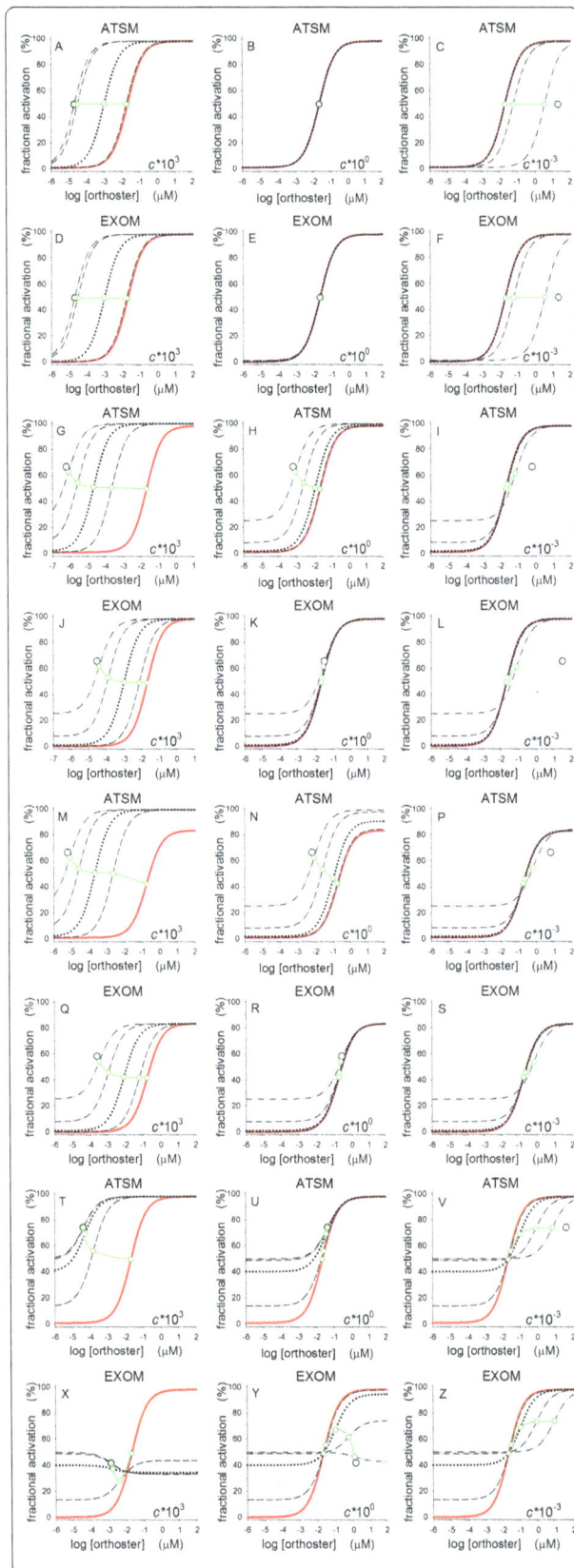

Figure 5 Simulations of concentration-response relations for **ATSM and EXOM.** The parameters A_s and A_m are both kept at unity, while parameter L is 10^{-2} for all ATSM simulations in order to keep spontaneous activity insignificant and n for all EXOM simulations is = 1. Parameter c, the binding cooperativity constant, is varied in three steps by multiplying with a factor 10^3 from 10^{-3} to 10^3 as indicated in the panels. Parameter a is 5000 in all ATSM panels except for panels M-P where it is 500. For EXOM, parameter a is 50 in all panels except for panels Q-S where it is 5. For ATSM, parameter b is 1 in panels A-C, and 50 in the rest of panels G-V. For EXOM, parameter b is 0.01 in panels D-F, and 0.5 in the rest of panels J-Z. Parameter d is 1 in all panels except in panels T-Z where it is 3×10^{-3}. All red curves have no alloster present, i.e., concentration of M = 0. M is varied in four steps. In panels A-F by a factor 100 from 2×10^{-4} to 2×10^2; in panels G-S by a factor 10 from 2×10^{-3} to 2×10^0; and in panels T-Z by a factor 10 from 2×10^{-1} to 2×10^2. Green curves with circles show the actual EC_{50} and the black circle represents the position of a limiting EC_{50} for M $\to \infty$. The black circle falls outside the orthoster concentration range, 10^{-6} to 10^2, in panels S and Z with limiting EC_{50} values of 250 and 1304.

values for compared simulations with L for ATSM chosen as 0.01 in order to suppress spontaneous activity, values for a and b in EXOM are chosen 100 fold higher in ATSM, Figure 5.

IntEffs for both ATSM and EXOM are always completely independent of A_s, a, c, and d. ATSM-IntEff is dependent on L and $b \cdot A_m \cdot M$. For more details see annotated Table 3. EXOM-IntEff only depends on $b \cdot A_m \cdot M$. Allo-agonism is a lift in the IntEff when supplying an alloster even before an orthoster is added. Various forms of allo-agonism are shown in Figure 5G-Z and with ceiling effects indicated by black circles for the limiting EC_{50} values as M $\to \infty$. Allo-agonism is often seen in studies with small molecule allosters [59]. Allo-agonism takes effect in both models when both b and $b \cdot A_m \cdot M$ are larger than unity. Furthermore, ATSM may simulate spontaneous activity before any ligand is added. Simulation of detectable spontaneous activity starts at values of L above 10^{-2}. This possibility is excluded from the EXOM theory.

MaxEff in ATSM is dependent on $L \cdot a$ and $b \cdot c \cdot d \cdot A_m \cdot M$, Table 3, while MaxEff in EXOM is dependent on a and $c \cdot d \cdot A_m \cdot M$. In comparison, EXOM-MaxEff demonstrates complete independence of b, which is somewhat inconsistent. The independence is due to the definition of parameter d (β) in EXOM, where an alloster only affects the efficacy of an orthoster with no reciprocity. Thus, synergy and mixed inhibition are different between ATSM and EXOM, since the MaxEff-ATSM has both parameter b and d involved while EXOM only depends on d.

As already indicated, more details on parameter influences on IntEff, enhancement, allo-agonism, allo-synergy, MaxEff, and mixed inhibition are given in comments to Table 3.

Table 3 Conditions for alloster effects on initial efficacy and maximal efficacy in ATSM

Assumptions for product parameters ·[M]	Reduced equation	Lower level product assumptions	Reduced equation at lower level product assumptions	IntEff / MaxEff, their dependence on product of
possible allo-agonism of **IntEff** for [orthoster] → 0: $L/[L+((1+A_m·M)/(1+b·A_m·M))]$				
$b·A_m·M \gg 1$	$L·b·A_m·M = X$ $X/(X+1+A_m·M)$	$A_m·M \gg 1$	$L·b/(L·b+1)$	$L·b$ vs 1
		$A_m·M = 1$	$L·b/(L·b+2)$	$L·b$ vs 2
		$A_m·M \ll 1$	$L·b/(L·b+1)$	$L·b$ vs 1
$b·A_m·M = 1$	$L·2/(L·2+1+A_m·M)$	$A_m·M \gg 1$	$L·2/(L·2+A_m·M)$	$L·2$ vs $A_m·M$
		$A_m·M = 1$	$L/(L+1)$	L vs 1
		$A_m·M \ll 1$	$L·2/(L·2+1)$	$L·2$ vs 1
$b·A_m·M \ll 1$	$L/(L+1+A_m·M)$	$A_m·M \gg 1$	$L/(L+A_m·M)$	L vs $A_m·M$
		$A_m·M = 1$	$L/(L+2)$	L vs 2
		$A_m·M \ll 1$	$L/(L+1)$	L vs 1
possible allo-synergy of **MaxEff** for [orthoster] →∞ : $L·a/[L·a+((1+c·A_m·M)/(1+b·c·d·A_m·M))]$				
$b·c·d·A_m·M \gg 1$	with $L·a·b·c·d·A_m·M =Y$ $Y/(Y+1+c·A_m·M)$	$c·A_m·M \gg 1$	$L·a·b·d/(L·a·b·d+1)$	$L·a·b·d$ vs 1
		$c·A_m·M = 1$	$L·a·b·d/(L·a·b·d+2)$	$L·a·b·d$ vs 2 $b·d \gg 1$
		$c·A_m·M \ll 1$	$Y/(Y+1)$	Y vs 1 $b·d \ggg 1$
$b·c·d·A_m·M = 1$	with $L·a·2 = Z$ $Z/(Z+1+c·A_m·M)$	$c·A_m·M \gg 1$	$Z/(Z+c·A_m·M)$	Z vs $c·A_m·M$
		$c·A_m·M = 1$	$L·a/(L·a+1)$	$L·a$ vs 1 $b·d = 1$
		$c·A_m·M \ll 1$	$L·a·2/(L·a·2+1)$	$L·a·2$ vs 1
$b·c·d·A_m·M \ll 1$	$L·a/(L·a+1+c·A_m·M)$	$c·A_m·M \gg 1$	$L·a/(L·a+c·A_m·M)$	$L·a$ vs $c·A_m·M$
		$c·A_m·M = 1$	$L·a/(L·a+2)$	$L·a$ vs 2 $b·d \gg 1$
		$c·A_m·M \ll 1$	$L·a/(L·a+1)$	$L·a$ vs 1

Initial and maximal response for ATSM with orthoster concentration as independent variable with an interfering alloster. M or [M] stands for alloster concentration. Conditions are listed with decreasing number of parameters from column 1 to 5 for products of M and parameters that affect the initial efficacy, IntEff, at very low concentrations of orthoster, S, and the final maximal efficacy, MaxEff, at very high concentrations of S.

All conclusions for IntEff and MaxEff of ATSM are similar for the EXOM with the following exceptions: for EXOM 1) parameter L is replaced with 1in all statements for ATSM and 2) parameter b disappears out of all MaxEff statements as listed for ATSM.

Below are further details about effects of parameters and alloster concentration on IntEff and MaxEff for ATSM and EXOM.

Initial efficacy. **IntEff** for ATSM or spontaneous activity:

For $b = 1$, IntEff = $L/(L+1)$ and independent of the value of $A_m·M$.

For $b > 1$, IntEff > $L/(L+1)$. With increasing values of $A_m·M$ above 1 the IntEff increases towards a ceiling value of $L·b/(L·b+1)$, equal allo-agonism. For decreasing values of $A_m·M$ below 1, the IntEff goes towards $L/(L+1)$.

For $b < 1$, IntEff < $L/(L+1)$. With increasing values of $A_m·M$ above 1 the IntEff reduces towards a ceiling value of $L·b/(L·b+1)$. For decreasing values of $A_m·M$ below 1, the IntEff increases towards $L/(L+1)$.

Allo-agonism above spontaneous activity in ATSM, $L/(L+1)$, is given by $L·b/[L·b+1+1/(A_m·M)]$, when both $b·A_m·M \gg 1$ and also parameter $b > 1$. The ceiling value of this allo-agonism is $L·b/(L·b+\#)$, where # is a value between 1 or 2, depending on the value of $A_m·M$.

IntEff for EXOM:

Allo-agonism in EXOM is always given by $b/[b+1+1/(A_m·M)]$, and going towards zero for $b → 0$, independent of the value for $b·A_m·M$, and with a ceiling level of $b/[b+¤]$, where ¤ is a value between 1 or 2, depending on the value of $A_m·M$. Examples of ceiling effects and their absence in ATSM and EXOM are shown in Figure 5. For $1/(A_m·M) \gg b+1$ in EXOM, IntEff goes towards 0 if $b < 1$, while for $1/(A_m·M) \ll b+1$, IntEff approaches $b/(b+1)$ as its ceiling level.

Maximal efficacy. **MaxEff** for ATSM:

When $b·c·d·A_m·M \gg 1$ and as long as $c·A_m·M \geq 1$, ATSM-MaxEff is always dependent on the product $b·d$ and independent of the value of $c·A_m·M$.

For $b·d = 1$, MaxEff = $L·a/(L·a+1)$, independent of $c·A_m·M$.

For $b·d > 1$, MaxEff > $L·a/(L·a+1)$, = synergy. With increasing values of $c·A_m·M$ above 1, the MaxEff increases towards a ceiling value of 100%, i.e., above $L·a/(L·a+1)$ if $L·a \gg 1$. For decreasing values of $c·A_m·M$ below 1, the MaxEff goes towards $L·a/(L·a+1)$.

For $b < 1$, MaxEff < $L·a/(L·a+1)$. With increasing values of $c·A_m·M$ above 1 the MaxEff reduces towards a ceiling value of $L·a/(L·a+1)$. For reducing values of $c·A_m·M$ below 1, the MaxEff increases towards $L·a/(L·a+1)$.

More details on dependence of MaxEff-ATSM on parameter combination are listed in the table.

As mentioned above, for $b·c·d·A_m·M \gg 1$, and $c·A_m·M \geq 1$, MaxEff is always independent of the value of $c·A_m·M$.

MaxEff for EXOM:

MaxEffs for EXOM are as well as for ATSM dependent on $c·d·A_m·M$. Further, for $c·A_m·M \gg 1$ when $d \gg 1$, EXOM-MaxEff goes to 100%, while for $c·A_m·M \gg 1$ but with $c·d·A_m·M \ll 1$, it is determined by $a/(a+c·A_m·M)$. When $c·A_m·M \leq 1$ and $c·d·A_m·M \gg 1$, EXOM-MaxEff goes to 1, while for $d \ll 1$, it goes to zero.

Ceiling effects of enhancement and allo-agonism by positive allosteric modulators (PAMs) are hallmarks and often detected in experiment [17,35-37]. These ceiling effects appear for $A_m \cdot M > 1$, panels A, D, G, J, M, Q, T, and X in Figure 5. Ceiling effects for competitive inhibition are determined by cooperative binding constant $c < 1$ and appears for $c \cdot A_m \cdot M > 10$, and best seen for $b \cdot d = 1$, panels C, F, I, L, P, S, V, and Z in Figure 5.

The ATSM was rejected as model for allo-competitive inhibition by gallamine at muscarinic subtype M2 receptors [20]. Meanwhile, both ATSM and EXOM can nicely simulate competitive inhibition with values of c low enough to keep the parameter products $b \cdot c \cdot d \cdot A_m \cdot M$ for ATSM and $c \cdot d \cdot A_m \cdot M$ for EXOM less than 10, exemplified in Figure 5C and F.

Allo-synergy, seen in the presence of allosters as a lift in MaxEff above MaxEff for othosters alone, is now commonly described for agonistic-PAMs as well [5,8,25,36]. In ATSM, these characteristics of PAMs with MaxEff above maximal response for endogenous ligands alone may be simulated with values of b and d when their product is > 1, Figure 5M-N, while EXOM can simulate allo-synergy for $d > 1$, not shown. Mixed inhibition, appearing as values of MaxEff lower than MaxEff with orthosters alone in the presence of NAMs, including pure non-competitive inhibition, may be simulated for $b \cdot d < 1$ in ATSM, Figure 5U, and for $d < 1$ in EXOM, Figure 5Y. Published examples of negative allosteric effects are now increasing as more interest is invested in development of NAMs [12,32,60].

In both allo-synergy and allo-inhibition, parameter c, as its value is lowered, will narrow the gap between MaxEff in the presence and absence of an alloster; compare panels M-P and panels T-Z in Figure 5.

The lack of effect of parameter b on MaxEff in EXOM clearly weakens the theory, even though additional details have been presented on the behaviour of EXOM [34]. A variant of EXOM has been developed with lumped parameters thus avoiding the problem of a missing effect of parameter b in MaxEff [24].

Comparison of best-fit analyses to experimental data for ATSM and EXOM

Results from analysis of experimental data with ATSM and EXOM are listed in Table 4. Ideally parameters in a theory should manage to stay constant when the theory is fitted to different data sets of the same experimental concentration-response system; for instance at increasing alloster concentrations. Therefore, the more the ratios in Table 4 for each single parameter deviate from unity in the present analysis, the worse is its model's credibility.

Both ATSM and EXOM have problems with a convincing determination of parameters fitted to data in data-figure 2. However, ATSM still seems to give the best result

Table 4 Parameter ratios from best-fits with ATSM and EXOM on three data sets

Model for analysis	Data-figure #	Parameters ratios from best fits to concentration-response curves for orthosters at three different concentrations of allosters			
		b	c	d	A_m
ATSM	1	4.9	3.4	3.2	1.8
EXOM		46	1.9	3.0	2.6
ATSM	2	2.8	97	11	15
EXOM *		50	17	3.0	84
ATSM	3	1.6	9.2	16	1.5
EXOM		26	35	33	3.8

Each single parameter ratio from best fits with ATSM or EXOM is adapted from analysis of three sets of data in the literature, data-figures 1 to 3, see last section in Methods for references. Each data set consists of four concentration-response curves, where one curve is an orthoster concentration-response curve without an alloster present and the three other curves are orthoster concentration-responses experimentally obtained at three different alloster concentrations.

Parameters a and A_s for both ATSM and EXOM were initially determined by model-fits to the basic orthoster concentration-response curves without an alloster present. Obtained values for a and A_s were inserted in the model equations, which were then use for fitting to experimental data of the parameters b, c, d, and A_m in the theories. Each number in the table is a ratio between best-fit values with the largest deviation between two of three results from fits for the single parameter to three concentration-response curves at different alloster concentrations.

* For responses indicating spontaneous activity as in data-figure 2, evaluation by EXOM theory was performed by assuming a level of 9% spontaneous activity, thus fitting the EXOM distribution equation to 91% activity for all three alloster concentrations, 0.03, 0.1, and 0.3 µM ([37]). For ATSM used on data-figure 2, spontaneous activity was implemented by setting $L/(1 + L) = 0.09$. For data-figures 1 and 3a value of 0.01 was selected for L.

For a more detailed explanation of how the presented parameter ratios are obtained, see last section in Methods.

based on an overall evaluation of ratios for all four parameters from the three data sets of data-figure 2, Table 4.

Although exponentiation in form of a Hill coefficient may also be invoked for both models, such exponentiation was omitted in the present analysis. Also, an interpretation and detailed discussion of the actually obtained parameter values are beyond the scope of this paper.

Thus, based on the ratios in Table 4, it may be concluded that ATSM seems to be better than EXOM at evaluating possible parameter values with a requirement of consistency when determined at 3 different alloster concentrations, since in general most of the ratios are closer to unity when employing the ATSM.

Conclusion

In a beautiful review, non-mechanistic EXOM against mechanistic ATSM is debated and further contrasted with an empirical general description of synagic behaviour of allosters in different experimental setups [17]. When system information is limited, analyses of allosteric behaviour by operational, empirical and mathematical approaches as Hill's exponentiation are still valid. Meanwhile, analysing systems of allosteric synagics as discussed here, the best description of allosteric effects is by Hall's millennium milestone mechanical model

[22] due to shortcomings of EXOM. Limitations of mechanistic models as the ATSM are given with its assumptions, which usually both exclude more than two binding sites and multi-steps or parallel pathways. The ATSM may still replace the EXOM as a phenomeno-logical model by applying assumptions similar to those for EXOM. For the future, allosteric models should be developed based on ATSM and implicating multi-binding and diverse pathways of receptor activation when needed. Thus, instead of switching to non-mechanistic approaches as EXOM or reduce require-ments for the basic TCM to analyse such systems [20,26], phenomenological or extended forms of the ATSM should be preferred (e.g., [25]).

Abbreviations

ATSM: Allosteric two-state model; EXOM: Extended operational model; cTSM: Cyclic two-state model; BLM: The Black & Leff operational model; *7TMRs /GPCRs*: 7 transmembrane helix G protein-coupled receptors; TCM: Ternary-complex model; ATCM: Allosteric ternary-complex model; EC_{50}: Apparent dissociation constant at 50% activity; IntEff: Initial efficacy; MaxEff: Maximal efficacy; PAMs and NAMs: Positive and negative allosteric modulators; *QSAR*: Quantitative structure-activity-relationship.

Competing interest

The author declares no conflicts of interest.

Authors' contribution

NB developed and wrote the MS.

Acknowledgments

I thank Dr. David A. Hall for helpful discussion on two-state and operational model approaches and for significant comments on previous versions of the MS.

References

1. Ledford H: **Drug buddies.** *Nature* 2011, **474**:433–434.
2. Macilwain C: **Pharmaceutical industry must take its medicine.** *Nature* 2011, **470**:141.
3. Scannell JW, Blanckley A, Boldon H, Warrington B: **Diagnosing the decline in pharmaceutical R&D efficiency.** *Nat Rev Drug Discov* 2012, **11**:191–200.
4. Elsinghorst PW, Härtig W, Gündisch D, Mohr K, Tränkle C, Gütschow M: **A hydrazide linker strategy for heterobivalent compounds as ortho- and allosteric ligands of acetylcholine-binding proteins.** *Curr Top Med Chem* 2011, **11**:2731–2748.
5. Gao ZG, Verzijl D, Zweemer A, Ye K, Göblyös A, Ijzerman AP, *et al*: **Functionally biased modulation of the A(3) adenosine receptor agonist efficacy and potency by imidazoquinolinamine allosteric enhancers.** *Biochem Pharmacol* 2011, **82**:658–668.
6. Jensen PC, Thiele S, Steen A, Elder A, Kolbeck R, Ghosh S, *et al*: **Reversed binding of a small molecule ligand in homologous chemokine receptors - differential role of extracellular loop 2.** *Br J Pharmacol* 2012, **166**:258–275.
7. Melancon BJ, Hopkins CR, Wood MR, Emmitte KA, Niswender CM, Christopoulos A, *et al*: **Allosteric modulation of seven transmembrane spanning receptors: theory, practice, and opportunities for central nervous system drug discovery.** *J Med Chem* 2012, **55**:1445–1464.
8. Valant C, Felder CC, Sexton PM, Christopoulos A: **Probe dependence in the allosteric modulation of a G protein-coupled receptor: Implications for detection and validation of allosteric ligand effects.** *Mol Pharmacol* 2012, **81**:41–52.
9. Audet M, Lagacé M, Silversides DW, Bouvier M: **Protein-protein interactions monitored in cells from transgenic mice using bioluminescence resonance energy transfer.** *FASEB J* 2010, **24**:2829–2838.
10. Chung KY, Rasmussen SG, Liu T, Li S, Devree BT, Chae PS, *et al*: **Conformational changes in the G protein Gs induced by the ß2 adrenergic receptor.** *Nature* 2011, **477**:611–615.
11. Comps-Agrar L, Kniazeff J, Nørskov-Lauritsen L, Maurel D, Gassmann M, Gregor N, *et al*: **The oligomeric state sets GABA(B) receptor signalling efficacy.** *EMBO J* 2011, **30**:2336–2349.
12. Henderson BJ, Orac CM, Maciagiewicz I, Bergmeier SC, McKay DB: **3D-QSAR and 3D-QSSR models of negative allosteric modulators facilitate the design of a novel selective antagonist of human a4ß2 neuronal nicotinic acetylcholine receptors.** *Bioorg Med Chem Lett* 2012, **22**:1797–1813.
13. Nygaard R, Valentin-Hansen L, Mokrosinski J, Frimurer TM, Schwartz TW: **Conserved water-mediated hydrogen bond network between TM-I, -II, -VI, and -VII in 7TM receptor activation.** *J Biol Chem* 2010, **285**:19625–19636.
14. Peeters MC, Wisse LE, Dinaj A, Vroling B, Vriend G, Ijzerman AP: **The role of the second and third extracellular loops of the adenosine A1 receptor in activation and allosteric modulation.** *Biochem Pharmacol* 2012, **84**:76–87.
15. Schelshorn DW, Joly F, Mutel S, Hampe C, Breton B, Mutel V, *et al*: **Lateral Allosterism in the Glucagon Receptor Family: GLP-1 Induces GPCR Heteromer Formation.** *Mol Pharmacol* 2012, **81**:309–318.
16. Van Eps N, Preininger AM, Alexander N, Kaya AI, Meier S, Meiler J, *et al*: **Interaction of a G protein with an activated receptor opens the interdomain interface in the alpha subunit.** *Proc Natl Acad Sci USA* 2011, **108**:9420–9424.
17. Keov P, Sexton PM, Christopoulos A: **Allosteric modulation of G protein-coupled receptors: a pharmacological perspective.** *Neuropharmacology* 2011, **60**:24–35.
18. Bindslev N: *Drug-Acceptor Interactions. Modeling Theoretical Tools to Test and Evaluate Experimental Equilibrium Effects.* 1st edition. Stockholm: Co-Action Publishing; 2008.
19. De Amici M, Dallanoce C, Holzgrabe U, Tränkle C, Mohr K: **Allosteric ligands for G protein-coupled receptors: a novel strategy with attractive therapeutic opportunities.** *Med Res Rev* 2010, **30**:463–549.
20. Ehlert FJ, Griffin MT: **Two-state models and the analysis of the allosteric effect of gallamine at the m2 muscarinic receptor.** *J Pharmacol Exp Ther* 2008, **325**:1039–1060.
21. Gomes I, Ijzerman AP, Ye K, Maillet EL, Devi LA: **G protein-coupled receptor heteromerization: a role in allosteric modulation of ligand binding.** *Mol Pharmacol* 2011, **79**:1044–1052.
22. Hall DA: **Modeling the functional effects of allosteric modulators at pharmacological receptors: an extension of the two-state model of receptor activation.** *Mol Pharmacol* 2000, **58**:1412–1423.
23. Jäger D, Schmalenbach C, Prilla S, Schrobang J, Kebig A, Sennwitz M, *et al*: **Allosteric small molecules unveil a role of an extracellular E2/ transmembrane helix 7 junction for G protein-coupled receptor activation.** *J Biol Chem* 2007, **30**:34968–34976.
24. Kenakin TP: **7TM receptor allostery: putting numbers to shapeshifting proteins.** *Trends Pharmacol Sci* 2009, **30**:460–469.
25. Stahl E, Elmslie G, Ellis J: **Allosteric modulation of the M3 muscarinic receptor by amiodarone and N-ethylamiodarone: application of the four-ligand allosteric two-state model.** *Mol Pharmacol* 2011, **80**:378–388.
26. Leach K, Sexton PM, Christopoulos A: **Allosteric GPCR modulators: taking advantage of permissive receptor pharmacology. Supplementary data.** *Trends Pharmacol Sci* 2007, **28**:382–389.
27. Black JW, Leff P: **Operational models of pharmacological agonism.** *Proc R Soc Lond B* 1983, **220**:141–162.
28. Ross EM, Maguire ME, Sturgill TW, Biltonen RL, Gilman AG: **Relationship between the beta-adrenergic receptor and adenylate cyclase.** *J Biol Chem* 1977, **252**:5761–5775.
29. De Lean A, Stadel JM, Lefkowitz RJ: **A ternary complex model explains the agonist specific binding properties of the adenylate cyclase coupled beta-adrenergic receptor.** *J Biol Chem* 1980, **255**:7108–7117.
30. Stockton JM, Birdsall NJ, Burgen AS, Hulme EC: **Modification of the binding properties of muscarinic receptors by gallamine.** *Mol Pharmacol* 1983, **23**:551–557.
31. Ehlert FJ: **Estimation of the affinities of allosteric ligands using radioligand binding and pharmacological null methods.** *Mol Pharmacol* 1988, **33**:187–194.
32. Bradley SJ, Langmead CJ, Watson JM, Challiss RA: **Quantitative analysis reveals multiple mechanisms of allosteric modulation of the mGlu5 receptor in rat astroglia.** *Mol Pharmacol* 2011, **79**:874–885.

33. Canals M, Lane JR, Wen A, Scammells PJ, Sexton PM, Christopoulos A: A Monod-Wyman-Changeux mechanism can explain G protein-coupled receptor (GPCR) allosteric modulation. *J Biol Chem* 2012, **287**:650–659.

34. Kenakin TP: Biased signaling and allosteric machines; new vistas and challenges for drug discovery. *Br J Pharmacol* 2012, **165**:1659–1669.

35. Leach K, Davey AE, Felder CC, Sexton PM, Christopoulos A: The role of transmembrane domain 3 in the actions of orthosteric, allosteric, and atypical agonists of the M4 muscarinic acetylcholine receptor. *Mol Pharmacol* 2011, **79**:855–865.

36. Smith NJ, Ward RJ, Stoddart LA, Hudson BD, Kostenis E, Ulven T, *et al*: Extracellular loop 2 of the free fatty acid receptor 2 mediates allosterism of a phenylacetamide ago-allosteric modulator. *Mol Pharmacol* 2011, **80**:163–173.

37. Suratman S, Leach K, Sexton P, Felder C, Loiacono R, Christopoulos A: Impact of species variability and 'probe-dependence' on the detection and in vivo validation of allosteric modulation at the M4 muscarinic acetylcholine receptor. *Br J Pharmacol* 2011, **162**:1659–1670.

38. Wootten D, Savage EE, Valant C, May LT, Sloop KW, Ficorilli J, *et al*: Allosteric modulation of endogenous metabolites as an avenue for drug discovery. *Mol Pharmacol* 2012, **82**:281–290.

39. Birdsall NJ: Class A GPCR heterodimers: evidence from binding studies. *Trends Pharmacol Sci* 2010, **31**:499–508.

40. Jakubík J, Janícková H, El-Fakahany EE, Dolezal V: Negative cooperativity in binding of muscarinic receptor agonists and GDP as a measure of agonist efficacy. *Br J Pharmacol* 2011, **162**:1029–1044.

41. Kiselyov VV, Versteyhe S, Gauguin L, De Meyts P: Harmonic oscillator model of the insulin and IGF1 receptors' allosteric binding and activation. *Mol Syst Biol* 2009, **5**:1–12.

42. Rovira X, Roche D, Serra J, Kniazeff J, Pin JP, Giraldo J: Modeling the binding and function of metabotropic glutamate receptors. *J Pharmacol Exp Ther* 2008, **325**:443–456.

43. Birnbaumer L, Bearer CF, Iyengar R: A two-state model of an enzyme with an allosteric regulator site capable of metabolizing the regulatory ligand. *J Biol Chem* 1980, **255**:3552–3557.

44. Leff P: The twostate model of receptor activation. *Trends Pharmacol Sci* 1995, **16**:89–97.

45. Stephenson RP: A modification of receptor theory. *Br J Pharmacol* 1956, **11**:379–393.

46. Changeux JP: Allosteric proteins: from regulatory enzymes to receptors - personal recollections. *Bioessays* 1993, **15**:625–634.

47. Monod J, Wyman J, Changeux J-P: On the nature of allosteric transitions: a plausible model. *J Mol Biol* 1965, **12**:88–118.

48. Changeux JP: 50th anniversary of the word "allosteric". *Protein Sci* 2011, **20**:1119–1124.

49. Koshland DE Jr: Application of a theory of enzyme specificity to protein synthesis. *Proc Natl Acad Sci* 1958, **44**:98–104.

50. Katz B, Thesleff S: A study of the desensitization produced by acetylcholine at the motor end-plate. *J Physiol* 1957, **138**:63–80.

51. Furchgott RF: Receptor mechanisms. *Ann Rev Pharmcol* 1964, **4**:21–50.

52. Furchgott RF: The use of β-haloalkylamines in the differentiation of receptors and in the determination of dissociation constants of receptor-agonist complexes. *Adv Drug Res* 1966, **3**:21–55.

53. Kenakin TP, Beek D: Is prenalterol (H133/80) really a selective beta 1 adrenoceptor agonist? Tissue selectivity resulting from differences in stimulus–response relationships. *J Pharmacol Exp Ther* 1980, **213**:406–413.

54. Slack RJ, Hall DA: Development of operational models of receptor activation including constitutive receptor activity and their use to determine the efficacy of the chemokine TARC at the CC-chemokine receptor CCR4. *Br J Pharmacol* 2012, **166**:1774–1792.

55. Ehlert FJ, Suga H, Griffin MT: Analysis of agonism and inverse agonism in functional assays with constitutive activity: estimation of orthosteric ligand affinity constants for active and inactive receptor states. *J Pharmacol Exp Ther* 2011, **338**:671–686.

56. Perdona E, Costantini VJ, Tessari M, Martinelli P, Carignani C, Valerio E, *et al*: In vitro and in vivo characterization of the novel GABAB receptor positive allosteric modulator, 2-{1-[2-(4-chlorophenyl)-5-methylpyrazolo[1,5-a]pyrimidin-7-yl]-2-piperidinyl}ethanol (CMPPE). *Neuropharmacology* 2011, **61**:957–966.

57. Hall DA, Langmead CJ: Matching models to data: a receptor pharmacologist's guide. *Br J Pharmacol* 2010, **161**:1276–1290.

58. Segel IH: *Enzyme kinetics. Behavior and analysis of rapid equilibrium and steady-state enzyme systems.* New York: Wiley & Sons; 1975. reissued 1993.

59. Holst B, Frimurer TM, Mokrosinski J, Halkjaer T, Cullberg KB, Underwood CR, *et al*: Overlapping binding site for the endogenous agonist, small-molecule agonists, and ago-allosteric modulators on the ghrelin receptor. *Mol Pharmacol* 2009, **75**:44–59.

60. Mueller R, Dawson ES, Meiler J, Rodriguez AL, Chauder BA, Bates BS, *et al*: Discovery of 2-(2-benzoxazoyl amino)-4-aryl-5-cyanopyrimidine as negative allosteric modulators (NAMs) of metabotropic glutamate receptor 5 (mGlu5): from an artificial neural network virtual screen to an in vivo tool compound. *ChemMedChem* 2012, **7**:406–414.

15

Evaluation of drug-induced tissue injury by measuring alanine aminotransferase (ALT) activity in silkworm hemolymph

Yoshinori Inagaki[1], Yasuhiko Matsumoto[1], Keiko Kataoka[2], Naoya Matsuhashi[2] and Kazuhisa Sekimizu[1,2]*

Abstract

Background: Our previous studies suggest silkworms can be used as model animals instead of mammals in pharmacologic studies to develop novel therapeutic medicines. We examined the usefulness of the silkworm larvae *Bombyx mori* as an animal model for evaluating tissue injury induced by various cytotoxic drugs. Drugs that induce hepatotoxic effects in mammals were injected into the silkworm hemocoel, and alanine aminotransferase (ALT) activity was measured in the hemolymph 1 day later.

Results: Injection of CCl_4 into the hemocoel led to an increase in ALT activity. The increase in ALT activity was attenuated by pretreatment with *N*-acetyl-$_L$-cysteine. Injection of benzoic acid derivatives, ferric sulfate, sodium valproate, tetracycline, amiodarone hydrochloride, methyldopa, ketoconazole, pemoline (Betanamin), *N*-nitroso-fenfluramine, and $_D$-galactosamine also increased ALT activity.

Conclusions: These findings indicate that silkworms are useful for evaluating the effects of chemicals that induce tissue injury in mammals.

Keywords: Silkworm, Alanine aminotransferase, Tissue injury, Animal model

Background

Tissue injury induced by chemicals in mammals, including humans, is associated with the rapid development of severe impairment of the organs involved in detoxification, e.g., fulminant hepatic failure [1]. Therefore, assessment of chemical-induced tissue injury is crucial in drug discovery.

In the development of novel therapeutic medicines, *in vivo* trials using animal models are essential for predicting toxicity and drug disposition in the human body. Mice and rats are used to evaluate the toxicity of synthesized compounds and natural medicines [2-4]. The use of mammals for experimental models, however, is associated with a number of problems, such as high cost and ethical issues. An alternative animal model is needed to overcome these problems.

Although invertebrate animals such as *Caenorhabditis elegans* (*C. elegans*) and *Drosophila* larvae have been proposed as model animals for evaluating bacterial pathogenicity and therapeutic effects of antibiotics, their body sizes are too small to inject a fixed amount of sample [5,6]. Large insect larvae can be easily injected into the midgut or subcutaneously with sample solution using a syringe. Silkworm hemolymph and tissue can be harvested separately and used in biochemical, haematological, and immunological analyses [7,8]. Thus, the silkworm is an invertebrate model that can relieve the issues related to the use of mammals and thus promote pharmaceutical studies [7,9-12]. We previously demonstrated that the lethal dose of various cytotoxic substances in silkworms is consistent with that in mammals [7]. Thus, silkworms are considered to be appropriate for evaluating the toxic effects of chemical compounds on animal bodies. In mammals, hepatotoxic substances induce increases in marker enzymes of tissue injury in the blood [13]. Increases in alanine aminotransferase (ALT) activity in mammalian blood are caused by leakage of this enzyme from injured tissue. ALT is conserved

* Correspondence: sekimizu@mol.f.u-tokyo.ac.jp
[1]Laboratory of Microbiology, Graduate School of Pharmaceutical Sciences, The University of Tokyo, 7-3-1 Hongo, Bunkyo-ku, Tokyo 113-0033, Japan
[2]Genome Pharmaceuticals Institute Co., Ltd., The University of Tokyo Entrepreneur Plaza, 7-3-1 Hongo, Bunkyo-ku, Tokyo 113-0033, Japan

throughout evolution [14] and is therefore considered to be a surrogate marker of tissue injury in insect larvae. To date, however, there has been no evidence that ALT activity is increased in the body fluid of the silkworm upon the induction of tissue injury.

The present study aimed to examine ALT activity in the body fluid of silkworm larvae injected with various hepatotoxic compounds. We also analyzed the effectiveness of using the silkworm model for evaluating drugs that have a protective effect against tissue injury induction.

Methods

Chemicals

Various cytotoxic drugs were purchased, as follows: carbon tetrachloride (CCl_4), salicylic acid, ferric sulfate, sodium valproate, N-nitroso-fenfluramine, and D-galactosamine were purchased from Wako Pure Chemical Industries, Osaka, Japan; acetaminophen was purchased from Tocris Biosciences, Ellisville, MO; acetylsalicylic acid was purchased from Cayman Chemical Co., Ann Arbor, MI; tetracycline was purchased from LKT Laboratories Inc., St Paul, MN; amiodarone hydrochloride was purchased from MP Biomedicals, Solon, OH; methyldopa was purchased from Sawai Pharmaceutical Co., Ltd., Osaka, Japan; ketoconazole was purchased from LKT Laboratories Inc.; and pemoline was purchased from Sanwa Kagaku Kenkyusho Co., Ltd., Nagoya, Japan. N-acetyl-L-cysteine (NAC), which acts to suppress increases in ALT activity, was purchased from Sigma-Aldrich, St. Louis, MO. Hydrosoluble and liposoluble compounds were dissolved in saline and dimethyl sulfoxide, respectively.

Animals

Fertilized silkworm eggs (*Bombyx mori*, Hu·Yo × Tukuba·Ne) were purchased from Ehime Sanshu Co., Ltd. (Ehime, Japan). Hatched larvae were fed artificial food, Silkmate 2S (Nosan Corporation, Yokohama, Japan) at 27°C.

Construction of cytotoxic induction model using silkworm larvae

Fifth-instar silkworm larvae on the first day were fed artificial food, Silkmate 2S, for 1 d. After the body weight increased to 1.8 to 2.2 g, they were fasted for 6 h, and solution containing a cytotoxic compound was injected into the hemocoel from the backside of the larvae. Liposoluble compounds were injected (25 μL/silkworm) using a glass syringe (MICROLITER™ #710, Hamilton Co., Reno, NV) with a 27G needle, and hydrosoluble compounds were injected (50 μL/silkworm) using a disposable syringe (Terumo Corporation, Tokyo, Japan) with a 27G needle. After incubation at 27°C for

1 d, the hemolymph was collected for measurement of ALT activity as described below.

Examination of suppressive effects against induced cytotoxicity

Fifth-instar silkworm larvae on the first day were fed Silkmate 2S for 1 d. After the body weight increased to 1.8 to 2.2 g, they were fasted for 6 h, and 50 μL of 0.9% saline or 0.4 M NAC was injected into hemocoel from the backside of the larvae using a disposable syringe. After 30 min, 25 μL of olive oil or 15% CCl_4 was injected into the hemocoel using a glass syringe. After incubation at 27°C for 1 d, the hemolymph was collected for measurement of ALT activity as described below.

Preparation of tissue homogenates from silkworm larvae

Fifth-instar silkworm larvae on the first day were fed Silkmate 2S for 1 d. After fasting for 6 h, the gut, fat body, silk gland, Malpighian tube, and outer coat were isolated. Each tissue was weighed and homogenized with insect physiologic saline (150 mM NaCl, 5 mM KCl, 1 mM $CaCl_2$). Samples were centrifuged at 3000 rpm for 5 min, and the supernatant was collected and stored at −80°C until measurement of ALT activity. The amount of protein in the supernatant was quantified using Lowry's method.

Measurement of ALT activity

Five μL of collected hemolymph or the supernatant of homogenized tissue was mixed with 550 μL of a reaction solution containing 0.5 M L-alanine, 0.2 mM NADH, 1.3 U/mL lactate dehydrogenase, and 0.9 mg/mL bovine serum albumin. After adding 50 μL of 180 mM 2-oxoglutarate solution, the reaction mixtures were incubated at 30°C for 90 min. Absorbance at 339 nm was recorded to detect decreases in NADH. The slope of the absorbance decrease is proportional to ALT activity. Final ALT activities were determined according to the standard curve drawn from the results of mouse liver homogenate. For ALT activity, 1U was defined as the enzyme activity that forms 1 μmol NAD/min under the assay conditions.

Statistical analysis

All experiments were performed at least twice and the data are shown as the mean ± standard deviation. The significance of differences was calculated using a 2-tailed Student's t-test at the significance level alpha = 0.05.

Results

Elevation of ALT activity in the hemolymph of silkworms injected with carbon tetrachloride (CCl_4)

CCl_4 is generally used as a model compound to evaluate hepatotoxic effects in mammals. Tissue injury induced by CCl_4 is considered to increase ALT activity in the body fluid. In this study, we examined changes in the ALT activity in silkworm hemolymph after injection of CCl_4. ALT activity in the silkworm hemolymph increased 8-fold following injection of CCl_4 compared with injection of olive oil (Figure 1). This finding suggests that tissue injury can be monitored in silkworms by measuring ALT activity. In the subsequent experiments, we used CCl_4 as a positive control and 0.9% saline or olive oil as a negative control.

Tissue distribution of ALT activity in silkworms

ALT localizes in the liver and muscles in mammals. Localization of ALT activity in the silkworm has not yet been reported. We determined the tissue distribution of ALT activity to determine which tissue produces ALT activity in the silkworm hemolymph. The total activity and specific activity of ALT in each tissue are shown in Table 1. The highest total activity and the highest specific activity were detected in the gut.

Suppressive effects on ALT activity increases by pretreatment with N-acetyl-L-cysteine (NAC)

As described above, CCl_4 that is hepatotoxic in mammals increased ALT activity in the silkworm hemolymph. Therefore, we considered the silkworm applicable as an animal model to evaluate drug-induced tissue injury. In mammals, radical scavengers such as NAC suppress the cytotoxic effects induced by hepatotoxic substances [15]. Pretreatment with NAC is useful for clarifying whether ALT activity in the silkworm hemolymph is increased

Table 1 Tissue distribution of ALT activity in silkworm

Tissue	Total activity (U/tissue)	Protein (mg)	Specific activity (U/mg)
Gut	7.0	4.7	1.5
Fat body	0.2	0.3	0.6
Silk grand	0.4	0.9	0.5
Malpighi grand	0.5	0.2	0.8
Outer coat	3.9	4.9	0.8

due to the production of radicals. In this study, we examined the effect of injecting the silkworm with NAC prior to injection of CCl_4 on ALT activity in the hemolymph. The ALT activity of CCl_4-injected silkworms that were preinjected with 0.4 M NAC was much lower than those of silkworms preinjected with 0.9% NaCl (Figure 2).

Increased ALT activity in the silkworm hemolymph following injection with cytotoxic drugs

Consistent with the results described above, CCl_4 was suggested to induce tissue injury via the production of radicals in the silkworm body. We then examined the influence of benzoic acid derivatives (acetaminophen, salicylic acid, and acetylsalicylic acid), which are known hepatotoxic agents due to the production of radicals by the catalytic reaction of P450 2E1 [16-18], on ALT activity in the silkworm hemolymph. ALT activity in the hemolymph increased in a dose-dependent manner following injection of each of these agents (Figure 3). Compared with the negative control, ALT activity was increased in groups treated with 6 mg acetaminophen (7-fold), 1.2 and 12 mg salicylic acid (9 and 10-fold, respectively), and 1.8 and 18 mg acetylsalicylic acid (3 and 11-fold, respectively). Based on the amount of each drug needed to increase ALT activity, salicylic acid was the most toxic among these three reagents.

Substances that produce toxic effects by the production of radicals were suggested to induce tissue injury in the silkworm body and to subsequently increase ALT activity in the silkworm hemolymph. It remains unclear, however, whether tissue injury induced by various biological mechanisms in mammals can be evaluated based on increased ALT activity in the silkworm. Other substances that induce tissue injury in mammals by different mechanisms were also examined to evaluate whether they would induce increases in ALT activity in the silkworm hemolymph. Excessive amounts of iron induce tissue injury by radical production [19]. Sodium valproate, tetracycline, and amiodarone induce tissue damage, probably via inhibiting the function of cell organelles such as mitochondria and lysosomes [20-22]. Compared with the negative control, ALT activity clearly increased in groups treated with 0.084 and 0.84 mg ferric acid (4 and 13-fold,

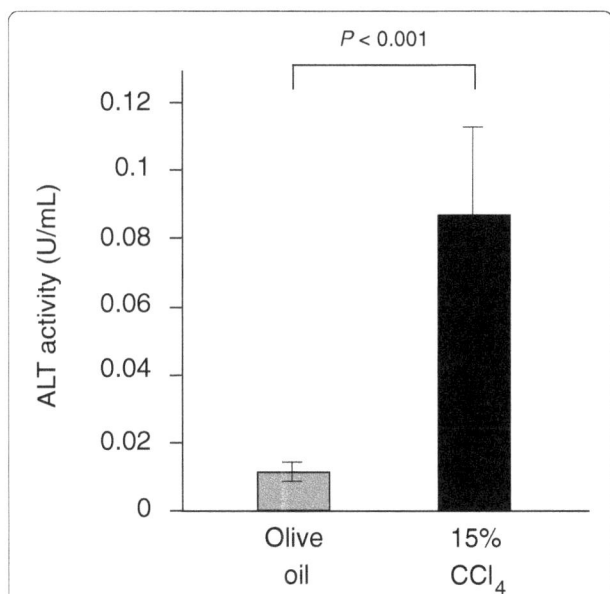

Figure 1 ALT activity in the silkworm hemolymph injected with CCl_4. Silkworms fasted for 6 h were injected with 15% CCl_4 or olive oil, and then ALT activity in the silkworm hemolymph was measured 1 d later. (n = 5).

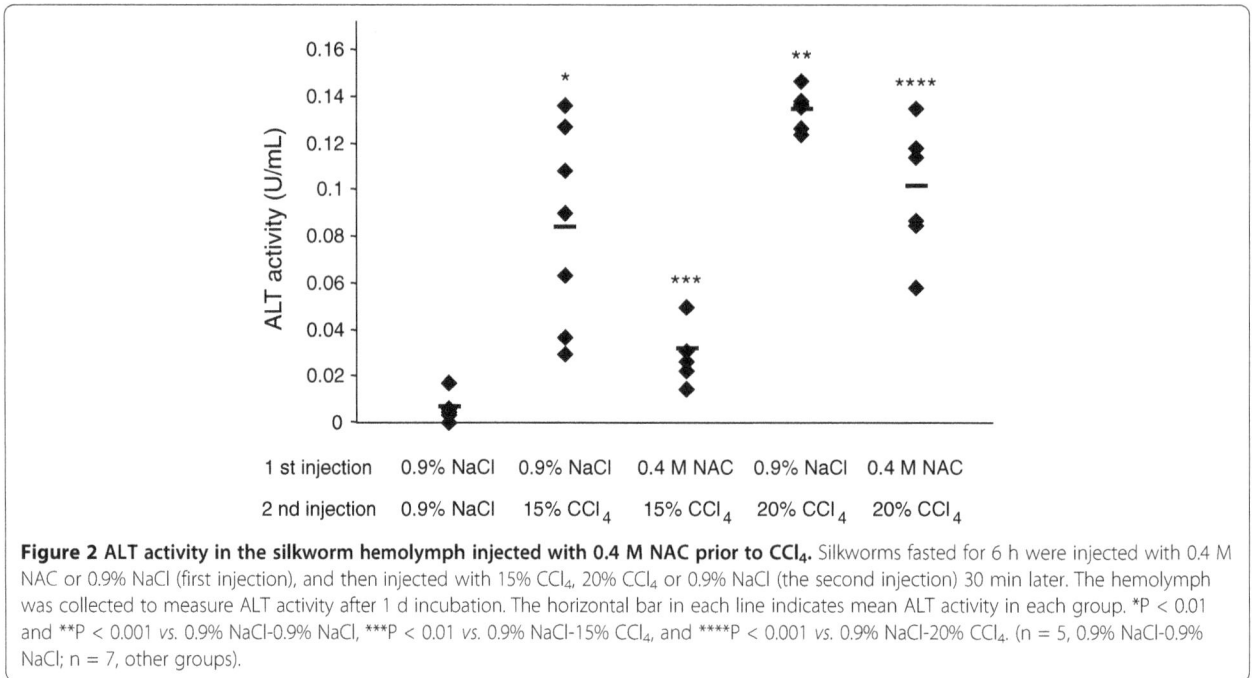

Figure 2 ALT activity in the silkworm hemolymph injected with 0.4 M NAC prior to CCl₄. Silkworms fasted for 6 h were injected with 0.4 M NAC or 0.9% NaCl (first injection), and then injected with 15% CCl₄, 20% CCl₄ or 0.9% NaCl (the second injection) 30 min later. The hemolymph was collected to measure ALT activity after 1 d incubation. The horizontal bar in each line indicates mean ALT activity in each group. *P < 0.01 and **P < 0.001 vs. 0.9% NaCl-0.9% NaCl, ***P < 0.01 vs. 0.9% NaCl-15% CCl₄, and ****P < 0.001 vs. 0.9% NaCl-20% CCl₄. (n = 5, 0.9% NaCl-0.9% NaCl; n = 7, other groups).

respectively), 4.8 mg sodium valproate (2-fold), 0.4 and 4 mg tetracycline (2 and 12-fold, respectively), and 0.16 and 1.6 mg amiodarone hydrochloride (2 and 13-fold, respectively; Figure 4A).

We then examined the induction of tissue injury by methyldopa, ketoconazole, and pemoline (Betanamin) in the silkworm. These agents are thought to induce hepatic injury in mammals by the formation of metabolites that cause immune hypersensitivity, such as eosinophilia [23-25]. All of the reagents increased ALT activity (3.9 mg methyldopa, 6-fold; 1.6 mg ketoconazole, 2-fold; and 5.6 mg pemoline, 2-fold; Figure 4B).

Excessive intake of N-nitroso-fenfluramine, which is generally used as a food supplement, has hepatotoxic effects [26,27]. Rapid depletion of ATP by impaired mitochondrial function and induction of DNA damage

by the production of alkyl cations are thought to be the mechanism of N-nitroso-fenfluramine-induced cell death [28]. We tested whether silkworms can be used to detect N-nitroso-fenfluramine-induced tissue injury by measuring ALT activity in the hemolymph. ALT activity in the hemolymph of silkworms injected with 450 μg N-nitroso-fenfluramine increased 3-fold (Figure 5A).

D-Galactosamine is a hepatotoxin that induces the depletion of uridine with subsequent necrosis [29]. This compound is frequently used for the construction of fulminant hepatic injury models [29]. Inhibition of the synthesis of nucleic acids, proteins, and lipids by UDP-glucosamine, which is derived from D-galactosamine, is the suggested mechanism of tissue damage [29]. We examined whether tissue injury was induced in silkworms by injection of D-galactosamine. ALT activity in

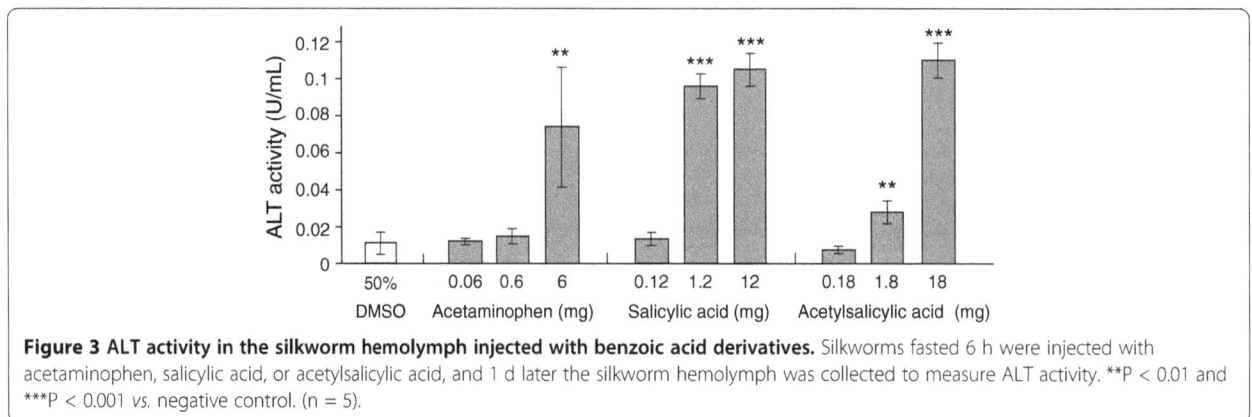

Figure 3 ALT activity in the silkworm hemolymph injected with benzoic acid derivatives. Silkworms fasted 6 h were injected with acetaminophen, salicylic acid, or acetylsalicylic acid, and 1 d later the silkworm hemolymph was collected to measure ALT activity. **P < 0.01 and ***P < 0.001 vs. negative control. (n = 5).

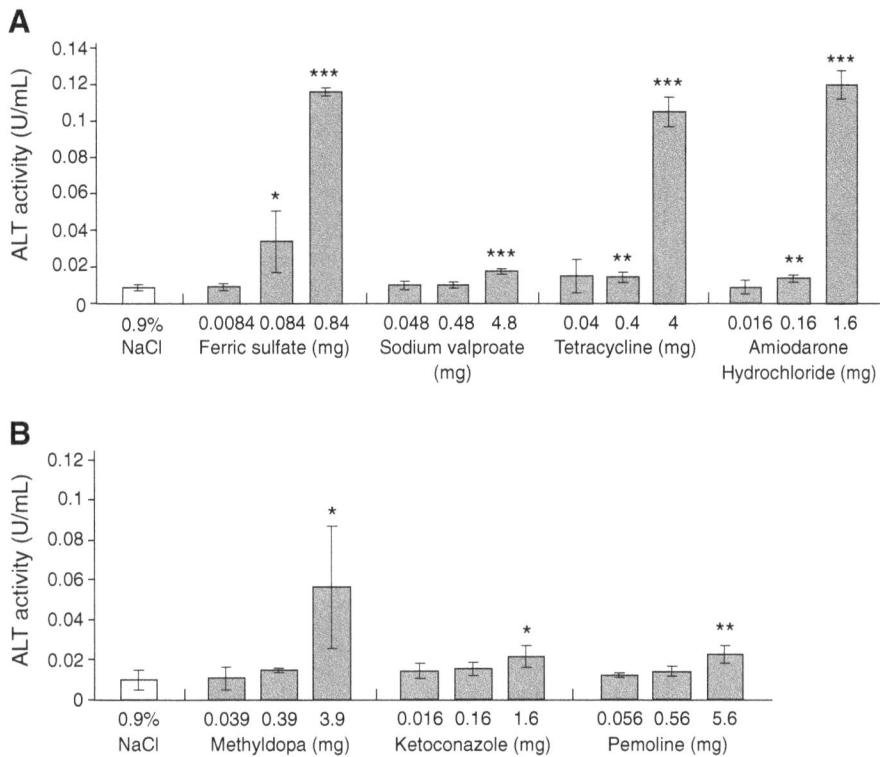

Figure 4 ALT activity in the silkworm hemolymph injected with various hepatotoxic drugs. Silkworms fasted 6 h were injected with ferric sulfate, sodium valproate, tetracycline, or amiodarone hydrochloride **(A)**, and with methyldopa, ketoconazole, or pemoline **(B)**, and 1 d later the silkworm hemolymph was collected to measure ALT activity. *P < 0.05, **P < 0.01 and ***P < 0.001 vs. negative control. (n = 5).

silkworm larvae injected with 7 mg D-galactosamine was increased compared with the negative control (injected 0.9% saline, 6-fold difference; Figure 5B).

Discussion

The findings of the present study demonstrate the applicability of silkworm larvae as an animal model for evaluating drug-induced tissue injury based on measurements of ALT activity in the hemolymph. ALT activity levels in human blood are considered to be a highly sensitive and fairly specific preclinical and clinical biomarker of cytotoxicity or hepatotoxicity [13]; therefore, ALT activity levels in the blood of mammals are measured in many pharmaceutical studies to evaluate the hepatotoxic effects induced by natural products or newly synthesized chemicals. Here, we demonstrated that ALT activity levels were increased

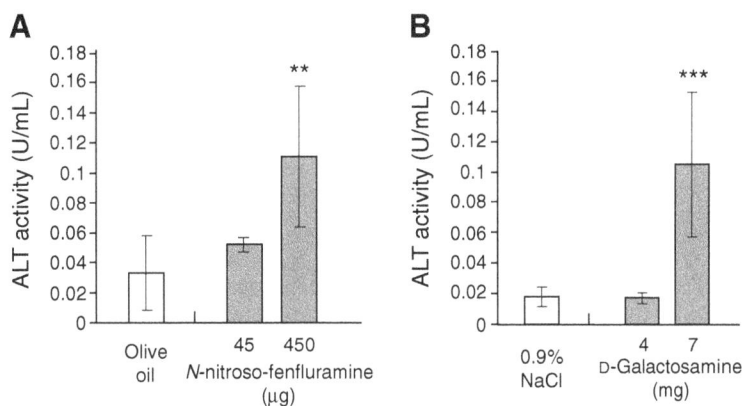

Figure 5 ALT activity in the silkworm hemolymph injected with *N*-nitroso-fenfluramine and D-galactosamine. Silkworms fasted 6 h were injected with *N*-nitroso-fenfluramine **(A)**, and with injected D-galactosamine **(B)**, and 1 d later the silkworm hemolymph was collected to measure ALT activity. **P < 0.01 and ***P < 0.001 vs. negative control. (n = 5).

in silkworm larvae by the injection of various cytotoxic drugs into the hemocoel. The results strongly suggest that we could establish a new experimental model to evaluate tissue injury effects using silkworm larvae.

The silkworm has been progressively developed as a scientifically useful experimental animal model [30]. Established silkworm models of infection with pathogenic bacteria and true fungi have been used to evaluate the effects of antibiotics and identify novel virulence genes [31-35]. The established hyperglycemic silkworm model is effective for developing antidiabetic drugs [36]. These studies suggest that silkworms can be used as model animals instead of mammals, such as mice and rats, in pharmacologic studies to develop novel therapeutic medicines. Furthermore, silkworms and mammals have common metabolic pathways involving cytochrome P450s and conjugation enzymes [7]. Cytotoxic effects on tissue and subsequent processes such as the release of marker enzymes from damaged cells occur similarly in silkworms and mammals. In the present study, we showed that ALT activity levels in the silkworm hemolymph were increased by the administration of CCl_4. In addition, the increase in ALT activity induced by CCl_4 administration was suppressed by pretreatment with NAC, suggesting that NAC suppressed CCl_4-induced tissue injury. NAC is a radical scavenger that attenuates hepatotoxic effects induced in the mammalian liver and is used to treat patients with acute acetaminophen hepatotoxicity [15,37]. The present result revealed that NAC has similar suppressive effects in the silkworm body. This silkworm model is thus considered to be useful not only for analyzing the histotoxicity of compounds, but also for the discovery of drugs that have protective effects against histotoxicity. Although we demonstrated the tissue distribution of ALT activity in the silkworm, the mechanism of tissue injury induction detected by elevated ALT levels remains unclear. The present silkworm model can be used to rapidly evaluate histotoxicity, but is not sufficient to elucidate the specific target of drugs. Further studies are needed to clarify the mechanism of tissue injury induction in silkworm.

The prediction of drug hepatotoxicity is crucial for drug discovery and development. Although small mammals such as mice and rats are generally used to evaluate hepatotoxicity, their use is associated with several problems, such as high experimental costs and ethical issues. *In vitro* assay systems using human hepatocytes have been developed in an attempt to solve these problems [38-40]. Toxicogenomic systems are suggested to be effective for predicting hepatotoxicity according to the varied expression of hepatotoxicity-responsive genes [41-43]. The collection of mammalian cells as a material and the conditional differences from *in vivo* examination, however, remain problems in these *in vitro* assay systems. The silkworm tissue injury model established in

the present study is a new animal model of histotoxicity. According to the tissue distribution of ALT activity, the gut had the highest ALT activity among other tissues in the silkworm. Thus, in the silkworm, increased ALT activity appears to be induced by tissue injury in the gut. This silkworm model would be extremely useful for evaluating the histotoxicity of newly synthesized chemicals prior to using mice or rats. We expect that the number of mammals needed for drug development can be reduced by first using the silkworm model.

Conclusions

The present study showed that ALT activity in the silkworm hemolymph is increased by the injection of various cytotoxic drugs. The present silkworm model is applicable for evaluating the toxicity of newly synthesized compounds. This method is more sensitive than toxicity assays based on counting the number of surviving silkworms after administration of test samples. Although further validation and applied research using other types of compounds must be performed, the use of this silkworm model prior to the use of mammals partially addresses the ethical and financial issues related to animal experiments using mammals.

Abbreviations
ALT: Alanine aminotransferase; *C. elegans*: *Caenorhabditis elegans*.

Competing interests
The authors and Genome Pharmaceuticals Institute Co., Ltd (Tokyo, Japan) declare that they have no competing interests. Employment costs for silkworm rearing were partially supported by Genome Pharmaceuticals Institute Co., Ltd (Tokyo, Japan).

Authors' contributions
KK and NM performed silkworm toxic assay. YI, YM and KS conceived the study and coordinated the writing of the manuscript. All authors read and approved the final manuscript.

Acknowledgements
This work was supported by a grant from the Ministry of Health, Labor, and Welfare (Research on Biological Resources and Animal Models for Drug Development) and Genome Pharmaceuticals Institute Co., Ltd (Tokyo, Japan).

References
1.   Bernuau J, Rueff B, Benhamou JP: **Fulminant and subfulminant liver failure: definitions and causes.** *Semin Liver Dis* 1986, **6**(2):97-106.
2.   Tanaka H, Uchida Y, Kaibori M, Hijikawa T, Ishizaki M, Yamada M, Matsui K, Ozaki T, Tokuhara K, Kamiyama Y, *et al*: **Na+/H+ exchanger inhibitor, FR183998, has protective effect in lethal acute liver failure and prevents iNOS induction in rats.** *J Hepatol* 2008, **48**(2):289-299.
3.   Itoh A, Isoda K, Kondoh M, Kawase M, Kobayashi M, Tamesada M, Yagi K: **Hepatoprotective effect of syringic acid and vanillic acid on concanavalin a-induced liver injury.** *Biol Pharm Bull* 2009, **32**(7):1215-1219.
4.   Girish C, Pradhan SC: **Drug development for liver diseases: focus on picroliv, ellagic acid and curcumin.** *Fundam Clin Pharmacol* 2008, **22**(6):623-632.
5.   Swem LR, Swem DL, O'Loughlin CT, Gatmaitan R, Zhao B, Ulrich SM, Bassler BL: **A quorum-sensing antagonist targets both membrane-bound and cytoplasmic receptors and controls bacterial pathogenicity.** *Mol Cell* 2009, **35**(2):143-153.

6. Limmer S, Haller S, Drenkard E, Lee J, Yu S, Kocks C, Ausubel FM, Ferrandon D: Pseudomonas aeruginosa RhlR is required to neutralize the cellular immune response in a Drosophila melanogaster oral infection model. *Proc Natl Acad Sci U S A* 2011, **108**(42):17378–17383.

7. Hamamoto H, Tonoike A, Narushima K, Horie R, Sekimizu K: **Silkworm as a model animal to evaluate drug candidate toxicity and metabolism.** *Comp Biochem Physiol C Toxicol Pharmacol* 2009, **149**(3):334–339.

8. Berger J: **Alternative haematotoxicological testing.** *J Appl Biomed* 2010, **8**:19–22.

9. Hamamoto H, Kurokawa K, Kaito C, Kamura K, Manitra Razanajatovo I, Kusuhara H, Santa T, Sekimizu K: **Quantitative evaluation of the therapeutic effects of antibiotics using silkworms infected with human pathogenic microorganisms.** *Antimicrob Agents Chemother* 2004, **48**(3):774–779.

10. Nagata M, Kaito C, Sekimizu K: **Phosphodiesterase activity of CvfA is required for virulence in Staphylococcus aureus.** *J Biol Chem* 2008, **283**(4):2176–2184.

11. Hanada Y, Sekimizu K, Kaito C: **Silkworm apolipophorin protein inhibits Staphylococcus aureus virulence.** *J Biol Chem* 2011, **286**(45):39360–39369.

12. Asami Y, Horie R, Hamamoto H, Sekimizu K: **Use of silkworms for identification of drug candidates having appropriate pharmacokinetics from plant sources.** *BMC Pharmacol* 2010, **10**:7.

13. Ozer J, Ratner M, Shaw M, Bailey W, Schomaker S: **The current state of serum biomarkers of hepatotoxicity.** *Toxicology* 2008, **245**(3):194–205.

14. Lindblom P, Rafter I, Copley C, Andersson U, Hedberg JJ, Berg AL, Samuelsson A, Hellmold H, Cotgreave I, Glinghammar B: **Isoforms of alanine aminotransferases in human tissues and serum–differential tissue expression using novel antibodies.** *Arch Biochem Biophys* 2007, **466**(1):66–77.

15. Galicia-Moreno M, Rodriguez-Rivera A, Reyes-Gordillo K, Segovia J, Shibayama M, Tsutsumi V, Vergara P, Moreno MG, Muriel P: **N-acetylcysteine prevents carbon tetrachloride-induced liver cirrhosis: role of liver transforming growth factor-beta and oxidative stress.** *Eur J Gastroenterol Hepatol* 2009, **21**(8):908–914.

16. Lee SS, Buters JT, Pineau T, Fernandez-Salguero P, Gonzalez FJ: **Role of CYP2E1 in the hepatotoxicity of acetaminophen.** *J Biol Chem* 1996, **271**(20):12063–12067.

17. Doi H, Horie T: **Salicylic acid-induced hepatotoxicity triggered by oxidative stress.** *Chem Biol Interact* 2010, **183**(3):363–368.

18. Damme B, Darmer D, Pankow D: **Induction of hepatic cytochrome P4502E1 in rats by acetylsalicylic acid or sodium salicylate.** *Toxicology* 1996, **106**(1–3):99–103.

19. Ramm GA, Ruddell RG: **Hepatotoxicity of iron overload: mechanisms of iron-induced hepatic fibrogenesis.** *Semin Liver Dis* 2005, **25**(4):433–449.

20. Fromenty B, Pessayre D: **Impaired mitochondrial function in microvesicular steatosis. Effects of drugs, ethanol, hormones and cytokines.** *J Hepatol* 1997, **26**(Suppl 2):43–53.

21. Labbe G, Fromenty B, Freneaux E, Morzelle V, Letteron P, Berson A, Pessayre D: **Effects of various tetracycline derivatives on in vitro and in vivo beta-oxidation of fatty acids, egress of triglycerides from the liver, accumulation of hepatic triglycerides, and mortality in mice.** *Biochem Pharmacol* 1991, **41**(4):638–641.

22. Fromenty B, Fisch C, Labbe G, Degott C, Deschamps D, Berson A, Letteron P, Pessayre D: **Amiodarone inhibits the mitochondrial beta-oxidation of fatty acids and produces microvesicular steatosis of the liver in mice.** *J Pharmacol Exp Ther* 1990, **255**(3):1371–1376.

23. Hubbard AK, Lohr CL, Hastings K, Clarke JB, Gandolfi AJ: **Immunogenicity studies of a synthetic antigen of alpha methyl dopa.** *Immunopharmacol Immunotoxicol* 1993, **15**(5):621–637.

24. Chien RN, Yang LJ, Lin PY, Liaw YF: **Hepatic injury during ketoconazole therapy in patients with onychomycosis: a controlled cohort study.** *Hepatology* 1997, **25**(1):103–107.

25. Berkovitch M, Pope E, Phillips J, Koren G: **Pemoline-associated fulminant liver failure: testing the evidence for causation.** *Clin Pharmacol Ther* 1995, **57**(6):696–698.

26. Kawaguchi T, Harada M, Arimatsu H, Nagata S, Koga Y, Kuwahara R, Hisamochi A, Hino T, Taniguchi E, Kumemura H, *et al*: **Severe hepatotoxicity associated with a N-nitrosofenfluramine-containing weight-loss supplement: report of three cases.** *J Gastroenterol Hepatol* 2004, **19**(3):349–350.

27. Shu L, Hollenberg PF: **Identification of the cytochrome P450 isozymes involved in the metabolism of N-nitrosodipropyl-, N-nitrosodibutyl- and N-nitroso-n-butyl-n-propylamine.** *Carcinogenesis* 1996, **17**(4):839–848.

28. Nakagawa Y, Tayama S, Ogata A, Suzuki T, Ishii H: **ATP-generating glycolytic substrates prevent N-nitrosofenfluramine-induced cytotoxicity in isolated rat hepatocytes.** *Chem Biol Interact* 2006, **164**(1–2):93–101.

29. Keppler DO, Rudigier JF, Bischoff E, Decker KF: **The trapping of uridine phosphates by D-galactosamine. D-glucosamine, and 2-deoxy-D-galactose. A study on the mechanism of galactosamine hepatitis.** *Eur J Biochem* 1970, **17**(2):246–253.

30. Banno Y, Shimada T, Kajiura Z, Sezutsu H: **The silkworm-an attractive BioResource supplied by Japan.** *Exp Anim* 2010, **59**(2):139–146.

31. Kaito C, Akimitsu N, Watanabe H, Sekimizu K: **Silkworm larvae as an animal model of bacterial infection pathogenic to humans.** *Microb Pathog* 2002, **32**(4):183–190.

32. Kaito C, Kurokawa K, Matsumoto Y, Terao Y, Kawabata S, Hamada S, Sekimizu K: **Silkworm pathogenic bacteria infection model for identification of novel virulence genes.** *Mol Microbiol* 2005, **56**(4):934–944.

33. Kaito C, Morishita D, Matsumoto Y, Kurokawa K, Sekimizu K: **Novel DNA binding protein SarZ contributes to virulence in Staphylococcus aureus.** *Mol Microbiol* 2006, **62**(6):1601–1617.

34. Kaito C, Sekimizu K: **A silkworm model of pathogenic bacterial infection.** *Drug Discov Ther* 2007, **1**(2):89–93.

35. Matsumoto Y, Miyazaki S, Fukunaga DH, Shimizu K, Kawamoto S, Sekimizu K: **Quantitative evaluation of cryptococcal pathogenesis and antifungal drugs using a silkworm infection model with Cryptococcus neoformans.** *J Appl Microbiol* 2012, **112**(1):138–146.

36. Matsumoto Y, Sumiya E, Sugita T, Sekimizu K: **An invertebrate hyperglycemic model for the identification of anti-diabetic drugs.** *PLoS One* 2011, **6**(3):e18292.

37. Prescott LF, Park J, Ballantyne A, Adriaenssens P, Proudfoot AT: **Treatment of paracetamol (acetaminophen) poisoning with N-acetylcysteine.** *Lancet* 1977, **2**(8035):432–434.

38. Butterworth BE, Smith-Oliver T, Earle L, Loury DJ, White RD, Doolittle DJ, Working PK, Cattley RC, Jirtle R, Michalopoulos G, *et al*: **Use of primary cultures of human hepatocytes in toxicology studies.** *Cancer Res* 1989, **49**(5):1075–1084.

39. Guillouzo A, Morel F, Langouet S, Maheo K, Rissel M: **Use of hepatocyte cultures for the study of hepatotoxic compounds.** *J Hepatol* 1997, **26**(Suppl 2):73–80.

40. Yeon JH, Na D, Park JK: **Hepatotoxicity assay using human hepatocytes trapped in microholes of a microfluidic device.** *Electrophoresis* 2010, **31**(18):3167–3174.

41. Martin R, Rose D, Yu K, Barros S: **Toxicogenomics strategies for predicting drug toxicity.** *Pharmacogenomics* 2006, **7**(7):1003–1016.

42. Suzuki H, Inoue T, Matsushita T, Kobayashi K, Horii I, Hirabayashi Y: **In vitro gene expression analysis of hepatotoxic drugs in rat primary hepatocytes.** *J Appl Toxicol* 2008, **28**(2):227–236.

43. Fan X, Lobenhofer EK, Chen M, Shi W, Huang J, Luo J, Zhang J, Walker SJ, Chu TM, Li L, *et al*: **Consistency of predictive signature genes and classifiers generated using different microarray platforms.** *Pharmacogenomics J* 2010, **10**(4):247–257.

16

Errors in medication history at hospital admission: prevalence and predicting factors

Lina M Hellström[1*], Åsa Bondesson[2], Peter Höglund[3] and Tommy Eriksson[3]

Abstract

Background: An accurate medication list at hospital admission is essential for the evaluation and further treatment of patients. The objective of this study was to describe the frequency, type and predictors of errors in medication history, and to evaluate the extent to which standard care corrects these errors.

Methods: A descriptive study was carried out in two medical wards in a Swedish hospital using Lund Integrated Medicines Management (LIMM)-based medication reconciliation. A clinical pharmacist identified each patient's most accurate pre-admission medication list by conducting a medication reconciliation process shortly after admission. This list was then compared with the patient's medication list in the hospital medical records. Addition or withdrawal of a drug or changes to the dose or dosage form in the hospital medication list were considered medication discrepancies. Medication discrepancies for which no clinical reason could be identified (unintentional changes) were considered medication history errors.

Results: The final study population comprised 670 of 818 eligible patients. At least one medication history error was identified by pharmacists conducting medication reconciliations for 313 of these patients (47%; 95% CI 43-51%). The most common medication error was an omitted drug, followed by a wrong dose. Multivariate logistic regression analysis showed that a higher number of drugs at admission (odds ratio [OR] per 1 drug increase = 1.10; 95% CI 1.06-1.14; p < 0.0001) and the patient living in their own home without any care services (OR = 1.58; 95% CI 1.02-2.45; p = 0.042) were predictors for medication history errors at admission. The results further indicated that standard care by non-pharmacist ward staff had partly corrected the errors in affected patients by four days after admission, but a considerable proportion of the errors made in the initial medication history at admission remained undetected by standard care (OR for medication errors detected by pharmacists' medication reconciliation carried out on days 4-11 compared to days 0-1 = 0.52; 95% CI 0.30-0.91; p=0.021).

Conclusions: Clinical pharmacists conducting LIMM-based medication reconciliations have a high potential for correcting errors in medication history for all patients. In an older Swedish population, those prescribed many drugs seem to benefit most from admission medication reconciliation.

Background

The problem of inaccurate medication lists at hospital admission and discharge is extensive [1-3] and has gained attention, specifically with regard to the issue of patient safety, in recent years [1,4]. An accurate medication list at hospital admission is essential for the evaluation and further treatment of patients, to prevent medication errors and adverse drug events in hospital and after discharge. Errors in the medication history are

sometimes identified and corrected early enough to prevent any harm to the patient and are then of no clinical importance, although the administrative work can waste valuable time for the health care staff involved. Unidentified errors, however, can result in the patient receiving potentially harmful, inaccurate treatment. Possible causes for the errors in medication histories are multifactorial, relating to the system, the patient, or the health care staff [1,5-7].

Medication reconciliation has been endorsed by patient safety organisations and authorities in a number of countries as a method of improving the accuracy of patients' medication lists [1,4,8]. The Institute for

* Correspondence: Lina.Hellstrom@lnu.se
[1]eHealth Institute and School of Natural Sciences, Linnaeus University, Kalmar, Sweden
Full list of author information is available at the end of the article

Healthcare Improvement in the United States has described medication reconciliation as being "the process of identifying the most accurate list of a patient's current medicines - including the name, dosage, frequency, and route - and comparing them to the current list in use, recognizing any discrepancies, and documenting any changes, thus resulting in a complete list of medications, accurately communicated" [1].

The Lund Integrated Medicines Management (LIMM) model offers a systematic approach for individualising and optimising drug treatment for inpatients [9]. The LIMM model has been continuously developed and implemented in a number of Swedish hospitals over more than ten years. This model includes a pharmacist intervention for medication reconciliation at admission, team interventions for medication reviews and monitoring during the hospital stay, and a discharge medication reconciliation procedure. Previous studies have associated the LIMM model with prescription of fewer inappropriate drugs [9,10] and reductions in the number of drug-related patient revisits to hospital [9,11] and primary care [11]. A smaller early study also suggested that using the LIMM medication reconciliation at admission would effectively identify errors in the medication history [12]. It is also important to carry out a more comprehensive evaluation of the subsequent actions of the pharmacists and medical practitioners. Evaluation of these actions (e.g. suggestions for change and changes made to the prescriptions) can provide insight into the factors responsible for the identified outcomes and suggestions for optimizing the intervention [13]. Furthermore, there is a need to determine whether it is possible to identify patients with the greatest risk of experiencing medication history errors at hospital admission. If those patients can be identified in clinical practice, it will enable better resource allocation, as interventions to prevent medication history errors can be directed towards the relevant groups. Results concerning which risk factors predict such errors in medication histories are currently contradictory [5-7,14-17].

The objective of this study was to describe the frequency and type of medication history errors identified by pharmacists performing medication reconciliations for patients admitted to a Swedish hospital, and to evaluate predictors for those medication errors. A secondary objective was to evaluate the degree to which standard care identifies errors in the medication history when the pharmacist's medication reconciliation is delayed.

Methods
Setting and population
This prospective study was conducted in two internal medicine wards (designated A and B) at the University hospital of Lund, Sweden. A LIMM-based clinical pharmacy service, including medication reconciliation at admission, was implemented in January and October, 2007, in the respective wards. All patients admitted to wards A and B after implementation of the service until the end of the year 2007, were eligible for inclusion in the study. Patients discharged or deceased before the pharmacist could conduct admission medication reconciliation were excluded from the study. There were 22 beds in each ward. The weekday staff in each ward comprised two junior physicians and two senior physicians, one clinical pharmacist, three nurses, three assistant nurses, one physiotherapist and one occupational therapist. Availability of beds alone decided the ward to which a patient was admitted. The wards used the standard hospital electronic health record (EHR) system (Melior®, Siemens Corp.); this was used in all hospital wards but was not used in primary care. The primary care centres in the region surrounding the hospital used either another EHR system or paper-based health records. Community care services used paper-based medication lists. The different levels of care (i.e. primary, secondary and community care) exchanged information about the patients' current medication lists by phone, fax, or mail. No electronic communications between the hospital and the primary care centres or community care services was possible at the time of the study. The regional ethical board of the University of Lund, Sweden, did not consider ethical approval to be necessary and had no objections to the study.

Collection of data
A two-step procedure was used to collect and classify data on medication discrepancies and errors in the medication histories. Firstly, clinical pharmacists conducted medication reconciliations and documented their work in a LIMM medication interview questionnaire form (Additional file 1). Five different pharmacists worked at the wards during the study period. Secondly, two pharmacy students and a research pharmacist classified the identified discrepancies and errors.

The medication reconciliation process in the LIMM model
The admission medication reconciliation process in the LIMM model is comprehensive and was developed over about 5 years and implemented on top of standard care [9,12]. Following a strict protocol, clinical pharmacists identified the patient's pre-admission medication list. For patients capable of participation and willing to participate, an initial medication interview was conducted. The pharmacist asked which medications and dosages the patient had been taking before admission. Specific questions were asked about the use of painkillers, heart medications, stomach medications, sleeping pills, antidiabetics, eye drops, inhalation drugs, over-the-counter

drugs and herbal drugs, in order to increase the probability of including all the patient's medications. Sometimes, a medical interview was conducted with a close relative instead of the patient. In addition (or otherwise, if an interview could not be conducted), the pharmacist consulted all available pre-admission lists, including drug lists from primary and community care, the national pharmacy register (all drugs dispensed within the past 15 months) [18], and prescription forms from the medication dispensing system ApoDos (a multi-dose system where all medications that the patient should be taking on one occasion are machine-packed together in small, fully labelled plastic bags at a pharmacy dispensing centre and delivered to the patient every second week) [19]. Based on this information, a list with the patient's prescribed medications was documented in the LIMM medication interview questionnaire, part 1 (Additional file 1). Parts 2 and 3 of the LIMM medication interview questionnaire were conducted with some patients; these parts comprised questions about knowledge of, practical handling of, adherence with, and beliefs about medications [9]. This paper reports the results from part 1 only.

The pre-admission medication list identified by the pharmacist was regarded as the most accurate list available since it was based on all available information sources and had been compiled according to a well established, systematic method [5,6,20-22]. Differences between this pharmacist-compiled pre-admission medication list and the medication list in the hospital EHR were documented in the LIMM medication interview questionnaire. The pharmacist consulted the patient's EHR to establish possible reasons for the differences. Discrepancies noted in the hospital medication list which the pharmacist judged relevant and possibly requiring correction were discussed with a ward physician. The pharmacist recommended corrections for the hospital EHR, and the physician then made the final decision and was responsible for correcting the hospital EHR list when necessary. The use of over-the-counter drugs and herbal drugs by the patients was also documented in the questionnaire and discussed with the physician when considered clinically relevant. The pharmacists' recommendations and the subsequent actions by the physician or pharmacist were documented in a medication review form.

It was ward policy that a clinical pharmacist should conduct the LIMM-based medication reconciliation within one day of admission to the ward or on Mondays for patients admitted on weekends. Medication reconciliation was conducted once for each patient and took on average 32 minutes per patient if a patient interview was conducted and 15 minutes if no interview was conducted [unpublished observations, personal communication Tommy Eriksson 27/03/2012]. This time included the face-to-face discussion with a physician about discrepancies in the hospital medication list.

Occasionally, it took longer than one day for the pharmacist to conduct the medication reconciliation. This was attributed to time constraints, lack of personnel, or temporarily closed wards because of an infection outbreak among the patients. If a clinical pharmacist was not available, physicians and/or nurses occasionally corrected errors in the medication history (standard care), but there were no instructions or forms for these changes, in contrast to the LIMM-based structured medication reconciliations.

Definition and classification of medication discrepancies and errors

The identified differences between the pharmacist-acquired medication list and the medication list in the EHR were classified retrospectively by reviewing the LIMM medication interview questionnaires and the EHR. A medication discrepancy was defined as an addition or withdrawal of a drug, or a change to the dose or dosage form. An incorrect dosage interval was not defined as a discrepancy if the total dosage/24 h had not been changed. Changes to an equivalent generic drug or withdrawal of drugs with a long dosage interval, e.g. once monthly, were also not regarded as medication discrepancies. The medication discrepancies were further classified by type: drug omitted (the drug had not been registered in the hospital EHR drug list), additional drug (a drug had been erroneously added to the hospital EHR drug list), dosage too high, dosage too low, or wrong dosage form.

Medication discrepancies for which the reviewing pharmacists could not identify any clinical reason (unintentional changes) were deemed to be medication errors. Our definition of a medication error was based on the definition proposed by Leape [23]: "A medication error is any error in the process of prescribing, dispensing or administering a drug, whether there are adverse consequences or not". There were two exceptions to this: that only errors in the medication history were included, and that discrepancies corrected before reaching the patient were not considered medication errors. For example, discrepancies concerning weekly doses that were identified before the dosing occasion or involving omission of drugs that were to be given as needed and which the patient had not yet required were not counted as errors. Over-the-counter drugs and herbal drugs were not included in the drug list in the EHR and hence could not result in medication discrepancies or errors.

Two pharmacy students (doing their Masters theses) were responsible for the classification of medication discrepancies and errors as described above. They were informed by a research pharmacist (ÅB) about the classification procedure and they continually discussed any lack of clarity with the research pharmacist. To evaluate the percent of cases which the raters agreed upon, 30 patients were classified independently by the two students and one research pharmacist (LH). The agreement with regard to the number and type of medication errors was 83%.

Statistics

An open source software based on the R language and environment for statistical computing (http://www.R-project.org) was used for all statistical analyses [24]. Descriptive statistics are shown as medians (interquartile range), means (95% confidence intervals, CI) and frequencies or percentages (95% CI) when appropriate. The denominator for calculating the error rate was the number of prescribed medications in the hospital EHR before medication reconciliation, plus any medications omitted. A multivariable binary logistic regression analysis was conducted where the response variable was the presence or absence of medication errors. The following model variables were pre-specified potential predictors: number of drugs at admission (every increase by one drug), age (every 10 years' increase), sex (0 = Female, 1 = Male), type of care service before admission (0 = Living in own home with no care service, 1 = Living in own home but enrolled in community home care services, 2 = Living in care home), and directly admitted to the study ward without transferral from another ward (0 = No, 1 = Yes). In addition, the extent to which standard care identified medication errors was evaluated by including the number of days from admission to the ward until medication reconciliation (0 = 0-1 days, 1 = 2-3 days, 2 = 4 days or more) in the model. This variable was not considered a potential predictor but was included in order to evaluate if the medication errors remained undetected by standard care if the LIMM admission medication reconciliation was delayed. The variables "2-3 days" and "4 days or more" were not targeted controls; the medication reconciliation was delayed because of time constraints or other factors and never deliberately. No variables were eliminated from the regression model. Eleven percent of the data for the variable "directly admitted to the study ward", and 10% for "number of days from admission to the ward until medication reconciliation" were missing. Data were complete for the other variables. In the multivariable regression model, missing data was imputed using a multiple imputation method [25]. The le Cessie-van Houwelingen-Copas-Hosmer unweighted sum of squares test for global goodness of fit was used to assess the fit of the model [25]. The significance level in the analysis was set to 0.05.

Results

Description of the study sample

In total, 818 patients were eligible for inclusion. Patients who did not receive a medication reconciliation (n = 137) and patients for whom important demographic and study data were missing (n = 11) were excluded. The final study population comprised 670 patients: 524 in ward A and 146 in ward B. The characteristics of the study population are summarised in Table 1. Most of the patients (62%) were aged over 80 years and 66% had been prescribed more than five drugs for regular use before admission to hospital. Seven percent were younger than 65 years. There were no differences in patient characteristics between wards A and B.

Description of the medication reconciliation process

The clinical pharmacists identified 1136 medication discrepancies between the lists for 420 of 670 patients (63%; 95% CI 59 to 66%). The mean of medication discrepancies in the total cohort was 1.7 (95% CI 1.6-1.8) per patient, and the mean per affected patient was 2.7 (95% CI 2.5-2.9). The actions of the pharmacists and physicians after the initial identification of discrepancies are summarised in Figure 1. The pharmacists recommended correction of 813 discrepancies (71%). For 567 of the 813 suggestions (70%), the medication list was corrected accordingly by the physician. In 193 cases (24%), it was unknown whether the medication list was corrected after the pharmacist's recommendation. Either the discrepancy was no longer relevant for the patient, or the pharmacist did not document the results because of lack of time, or the physician never decided on an eventual correction.

Frequency and types of errors in medication history

Of the 1136 identified medication discrepancies, 672 (59%) were classified as medication errors. These errors affected 313 patients, representing a frequency of 47% (95% CI 43 to 51%). The error rate was 10.2% (672/6582) of the total number of prescribed drugs at

Table 1 Characteristics of the study participants (n = 670)

Age, mean, in years (SD)	81 (10)
Sex, % female	53%
Number of drugs at admission, median (IQR)	
Regular use	7 (5-11)
As needed	1 (0-2)
Patients using a multi-dose system (ApoDos®), % of patients	21%
Length of stay in the ward, median days (IQR)	8 (4-12)
Number of drugs at discharge, median (IQR)	
Regular use	8 (5-11)
As needed	1 (1-3)

SD, standard deviation. IQR, interquartile range

Activities by clinical pharmacists

Activities by physicians

| Correction of medication list after pharmacist's recommendation N=567 MD (549 ME) |

| Identification of medication discrepancies N=1139 MD (672 ME) | → | Correction of medication list recommended N=813 MD (582 ME) |

| No correction of medication list necessary according to discussion between physician and pharmacist N=41 MD (3 ME) |

| No correction of medication list recommended N=326 MD (90 ME) | | No further documentation N=193 MD (18 ME) |

| Medication list corrected by physician before the recommendation was discussed N=12 MD (12 ME) |

Reasons for not recommending correction

• No correction of medication list necessary according to pharmacist N=78 MD (6 ME)
• Medication list corrected by physician before the recommendation was discussed N=68 MD (66 ME)
• Reason not documented N=180 MD (18 ME)

Figure 1 Illustration of the medication reconciliation process. The figure includes the number of identified medication discrepancies (MD), the number of pharmacist-suggested changes, and the number of corrected drug prescriptions. The number of discrepancies that were later classified as medication errors (ME) by the reviewing pharmacists is also given.

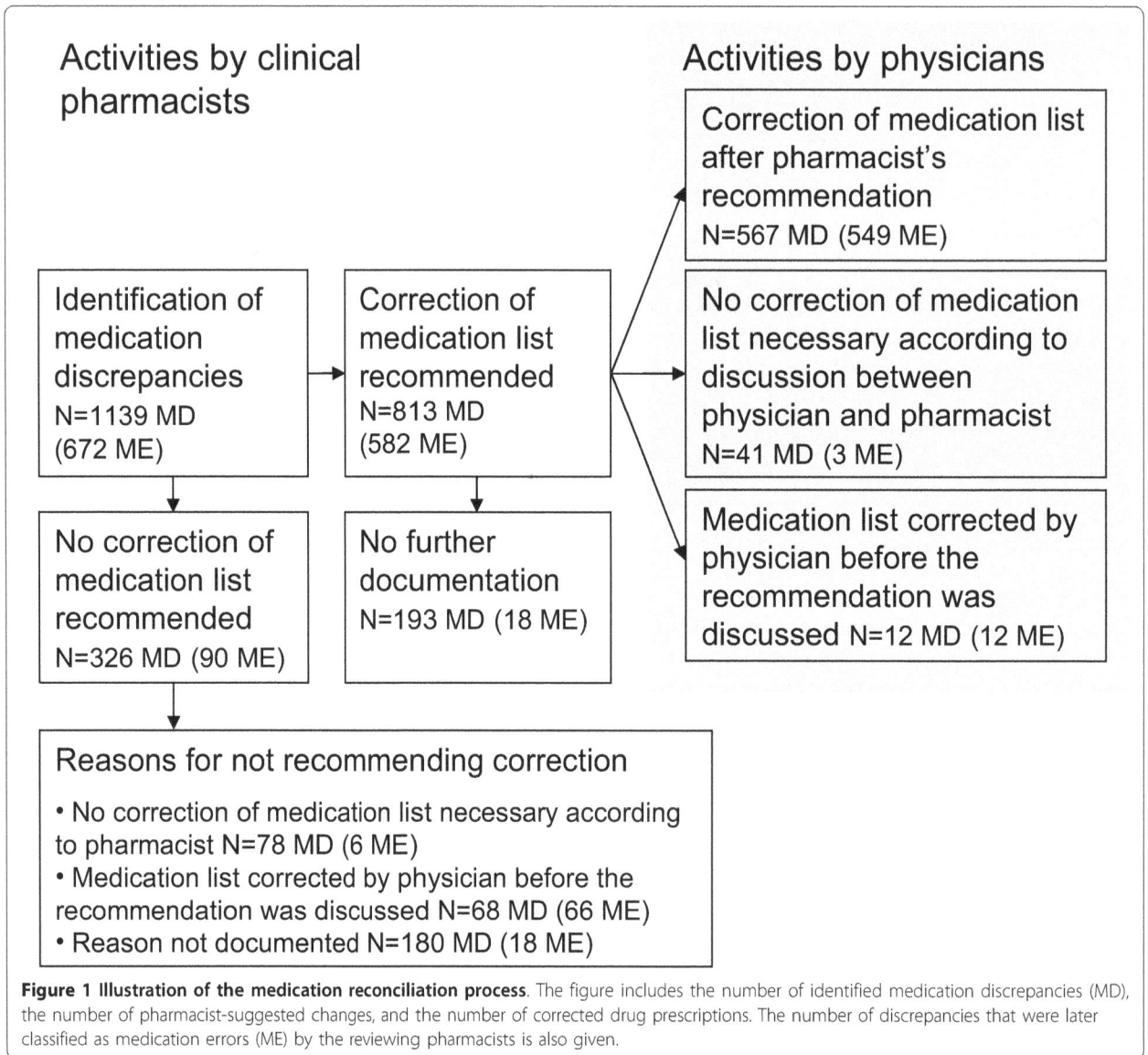

hospital admission. The overall mean (in the total cohort) was 1.0 (95% CI 0.9-1.1) medication error per patient, and the mean per affected patient was 2.1 (95% CI 1.9-2.3). Twenty-three percent of the patients had one error, 11% had two errors and 13% had between three to nine errors. The most common medication error was omission of a drug, followed by a wrong dose. The frequencies of the various types of medication error and the most commonly associated drug classes are shown in Table 2. Overall, 93% (n = 627) of the medication errors resulted in correction of the EHR medication lists, as a result of either the pharmacist's suggestion (n = 549) or the physician's initiative before the pharmacist's suggestion (n = 78) (Figure 1).

Predicting errors in medication history

In the multivariable logistic regression model, an increased number of drugs at admission and absence of any care service before hospital admission (i.e. patients living in their own homes without community care service) were significant predictors for medication errors (Table 3). The odds for a patient experiencing at least one medication error increased by 10% for every additional medication at admission (OR 1.10; 95% CI 1.06-1.14). Among patients living in their own homes without any care service, 48% experienced at least one error compared to 47% of those living in a care home (OR 1.58; 95% CI 1.02-2.45). The remaining prediction factors included in the regression model showed no correlation with the risk of experiencing medication errors.

Table 2 Number of medication errors by type, and most frequent ATC codes for each type of error.

Type of error	Medication errors; numbers (%)	The three most frequent ATC codes by type of error; number of errors					
		B03	C07	N02	N05	N06	R03
Omission of drug	417 (62)			37	37		47
Dose too high	86 (13)	8		9	11		
Dose too low	82 (12)			11	12	7	
Additional drug	79 (12)			7	8		8
Wrong dosage form	8 (1)		3	3			2
Total	672 (100)			67	68		57

ATC-codes: B03, Antianemic preparations; C07, Beta-blocking agents; N02, Analgesics; N05, Psycholeptics; N06, Psychoanaleptics; R03, Drugs for obstructive pulmonary disease
ATC, Anatomic Therapeutic Chemical

Correction of errors in medication history by standard care

As the variable for the number of days until medication reconciliation was included in the regression model, it can be assumed that the patients reconciled on days 4-11 had the same adjusted rate of medication error when they were admitted to hospital as the rest of the patients. The odds ratio for medication errors detected by pharmacist medication reconciliation was 0.52 (95% CI 0.30-0.91) on days 4-11 (Table 3). The results thus suggest that, in a statistically significant proportion of the patients reconciled on days 4-11 who had medication errors at admission, the errors had already been corrected at the time of pharmacist medication reconciliation and that standard care was responsible for these corrections. In the remaining patients who had medication errors in their EHRs at admission, the errors were still undetected by standard care after 4-11 days and instead identified by the pharmacist medication reconciliation. Within 2-3 days after admission, the probability that a pharmacist would detect the errors was as high as that on days 0-1 (Table 3), i.e. standard care did not correct significantly more errors when the pharmacist's medication reconciliation was moderately delayed.

Discussion

In our study population of mainly older patients, approximately 50% were affected by errors in the medication history at admission to hospital. The most common error was the erroneous omission of a drug from the hospital EHR medication list. Predictors of the

Table 3 Predictors of errors in the medication history at admission to hospital.

Potential predictors		Number of patients with an error (%)	Odds ratio (95% CI)
Number of drugs at admission	For each 1-drug increase	313 (47)	1.10 (1.06-1.14)*
Age	For each 10-yr increase	313 (47)	1.08 (0.92-1.27)
Ward	A	250 (48)	Reference
	B	63 (43)	0.82 (0.56-1.21)
Sex	Male	135 (43)	Reference
	Female	178 (50)	1.33 (0.96-1.83)
Type of care service before admission	Care home	63 (47)	Reference
	Own home with community care services	74 (45)	1.08 (0.67-1.75)
	Own home, no care service	176 (48)	1.58 (1.02-2.45)*
Directly admitted to study ward [a]	Yes	155 (47)	Reference
	No; transferred from another ward	131 (49)	1.12 (0.80-1.57)
Days until medication reconciliation			
Number of days until the pharmacist's medication reconciliation [a]	0-1 days	168 (51)	Reference
	2-3 days	101 (49)	0.85 (0.59-1.23)
	4-11 days	24 (38)	0.52 (0.30-0.91)*

Odds ratios were derived from a multivariable binary logistic regression model
* p < 0.05
[a]Number (%) of patients is reported only for those with complete data. In the logistic regression model missing data was imputed

occurrence of medication errors included an increased number of preadmission drugs and living in one's own home without community care service.

Our findings are similar to those of other studies [2,17,20], but there are also reports of lower [15] or higher [2,6] rates of error in medication histories at hospital admission. Different definitions of medication discrepancies and errors and variability in methods of data collection could explain the differences between studies and make it difficult to compare rates of error across studies.

The association between the number of prescribed drugs at admission and the occurrence of medication errors was not surprising. Previously, some researchers have found associations between errors in the medication history and the number of drugs at admission [5,14], but some have not [6,15,16]. To the best of our knowledge, the association between absence of any care service before admission and medication errors has not been previously suggested. It is likely that the type of care service is not, in itself, important. Rather, the availability of a current medication list at hospital admission might be the important underlying factor. Patients in community care or care homes often take a current medication list with them to hospital, possibly facilitating the recording of the initial medication history by a physician or nurse and subsequently lowering the risk for medication errors. However, the absolute difference between the groups (48% vs 47% of patients with an error, as seen in Table 3) was small and the value of this predictor in clinical practice would be limited. Also, the influence of this predictor is likely to vary substantially between settings and above all between countries; it will depend on the level of communication between community care services and the hospital, and on the routines for the patient taking their medication lists or medications with them when attending the emergency department.

There are varying results from other research on predictors for errors in the medication history. In accordance with our results, Gleason and colleagues found that there were few predictors associated with medication errors at admission and they suggested that well-designed processes for medication history verification were more important than patient characteristics [5]. In contrast to our results, some researchers have found that higher age [5,14,15] is a significant predictor. However, the patients in our study wards were older than those in previous studies [5,14,15], and our results might have differed if the patient cohort had been younger. Previous studies have identified significant predictors for errors in the medication history which were not included in our regression model, e.g. certain "high-

risk" drugs, many outpatient visits during the previous year, and staffing levels [6,7].

The relative importance of the medication reconciliation by a pharmacist in terms of added value compared to standard care was also of interest. Optimally, this should be studied in a randomized, controlled trial. Because we were unable to carry out a randomized trial, we used an indirect measure to evaluate the degree to which standard care corrected medication errors. The pharmacists did not conduct the medication reconciliation until 4-11 days after admission for 20% of the patients due to time constraints or lack of personnel. If standard care had not identified and corrected any medication errors at all, the probability that the pharmacists identified medication errors on days 4-11 would have been as high as that on days 0-1. However, regression analysis suggested that the probability that there would still be an error in a patient's medication history after 4 or more days in the ward was lower compared to days 0-1. This implies that standard care had had partly corrected the errors in affected patients by that time, but a considerable proportion of the errors made in the initial EHR medication history at admission remained undetected by standard care. Two to three days after admission, the probability that patients would still be prescribed the wrong drug or dose was as high as the first day after admission. The potentially severe nature of some of the errors in medication history [5,17,21] underlines the importance of reconciling the medication list soon after admission to avoid patient harm as a consequence of error, preferably within 24 hours of admission.

We believe it is necessary for medication reconciliation processes to be well designed and systematic, and aided by structured forms and detailed guidelines. Clinical pharmacists, as key members of a multidisciplinary team, are very well suited to perform such systematic medication reconciliations. A review by the British National Institute for Health and Clinical Excellence [1] showed that there is evidence that pharmacist interventions are the most effective among the studied medication reconciliation interventions. However, it was commented that the current evidence is poor and further comparative studies of different medication reconciliation programs will be needed to reveal which approach is most effective from a clinical and economic perspective. There are many promising and emerging technologies that may be effective in medicines reconciliation as well. Nonetheless, our results highlight the benefits of structured reconciliations by pharmacists over occasional reconciliations as part of standard care.

The physicians' acceptance of the pharmacists' recommended changes to drug therapy is often used in studies of clinical pharmacy services as a measure of quality. In this study, 94% of the recommendations from the pharmacist concerning errors in medication history were accepted and implemented by the physicians, which suggests that the process was effective. In a number of cases, there was no information about the measures taken by the physicians after the pharmacists' recommendations, or about the pharmacists' reasons for not recommending changes to the medication list. More precise documentation might have provided even better insight into the effectiveness of the process.

This study adds to the evidence that LIMM-based patient care in hospital offers a positive contribution. We detected and corrected medication errors in almost half of the study patients. Although this study did not evaluate possible harm from these errors, a study including a sample of our study patients reported the clinical significance of pharmacists' recommendations [26]. Recommendations were ranked by two physicians on a six-point scale from 1 (adverse significance) to 6 (extremely significant). Of 70 recommendations, 59% were ranked somewhat significant, 23% significant and 10% very significant. Seven percent had no significance and one recommendation was judged to have adverse significance. However, this case did not result in documented patient harm. Fifty-six of our study patients were also followed up as part of an intervention study [9]. That study showed that LIMM-based medication reconciliation at admission and medication reviews in hospital improve the appropriateness of drug therapy and may also decrease drug-related revisits to hospital. The results of the admission process (i.e. the correction of medication errors) in the present study are therefore very likely to be at least partly responsible for these positive clinical outcomes [9].

This study had several limitations. Firstly, it was conducted in an internal medicine population in a single hospital, which limits the generalisability. Secondly, acceptance of the pharmacist-acquired medication list as the most accurate preadmission drug list available could be questioned. It is possible that some medication discrepancies escaped our detection. However, studies have shown that pharmacists appear to be especially suited and more effective than physicians when obtaining medication histories [22] and the methods used by pharmacists to obtain medication histories are well established [5,6,20,21]. Our method was strengthened by the fact that the pharmacists used a number of different information sources apart from the patient interview; for example, pharmacy records are known to improve the accuracy of medication lists [27]. The pharmacists were also well informed of the requirements and followed a strict protocol for the medication reconciliation process. Thirdly, the classification of discrepancies into

medication errors partly relies on subjective judgment and is therefore subject to bias.

Conclusions

We conclude that medication history errors at hospital admission are common, which highlights the importance of introducing processes for ensuring that the medication lists are accurate and complete as soon as possible after admission. Clinical pharmacists can be valuable in performing structured medication reconciliations to reduce the risk of medication errors. Our findings suggest that there is limited potential for predicting which patients are at highest risk of experiencing errors in their medication history. More research is needed, particularly to uncover the reasons for the possible impact of pre-admission care services on medication errors. In general, we believe that systematic medication reconciliations should be conducted in all patients admitted to hospital. Among older patients admitted to Swedish hospitals, those being prescribed many drugs could benefit the most from admission medication reconciliations by clinical pharmacists.

Additional material

> **Additional file 1: LIMM Medication Interview Questionnaire.** The LIMM Medication Interview Questionnaire used by the clinical pharmacists when conducting admission medication reconciliation.

Acknowledgements
The authors thank the pharmacists Kristin Holmqvist and Nedal Ahmad for skilful help with the collection and classification of data, all staff of the study wards, and the clinical pharmacists who were members of the team. The contributions of the Hospital pharmacy, Skåne University Hospital in Lund, Sweden, former employer of Lina Hellström and Åsa Bondesson, are gratefully acknowledged. The study was funded by Apoteket AB (a national corporation of Swedish pharmacies), Skåne Regional Council and Linnaeus University, Sweden.

Author details
[1]eHealth Institute and School of Natural Sciences, Linnaeus University, Kalmar, Sweden. [2]Department of Medicines Management and Informatics, Skåne Regional council, Malmö, Sweden. [3]Department of Clinical Pharmacology, Lund University, Lund, Sweden.

Authors' contributions
All authors were involved in designing the study. ÅB, TE and LH were involved in the collection of data. ÅB, TE, PH and LH interpreted the data. LH and PH were responsible for the statistical analysis. LH drafted the first version of the manuscript and all authors made critical revisions to the manuscript. All authors gave final approval to the manuscript.

Competing interests
The authors declare that they have no competing interests.

References
1.   Campbell F, Karnon J, Czoski-Murray C, Jones R: A systematic review of the effectiveness and cost-effectiveness of interventions aimed at

preventing medication error (medicines reconciliation) at hospital admission. *The University of Sheffield, School of Health and Related Research: Sheffield* 2007.

2. Tam VC, Knowles SR, Cornish PL, Fine N, Marchesano R, Etchells EE: **Frequency, type and clinical importance of medication history errors at admission to hospital: a systematic review.** *CMAJ* 2005, **173**:510-515.

3. Chhabra PT, Rattinger GB, Dutcher SK, Hare ME, Parsons KL, Zuckerman IH: **Medication reconciliation during the transition to and from long-term care settings: A systematic review.** *Res Social Adm Pharm* 2012, **8**:60-75.

4. World Health Organization: **Assuring medication accuracy at transitions in care.** *Standard operating protocol fact sheet* , Retrieved March 14, 2012 from http://www.who.int/patientsafety/implementation/solutions/high5s/ps_medication_reconciliation_fs_2010_en.pdf.

5. Gleason KM, McDaniel MR, Feinglass J, Baker DW, Lindquist L, Liss D, Noskin GA: **Results of the medications at transitions and clinical handoffs (MATCH) study: an analysis of medication reconciliation errors and risk factors at hospital admission.** *J Gen Intern Med* 2010, **25**:441-447.

6. Pippins JR, Gandhi TK, Hamann C, Ndumele CD, Labonville SA, Diedrichsen EK, Carty MG, Karson AS, Bhan I, Coley CM, *et al*: **Classifying and predicting errors of inpatient medication reconciliation.** *J Gen Intern Med* 2008, **23**:1414-1422.

7. Picone DM, Titler MG, Dochterman J, Shever L, Kim T, Abramowitz P, Kanak M, Qin R: **Predictors of medication errors among elderly hospitalized patients.** *Am J Med Qual* 2008, **23**:115-127.

8. The Joint Comission: *National Patient Safety Goals Effective July 1, 2011. Hospital Accreditation Program* , Retrieved March 14, 2012 from http://www.jointcommission.org/assets/1/6/NPSG_EPs_Scoring_HAP_20110706.pdf.

9. Hellstrom LM, Bondesson A, Hoglund P, Midlov P, Holmdahl L, Rickhag E, Eriksson T: **Impact of the Lund integrated medicines management (LIMM) model on medication appropriateness and drug-related hospital revisits.** *Eur J Clin Pharmacol* 2011, **67**:741-752.

10. Bergkvist A, Midlov P, Hoglund P, Larsson L, Eriksson T: **A multi-intervention approach on drug therapy can lead to a more appropriate drug use in the elderly. LIMM-Landskrona Integrated Medicines Management.** *J Eval Clin Pract* 2009, **15**:660-667.

11. Midlov P, Deierborg E, Holmdahl L, Hoglund P, Eriksson T: **Clinical outcomes from the use of medication report when elderly patients are discharged from hospital.** *Pharm World Sci* 2008, **30**:840-845.

12. Bondesson A, Hellstrom L, Eriksson T, Hoglund P: **A structured questionnaire to assess patient compliance and beliefs about medicines taking into account the ordered categorical structure of data.** *J Eval Clin Pract* 2009, **15**:713-723.

13. Craig P, Dieppe P, Macintyre S, Michie S, Nazareth I, Petticrew M: **Developing and evaluating complex interventions: the new medical research council guidance.** *BMJ* 2008, **337**:a1655.

14. Climente-Marti M, Garcia-Manon ER, Artero-Mora A, Jimenez-Torres NV: **Potential risk of medication discrepancies and reconciliation errors at admission and discharge from an inpatient medical service.** *Ann Pharmacother* 2010, **44**:1747-1754.

15. Unroe KT, Pfeiffenberger T, Riegelhaupt S, Jastrzembski J, Lokhnygina Y, Colon-Emeric C: **Inpatient medication reconciliation at admission and discharge: a retrospective cohort study of age and other risk factors for medication discrepancies.** *Am J Geriatr Pharmacother* 2010, **8**:115-126.

16. Andersen SE, Pedersen AB, Bach KF: **Medication history on internal medicine wards: assessment of extra information collected from second drug interviews and GP lists.** *Pharmacoepidemiol Drug Saf* 2003, **12**:491-498.

17. Cornish PL, Knowles SR, Marchesano R, Tam V, Shadowitz S, Juurlink DN, Etchells EE: **Unintended medication discrepancies at the time of hospital admission.** *Arch Intern Med* 2005, **165**:424-429.

18. Astrand B, Hovstadius B, Antonov K, Petersson G: **The Swedish national pharmacy register.** *Stud Health Technol Inform* 2007, **129**:345-349.

19. Larsson A, Åkerlund M: **Apodos: the Swedish model of multi-dose.** *EJHP Practice* 2007, **13**:51.

20. De Winter S, Spriet I, Indevuyst C, Vanbrabant P, Desruelles D, Sabbe M, Gillet JB, Wilmer A, Willems L: **Pharmacist- versus physician-acquired medication history: a prospective study at the emergency department.** *Qual Saf Health Care* 2010, **19**:371-375.

21. Slee A, Farrar K, Hughes D, Constable S: **Optimising medical treatment - how pharmacist-acquired medication histories have a positive impact on patient care.** *Pharm J* 2006, **277**:737-739.

22. Reeder TA, Mutnick A: **Pharmacist- versus physician-obtained medication histories.** *Am J Health Syst Pharm* 2008, **65**:857-860.

23. Leape LL: **Preventing adverse drug events.** *Am J Health Syst Pharm* 1995, **52**:379-382.

24. R Development Core Team: *R: a language and environment for statistical computing* Vienna, Austria: R Foundation for Statistical Computing; 2009.

25. Harrell FE: *Regression Modeling Strategies with Applications to Linear Models, Logistic Regression, and Survival Analysis* New York: Springer-Verlag; 2001.

26. Bondesson A, Holmdahl L, Midlov P, Hoglund P, Andersson E, Eriksson T: **Acceptance and importance of clinical pharmacists' LIMM-based recommendations.** *Int J Clin Pharm* 2012.

27. Glintborg B, Poulsen HE, Dalhoff KP: **The use of nationwide on-line prescription records improves the drug history in hospitalized patients.** *Br J Clin Pharmacol* 2008, **65**:265-269.

Pre-publication history

The pre-publication history for this paper can be accessed here:
http://www.biomedcentral.com/1472-6904/12/9/prepub

17

The association between prescription change frequency, chronic disease score and hospital admissions: a case control study

Carolien GM Sino[1*], Rutger Stuffken[2,3], Eibert R Heerdink[2], Marieke J Schuurmans[1,4], Patrick C Souverein[2] and Toine (A) CG Egberts[2,5]

Abstract

Background: The aim of this study was to assess the association between prescription changes frequency (PCF) and hospital admissions and to compare the PCF to the Chronic Disease Score (CDS). The CDS measures comorbidity on the basis of the 1-year pharmacy dispensing data. In contrast, the PCF is based on prescription changes over a 3-month period.

Methods: A retrospective matched case–control design was conducted. 10.000 patients were selected randomly from the Dutch PHARMO database, who had been hospitalized (index date) between July 1, 1998 and June 30, 2000. The primary study outcome was the number of prescription changes during several three-month time periods starting 18, 12, 9, 6, and 3 months before the index date. For each hospitalized patient, one nonhospitalized patient was matched for age, sex, and geographic area, and was assigned the same index date as the corresponding hospitalized patient. We classified four mutually exclusive types of prescription changes: change in dosage, switch, stop and start.

Results: The study population comprised 8,681 hospitalized patients and an equal number of matched nonhospitalized patients. The odds ratio of hospital admission increased with an increase in PCF category. At 3 months before the index date from PCF=1 OR 1.4 [95% CI 1.3-1.5] to PCF= 2–3 OR 2.2 [95% CI 1.9-2.4] and to PCF ≥ 4 OR 4.1 [95% CI 3.1-5.1]. A higher CDS score was also associated with an increased odds ratio of hospitalization: OR 1.3 (95% CI 1.2-1.4) for CDS 3–4, and OR 3.0 (95% CI 2.7-3.3) for CDS 5 or higher.

Conclusion: The prescription change frequency (PCF) is associated with hospital admission, like the CDS. Pharmacists and other healthcare workers should be alert when the frequency of prescription changes increases. Clinical rules could be helpful to make pharmacists and physicians aware of the risk of the number of prescription changes.

Keywords: Prescription changes, Prescription change frequency, Hospital admission, Chronic disease score

Background

Medication-related problems are responsible for 3–10% of acute hospital admissions, of which approximately half are potentially preventable [1-11]. Hospital admissions can lead to additional functional decline [12,13], unintentional harm [14], and increased costs. Medication monitoring and management are methods used to avoid medication-related complications.

In 2008, the Dutch HARM study group established seven independent risk factors for medication-related hospital admissions: (a) impaired cognition, (b) four or more diseases in the patient's medical history, (c) dependent living situation, (d) impaired renal function before hospitalization, (e) non-adherence to medication regimen, (f) the use of five or more medications at the time of admission (polypharmacy), and (g) age over 65 [11]. In the industrialized world, the proportion of the population that is 65 years or older is rapidly increasing. Elderly patients more often suffer from multiple morbidities, use more medications, and are treated by more healthcare

* Correspondence: Carolien.sino@hu.nl
[1]University of Applied Sciences Utrecht, Research Centre for Innovation in Healthcare, Bolognalaan 101, 3584 Utrecht, CJ, The Netherlands
Full list of author information is available at the end of the article

professionals than younger patients [15]. Drug consumption is three times higher among people aged 65 years or older, and four times higher in people aged 75 years or older, than it is in people younger than 65 years. The majority of these drugs are taken chronically (www.SFK.nl). The increased use of prescription drugs by the elderly is a consequence of their longer lifespan, their increasing use of health services, and the availability of new drugs [16]. From a clinical perspective, prescription changes are a risk factor for medication-related hospital admission. During the course of a disease, it may be necessary to change the dosage of medication, to switch to a similar medication, to temporarily withdraw the drug, or to start a new drug. With the exception of the study of Koecheler [17], who reported 'medication regimen changes in four or more times during the past 12 months' to be one of the six prognostic indicators for identifying ambulatory patients who need pharmacist monitoring, there have been no other studies that evaluated the association between the number of prescription changes and hospital admission. For this reason, we investigated whether the frequency of prescription changes is associated with hospital admission, and, if so, whether the strength of this association changes in the months before hospital admission.

The Chronic Disease Score (CDS), a well-established instrument to predict hospital admission, measures comorbidity on the basis of the 1-year pharmacy dispensing data for 17 therapeutic groups of somatic medications intended for chronic use [18]. The latter makes the CDS a static instrument. In contrast, the Prescription Changes Frequency (PCF) is based on prescription changes over a 3-month period.

The objectives of this study were (1) to assess the association between the PCF and hospital admission at different times before admission and (2) to compare the PCF with the CDS for predicting hospital admission.

Methods

Study design and setting

This retrospective, matched case–control study used with permission data from the Dutch PHARMO Record Linkage System (RLS) (www.pharmo.nl). The PHARMO RLS includes the dispensing records of community pharmacies linked to hospital discharge records. It consists of a representative sample of more than 200 community pharmacies in more than 50 regions throughout the Netherlands and is representative for the Netherlands [19]. It currently includes data for more than 2 million residents (12% of the Dutch population) regardless of the type of medical insurance. The computerized pharmacy dispensing records contain information about drugs dispensed, dispensing date, prescribing physician, amount of drug dispensed, and prescribed dosage regimen. Patient information includes sex and date of birth. Each patient is assigned an anonymous unique patient identification code and each medication is also given a unique code, according to the Anatomical Therapeutic Chemical (ATC) classification system. This makes it possible to track drug therapy and changes in drug therapy over time. The database does not record the indication for which a medicine is prescribed and neither does it include all medications used because non-prescription products can be purchased over-the-counter.

Cases and controls

Initially, 10,000 patients who had been hospitalized for the first time of possible repeated hospitalizations between July 1998 and June 2000 were randomly selected from the PHARMO RLS. The date of hospital admission was considered the index date. Each hospitalized patient was matched by age on birthday, sex, geographic area per pharmacy catchment area with a control patient who was assigned the same index date. Patients were

Table 1 Classification of prescription changes

Classification	Definition
1. Change in dosage	Change in dosage means that, for the same drug, the daily dosage is increased or decreased (e.g., amitriptyline 25 mg changes in amitriptyline 10 mg or vv).
2a. Product formulation switch	Metoprolol 50 mg plain tablet instead of metoprolol slow release tablet (Selokeen ZOC®).
2b. Generic brand switch	Change to another product containing the same active substance with the same strength and the same dosage (e.g., atenolol 50 mg tablet (generic product) instead of Tenormin® 50 mg tablet (brand) or Renitec® 10 mg tablet (brand) instead of enalapril 10 mg tablet).
2c. Therapeutic switch	Change to another active substance within the same therapeutic group; the first four characters of the ATC classification are the same (e.g. amitriptyline (N06AA09) instead of citalopram (N06AB04) or fluoxetine (N06AB03) instead of citalopram (N06AB04)).
3. Stop	No continuation 90 days after one of the five control time points and no generic-brand substitution (1), product formulation switch (2) ortherapeutic switch (3).
4. Start	Start of a drug means prescription of a drug which had not been prescribed during the previous six months and which is not a generic brand substitution (1), product formulation switch (2) or therapeutic switch (3).

included if medication data were available for at least 24 months before the index date.

Prescription change frequency

A prescription is defined as one medication order. PCF is defined as the number of prescription changes made during a 3-month period, without distinguishing between intentional and unintentional changes. Four different types of prescription changes were distinguished: (1) change in dosage, (2a) product switch, (2b) generic brand switch, (2c) therapeutic switch, (3) stopping medication, and (4) starting medication (Table 1). As we were interested in whether the PCF affects hospitalization over time, we calculated the PCF score for both patients and controls at 18, 12, 9, 6, and 3 months before the index date. The duration of use of each drug was estimated by dividing the number of dispensed units by the prescribed daily dose. Drugs that had a theoretical end date beyond 18, 12, 9, 6, or 3 months before the index date were considered as being in use on these dates. Only drugs intended for systemic use were taken into account. PCF scores were categorized into 0 prescription changes (PCF 0), 1 prescription change (PCF 1), 2 or 3 prescription changes (PCF 2 or 3), and 4 or more prescription changes (PCF≥ 4).

Chronic disease score

The CDS is calculated on the basis of the use over 1 year of medications for 17 therapeutic groups of somatic medications. The CDS has been shown to be a valid measure of complications related to an individual patient's burden of chronic somatic diseases and is clearly associated with the probability of being hospitalized [20-22]. To compare the PCF with the CDS, we calculated and categorized the CDS for the year preceding the index date into four categories: CDS score = 0, CDS score = 1 or 2, CDS score = 3 or 4, and CDS score 5 or higher.

Statistical analysis

The strength of the association between the PCF score and hospital admission was calculated by comparing the number of patients and controls in each PCF category at 18, 12, 9, 6 and 3 months before the index date with forced entry univariate logistic regression analysis; outcomes are expressed as the odds ratio (95% CI), using PCF 0 as reference. To assess the effects of other patient or hospitalization characteristics, we performed stratified analyses with age (< 65 years ≥ 65 years), admission type (emergency or planned), CDS score, and polypharmacy (the use of five or more drugs concomitantly) as variables. To assess the strength of the association between the CDS score and hospital admission, the number of patients and controls per CDS category were compared (expressed as OR 95% CI), taking CDS 0 as reference.

The nature of prescription changes was determined for each time period. The correlation between the PCF and the CDS was measured with a two-tailed Spearman's correlation coefficient. Statistical analyses were performed using SPSS 16.0 (SPSS, Chicago, IL).

Results

The source population was a random sample of 10,000 patients admitted to a hospital and an equal number of matched non-admitted individuals (controls). Because 1319 matched patients had less than 24 months of exposure history available in PHARMO RLS, the final

Table 2 Characteristics of hospitalized and non-hospitalized patients at the index date

Characteristics	Hospitalized N=8681	%	Non-Hospitalized N=8681	%
Sex				
Male	3588	41.3	3588	41.3
Female	5093	58.7	5093	58.7
Age (years at index date)				
0 - ≥ 18	574	6.6	574	6.6
>18 - ≥ 45	2737	31.5	2737	31.5
> 45 - ≥ 65	2246	25.9	2246	25.9
> 65 - ≥ 79	2218	25.6	2218	25.6
> 79	906	10.4	906	10.4
Number of medications				
0	3416	39.4	4534	52.2
1	1794	20.7	2121	24.4
2	985	11.3	872	10.0
3	767	8.8	535	6.2
4	544	6.3	302	3.5
≥5	1175	13.5	317	3.7
CDS category				
CDS score 0	3671	42.3	5206	60.0
CDS score 1-2	1331	15.3	1287	14.3
CDS score 3-4	1731	19.9	1415	16.3
CDS score ≥5	1948	22.4	773	8.9
Duration of hospitalization				
1 day	417	4.8		
2-5 days	4374	50.4		
> 5days	3890	44.8		
Admission type				
Emergency	3966	45.7		
Planned	4715	54.3		
Admission for surgery				
Yes	4360	50.2		
No	4321	49.8		

Table 3 The association between prescription change TYPE and hospital admission at different time points before index date

	-18				-12				-9				-6				-3			
	H	NH	OR	CI 95%	H	NH	OR	CI 95%	H	NH	OR	CI 95%	H	NH	OR	CI 95%	H	NH	OR	CI 95%
PC TYPE																				
Change in Dosage	946	521	*1.4*	1.3 1.6	1183	699	*1.3*	1.2 1.4	1093	597	*1.4*	1.3 1.6	1162	639	*1.4*	1.3 1.5	1405	656	*1.5*	1.4 1.6
Product Switch	211	127	*1.6*	1.3 2.0	329	187	*1.6*	1.3 1.9	325	202	*1.5*	1.3 1.8	349	217	*1.5*	1.3 1.8	422	245	*1.6*	1.4 1.8
Generic Brand Switch	114	67	*1.7*	1.2 2.2	180	93	*1.8*	1.4 2.3	192	103	*1.8*	1.4 2.3	219	101	*2.1*	1.6 2.6	274	91	*2.8*	2.2 3.5
Therap. Switch	221	100	*1.9*	1.5 2.4	230	117	*1.7*	1.4 2.1	256	96	*2.3*	1.8 2.9	300	111	*2.3*	1.8 2.8	345	117	*2.6*	2.1 3.1
Stop	2735	1923	*1.3*	1.2 1.3	2961	1910	*1.3*	1.3 1.4	3122	1950	*1.4*	1.3 1.4	3122	1943	*1.4*	1.3 1.4	3102	2005	*1.3*	1.3 1.4
Start	162	61	*2.3*	1.7 3.0	136	76	*1.6*	1.3 2.1	157	61	*2.3*	1.8 3.1	186	75	*2.2*	1.7 2.8	227	71	*2.9*	2.2 3.7

H=hospitalized patients (N=8681), NH=Non=Hospitalized Patients (N=8681), OR=Odds Ratio, CI 95%= Confidence Interval 95%.
PC Type=Prescription Change Type.

study population comprised 8681 patients and 8681 controls. The characteristics of the study population are displayed in Table 2. The mean age was 52.6 years (SD 21.8) and 58.7% of the participants were women. At the index date, 60.6% of the patients and 47.8% of the controls were using systemic medication; the mean number of drugs used at the index date was 3.0 for patients and 2.1 for controls. In both groups, the number of drugs used increased with age. The CDS was higher in the patients than in the controls. The most frequent reasons for prescription changes at all time points before the index date were stopping medication and changes in dosage (Table 3).

The risk of hospital admission increased with the number of prescription changes. At 3 months before the index date, the likelihood of hospitalization increased with increasing PCF category: the odds ratio (OR) between patients and controls was 1.4 (95% CI 1.3-1.5) in the lowest PCF category (PCF 1) and 4.1 (95% CI 3.1-5.1) in the highest PCF category (PCF 4). This was also true for comparisons for 18, 12, 9, and 6 months before index date (Tables 4 and 5).

The risk of hospital admission also increased per CDS category. A higher CDS score was associated with an increased risk of hospitalization: OR 1.5 (95% CI 1.4-1.6]) for CDS 1–2, OR 1.7 (95% CI 1.6-1.9) for CDS 3–4, and OR 3.6 (95% CI 3.3-3.9) for CDS 5 or higher.

Stratification by age (< 65 years ≥ 65 years), admission type (planned or emergency admission), CDS score, and polypharmacy resulted in comparable increases in OR with increasing PCF score. For participants on polypharmacy, the OR of PCF 4 or more decreased between 9 and 3 months before the index date, from 3.5 (95% CI 1.9-6.67) to 2.2 (95% CI 1.0-5.4). When stratified by CDS, the likelihood of being hospitalized also increased with increasing PCF score (Figure 1).

A two-tailed Spearman' correlation coefficient showed a significant but poor correlation between CDS 0 and PCI 0 (0.019, p= 0.01) and CDS 5 or higher and PCI 4 or higher (0.027, p=0.01) and no significant correlation between CDS 1 or 2 and PCF 1 and CDS 3 or 4 and PCF 2 or 3 at 3 months before the index date.

Table 4 The association between prescription change frequency and hospital admission at different time points before index date

	-18				-12				-9				-6				-3			
	H	NH	OR	CI 95%	H	NH	OR	CI 95%	H	NH	OR	CI 95%	H	NH	OR	CI 95%	H	NH	OR	CI 95%
PCF Cat																				
0	**6086**	6736	*1*	ref	5844	6524	*1*	ref	5788	6556	*1*	ref	5723	6570	*1*	ref	5591	6537	*1*	ref
1	1631	1418	*1.3*	1.2 1.4	1731	1564	*1.2*	1.2 1.3	1720	1561	*1.3*	1.2 1.4	1751	1483	*1.4*	1.3 1.5	5591	1493	*1.4*	1.3 1.5
2 or 3	760	451	*1.9*	1.7 2.1	853	514	*1.9*	1.7 2.1	899	490	*2.1*	1.9 2.3	923	542	*2.0*	1.8 2.2	1031	560	*2.2*	1.9 2.4
≥ 4	204	76	*3.0*	2.3 2.4	253	79	*3.6*	2.8 4.6	274	74	*4.2*	3.3 5.4	284	86	*3.8*	3.0 4.8	316	91	*4.1*	3.1 5.1

H=hospitalized patients (N=8681), NH=Non=Hospitalized Patients (N=8681).
OR=Odds Ratio, CI 95%= Confidence Interval 95%.
PCF Cat=Prescription Change Frequency Category.

Table 5 The association between the chronic disease score and hospital admission

| | Indexdate | | | |
	Hospitalized patients N=8681	Non Hospitalized patients N=8681)	OR	CI 95%
CDS score				
0	3671	5206	*1*	ref
1 or 2	1331	1287	*1.04*	0.96 1.13
3 or 4	1731	1415	*1.27*	1.18 1.38
≥ 4	1948	773	*2.95*	2.71 3.23

OR=Odds Ratio,

CI 95%= Confidence Interval 95%,

CDS =Chronic Disease Score
at indexdate

ref= reference

Discussion

The main finding of this study is that the frequency of prescription changes (PCF) is associated with an increased risk of hospital admission. We also confirmed the known association between the Chronic Disease Score (CDS) and hospital admission. While the PCF and CDS were both associated with hospital admission, the correlation between the two instruments was poor. The CDS measures comorbidity on the basis of the 1-year pharmacy dispensing data. In contrast, the PCF is based on prescription changes over a 3-month period. The results showed that the PCF within a three month period is comparable with the one year period of the CDS. Therefore, the PCF is more useful in practice.

We found that among patients with a low CDS score, an increasing number of prescription changes was associated with an increased risk of hospital admission. Stratified analysis of the CDS scores into the four categories confirmed this finding: at each CDS category, we found a comparable increase in the risk of hospitalization caused by the number of prescription changes.

Stratification by age (<65 or ≥65 year) and medication use (< 5 or ≥5 medications used) showed an increasing risk of hospitalization with increasing PCF (Figure 1). Several studies have reported age and polypharmacy as risk factors for hospital admission. We found that, based on PCF scores, even patients younger than 65 years and patients without polypharmacy were at increased risk of hospital admission. It is plausible that the risk was lower for planned than for emergency admissions, but this was not confirmed after stratification by type of hospitalization. Unexpectedly, patients on polypharmacy had a decreased risk of hospital admission: PCF 4 or higher decreased between 9 and 3 months before the index date. On the basis of this finding, the most common reason for prescription changes, namely, stopping medication, would appear to be protective against

hospital admission in patients on polypharmacy. As we do not know which medications were stopped, this finding does not mean that stopping specific medications is protective.

The CDS has the disadvantage that it is based on information about medication history collected for at least 1 year prior to the event under investigation. We showed that it is possible to predict the risk of hospitalization on the basis of the number of prescription changes in 3 months. On the other hand, the CDS is based on the use for 17 therapeutic groups of somatic medications, whereas the PCF is based on all medications and thus requires detailed medication histories. The CDS was developed to measure a patient's overall health status, but the PCF is not suitable for this. A potential weakness of the CDS, which was developed in 1992, is that it has never been adjusted to accommodate new medication classes, unlike the PCF, which is based on all medications used. Despite this, the CDS is still associated with hospital admissions.

Limitations

This study has a number of limitations. The database does not provide information about the indication for which a drug is prescribed, so we cannot comment about the frequency of medication changes for specific indications. One could argue that more ill patients will have more prescription changes. However, this was not the aim of the study. The use of non-prescription medicines is not known as patients could also buy medications OTC. In addition, prescribers might not write out a new prescription each time drug use is changed. Because the PCF is based on dispensing data from community pharmacies, this would mean that the association between PCF and hospital admission might have been underestimated. As the data set used in this study covered the period between July 1998 and June 2000, it is possible, but unlikely, that since then the prescribing behavior of doctors has changed, influenced by medication reconciliation programmes, or indications for hospital admission might have become stricter, both of which would have led to overestimation of the association between PCF and hospitalization. While the Dutch PHARMO database is complete, it does not provide information about the socioeconomic status or compliance of patients or their health status (the controls might have been ill less often than the patients); however, as the controls were sampled independently of exposure status, these factors would not influence our results. Lastly, it was outside the scope of this study to distinguish between the different reasons for changing medication in greater detail. To our knowledge, besides the study of Koecheler *et al.* [17], no other studies have investigated prescription changes and the risk of hospital admission. Several other studies, like the HARM study,

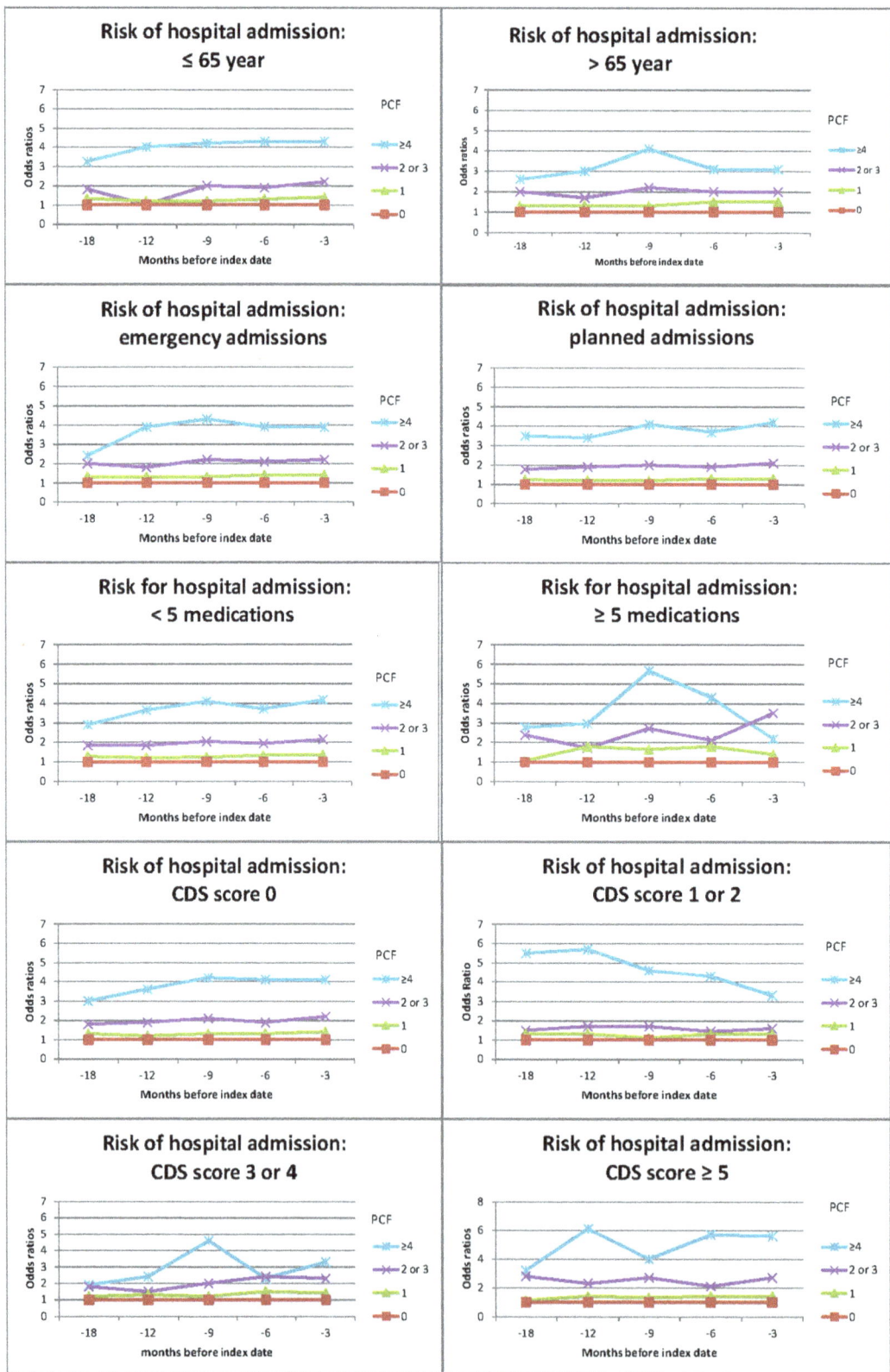

Figure 1 Stratification on age category, admission type, polypharmacy and CDS score.

have described risk factors for medication-related hospital admission, but did not focus on prescription changes.

Further research should consider more detailed variables of the prescription changes like types of medications involved. In addition, it should be interesting to test the PCF model in a follow up study.

Conclusion

This longitudinal study of a large group of patients over 24 months demonstrated that the frequency of prescription changes (PCF) over a 3-month period is associated with hospital admission, which suggests that the PCF could be used as an alternative to the CDS for predicting hospital admission. In the ambulant setting, the PCF score could function as a warning signal for an increased risk of hospitalization and as such contribute to medication safety programmes. The PCF might be particularly useful for older patients, who tend to use more medications. District nurses and social workers care should be alerted if the frequency of prescription changes increases in their patients. Community pharmacists can use the PCF as a clinical rule to facilitate early identification of potential drug-related problems. Further research is needed to determine the predictive value of the PCF in practice as a clinical rule.

Competing interests

Possible conflict of interest: nothing to disclose.The department of Pharmacoepidemiology & Pharmacology has received unrestricted funding for pharmacoepidemiological research from GlaxoSmithKline, Novo Nordisk, the private-public funded Top Institute Pharma (www.tipharma.nl, includes co-funding from universities, government and industry), the Dutch Medicines Evaluation Board and the Dutch Ministry of Health.

Authors' contributions

All authors contribute the study conception and design and the study's analytic strategy (CS-RS-EH-MS-PS-TE). PS prepared the database for analysis. CS has done the statistical data analysis, supported by EH and PS. CS and RS conduct the literature review and have written the drafting of the manuscript. Author MS and TE supervised the study and helped with critical revisions of the manuscript for important intellectual content. All authors read and approved the final manuscript.

Acknowledgments

No special funding was received for this study.

Author details

[1]University of Applied Sciences Utrecht, Research Centre for Innovation in Healthcare, Bolognalaan 101, 3584 Utrecht, CJ, The Netherlands. [2]Department of Pharmacoepidemiology and Clinical Pharmacology, Utrecht University, Faculty of Science, Utrecht, The Netherlands. [3]Department of Clinical Pharmacy, Tergooi Hospitals, Blaricum/Hilversum, The Netherlands. [4]Department of Rehabilitation, University Medical Centre Utrecht, Nursing Science and Sports, Utrecht, The Netherlands. [5]Department of Clinical Pharmacy, University Medical Centre Utrecht, Utrecht, The Netherlands.

References

1. Lazarou J, Pomeranz BH, Corey PN: Incidence of adverse drug reactions in hospitalized patients: a meta-analysis of prospective studies. *JAMA* 1998, **279**(15):1200–1205.

2. Roughead EE, Gilbert AL, Primrose JG, Sansom LN: Drug-related hospital admissions: a review of Australian studies published 1988–1996. *Med J Aust* 1998, **168**(8):405–408.

3. Green CF, Mottram DR, Rowe PH, Pirmohamed M: Adverse drug reactions as a cause of admission to an acute medical assessment unit: a pilot study. *J Clin Pharm Ther* 2000, **25**(5):355–361.

4. Pouyanne P, Haramburu F, Imbs JL, Begaud B: Admissions to hospital caused by adverse drug reactions: cross sectional incidence study. French pharmacovigilance centres. *BMJ* 2000, **320**(7241):1036.

5. Beijer HJ, de Blaey CJ: Hospitalisations caused by adverse drug reactions (ADR): a meta-analysis of observational studies. *Pharm World Sci* 2002, **24**(2):46–54.

6. Onder G, Pedone C, Landi F, Cesari M, Della Vedova C, Bernabei R, *et al*: Adverse drug reactions as cause of hospital admissions: results from the Italian group of pharmacoepidemiology in the elderly (GIFA). *J Am Geriatr Soc* 2002, **50**(12):1962–1968.

7. Waller P, Shaw M, Ho D, Shakir S, Ebrahim S: Hospital admissions for 'drug-induced' disorders in England: a study using the hospital episodes statistics (HES) database. *Br J Clin Pharmacol* 2005, **59**(2):213–219.

8. Klarin I, Wimo A, Fastbom J: The association of inappropriate drug use with hospitalisation and mortality: a population-based study of the very old. *Drugs Aging* 2005, **22**(1):69–82.

9. van der Hooft CS, Dieleman JP, Siemes C, Aarnoudse AJ, Verhamme KM, Stricker BH, *et al*: Adverse drug reaction-related hospitalisations: a population-based cohort study. *Pharmacoepidemiol Drug Saf* 2008, **17**(4):365–371.

10. Kongkaew C, Noyce PR, Ashcroft DM: Hospital admissions associated with adverse drug reactions: a systematic review of prospective observational studies. *Ann Pharmacother* 2008, **42**(7):1017–1025.

11. Leendertse AJ, Egberts AC, Stoker LJ, van den Bemt PM, HARM Study Group: Frequency of and risk factors for preventable medication-related hospital admissions in the Netherlands. *Arch Intern Med* 2008, **168**(17):1890–1896.

12. Boyd CM, Ricks M, Fried LP, Guralnik JM, Xue QL, Xia J, *et al*: Functional decline and recovery of activities of daily living in hospitalized, disabled older women: the Women's health and aging study I. *J Am Geriatr Soc* 2009, **57**(10):1757–1766.

13. Hoogerduijn JG, Schuurmans MJ, Duijnstee MS, de Rooij SE, Grypdonck MF: A systematic review of predictors and screening instruments to identify older hospitalized patients at risk for functional decline. *J Clin Nurs* 2007, **16**(1):46–57.

14. Zegers M, de Bruijne MC, Wagner C, Hoonhout LH, Waaijman R, Smits M, *et al*: Adverse events and potentially preventable deaths in Dutch hospitals: results of a retrospective patient record review study. *Qual Saf Health Care* 2009, **18**(4):297–302.

15. Higashi T, Shekelle PG, Solomon DH, Knight EL, Roth C, Chang JT, *et al*: The quality of pharmacologic care for vulnerable older patients. *Ann Intern Med* 2004, **140**(9):714–720.

16. Linjakumpu T, Hartikainen S, Klaukka T, Veijola J, Kivela SL, Isoaho R: Use of medications and polypharmacy are increasing among the elderly. *J Clin Epidemiol* 2002, **55**(8):809–817.

17. Koecheler JA, Abramowitz PW, Swim SE, Daniels CE: Indicators for the selection of ambulatory patients who warrant pharmacist monitoring. *Am J Hosp Pharm* 1989, **46**(4):729–732.

18. Von Korff M, Wagner EH, Saunders K: A chronic disease score from automated pharmacy data. *J Clin Epidemiol* 1992, **45**(2):197–203.

19. RMC Herings: *PHARMO: a record linkage system for postmarketing surveillance of prescription drugs in the Netherlands.* The Netherlands: Department of Pharmacoepidemiology and Pharmacotherapy, Thesis Utrecht University; 1993.

20. Clark DO, Von Korff M, Saunders K, Baluch WM, Simon GE: A chronic disease score with empirically derived weights. *Med Care* 1995, **33**(8):783–795.

21. Fishman PA, Shay DK: Development and estimation of a pediatric chronic disease score using automated pharmacy data. *Med Care* 1999, **37**(9):874–883.

22. Putnam KG, Buist DS, Fishman P, Andrade SE, Boles M, Chase GA, *et al*: Chronic disease score as a predictor of hospitalization. *Epidemiology* 2002, **13**(3):340–346.

18

Computational analysis of protein-protein interfaces involving an alpha helix: insights for terphenyl–like molecules binding

Adriana Isvoran[1,2†], Dana Craciun[3†], Virginie Martiny[4,5], Olivier Sperandio[4,5] and Maria A Miteva[4,5*]

Abstract

Background: Protein-Protein Interactions (PPIs) are key for many cellular processes. The characterization of PPI interfaces and the prediction of putative ligand binding sites and hot spot residues are essential to design efficient small-molecule modulators of PPI. Terphenyl and its derivatives are small organic molecules known to mimic one face of protein-binding alpha-helical peptides. In this work we focus on several PPIs mediated by alpha-helical peptides.

Method: We performed computational sequence- and structure-based analyses in order to evaluate several key physicochemical and surface properties of proteins known to interact with alpha-helical peptides and/or terphenyl and its derivatives.

Results: Sequence-based analysis revealed low sequence identity between some of the analyzed proteins binding alpha-helical peptides. Structure-based analysis was performed to calculate the volume, the fractal dimension roughness and the hydrophobicity of the binding regions. Besides the overall hydrophobic character of the binding pockets, some specificities were detected. We showed that the hydrophobicity is not uniformly distributed in different alpha-helix binding pockets that can help to identify key hydrophobic hot spots.

Conclusions: The presence of hydrophobic cavities at the protein surface with a more complex shape than the entire protein surface seems to be an important property related to the ability of proteins to bind alpha-helical peptides and low molecular weight mimetics. Characterization of similarities and specificities of PPI binding sites can be helpful for further development of small molecules targeting alpha-helix binding proteins.

Background

Protein-Protein Interactions (PPIs) are key to many cellular processes. Abnormal PPIs contribute to many disease states and as such, PPIs represent today a new class of drug targets essentially unexploited for drug discovery. Indeed, the size of the human interactome has been estimated to be between 300,000 [1] and 650,000 interactions [2]. In the last decade many studies have been performed in order to target PPIs [3]. Several small-molecule inhibitors of PPIs have been demonstrated therapeutic potential [4-8]. However, efficient targeting of PPIs is still being

considered as an important challenge [3,9,10]. In contrast to enzyme-substrate interactions, protein-protein recognition often occurs through flat surfaces or wide shallow grooves. Recent structural analyses of PPI interfaces and small molecules disrupting PPIs suggested that such ligands might mimic the structural characteristics of the protein partner [6,11]. To facilitate the discovery of new PPI small-molecule inhibitors, the characterization of PPI interfaces [12,13] and the prediction of putative ligand binding sites are essential. Physicochemical properties of both ligand and protein are key to mediate the binding [14], such as cavity sizes, shape complementarity, electrostatic potential and hydrophobicity [12,15].

The role of alpha-helical peptides in mediating many PPIs is well demonstrated and development of small organic molecules mimicking such peptides becomes important [16]. Recent studies have been carried out on

* Correspondence: maria.miteva@univ-paris-diderot.fr
†Equal contributors
4Université Paris Diderot, Sorbonne Paris Cité, Molécules Thérapeutiques in silico, Inserm UMR-S 973, 35 rue Helene Brion, Paris 75013, France
5INSERM, U973, Paris F-75205, France
Full list of author information is available at the end of the article

the whole Protein Data Bank (PDB) in order to establish a druggability profile of alpha-helix mediated PPIs and to predict which of them could bind a small molecule [17]. More specifically, terphenyl and its derivates are small organic molecules [18-26] mimicking one face of an alpha-helical peptide, *i.e.* the side chains of three key residues occupying positions *i, i+3* and *i+7* [25,26] or *i, i+4* and *i+7* [20] of the bound helix. It has been suggested that terphenyl compounds can serve as pharmacological probes because they are membrane permeable [22]. Terphenyl 1 and 2, which mimic the calmodulin binding face of smooth muscle myosin light chain kinase (smMLCK), have been shown to inhibit the interactions of calmodulin (CaM) with the enzyme 3'-5'-cyclic nucleotide phosphodiesterase (PDE) and with the helical peptide C20W of the plasma membrane calcium pumps [18]. Following the similarity between the calmodulin and human centrin 2 (HsCen2) alpha-helix binding sites, we recently suggested that terphenyl 2 might also inhibit the interaction between HsCen2 and a 17 residues peptide of *Xeroderma Pigmentosum Group C* (XPC) protein

[27]. Terphenyl derivates mimicking the alpha-helical structure of p53 N-terminal peptide inhibit the p53-MDM2 [22] and the p53-HDM2 interactions [21]. These molecules also mimic the alpha-helical region of Bak BH3 domain, which binds BCL-X_2, thus disrupting the BCL-X_2/Bak interaction [19,20,24].

In this work we performed a computational analysis in order to evaluate several key physicochemical and surface properties of proteins known to interact with alpha-helical peptides or to bind terphenyl and its derivatives. We calculated the binding pocket volumes and the fractal dimensions of the surface cavities for the entire protein and for the binding pockets. We identified several similarities and specificities characterizing such protein binding sites that can be helpful for future development of more efficient small-molecule inhibitors targeting alpha-helix binding proteins.

Methods

In this study we compared the sequence and surface properties of the investigated proteins. In order to analyze the

Table 1 Protein – alpha-helical peptide complexes

Protein complex	PDB code Resolution	SwissProt code	Interacting residues of the bound alpha-helix
Chicken calmodulin in complex with smooth muscle myosin light chain kinase (smMLCK)	2O5G* 1.08 Å	P62149	TRP5, THR8, VAL12
Human calmodulin in complex with a mutant peptide of human DRP-1 kinase	1ZUZ 1.91 Å	P62158	TRP305, PHE309, VAL312
Human calmodulin in complex with CAV1.1 IQ peptide	2VAY* 1.94 Å	P62158	THR526, ILE529, PHE533
Human calmodulin in complex with CAV2.2 IQ peptide	3DVE 2.35 Å	P62158	MET854, VAL857, MET161
E Coli calmodulin in complex with RS20 peptide of smMLCK	1QTX 1.65 Å	-	TRP5, THR8, VAL12
Rat calmodulin in complex with NMDA receptor NR1C1peptide	2HQW 1.90 Å	P62161	PHE880, THR884, LEU887
Human centrin 2 in complex with the centrin binding region of XPC protein	2GGM 2.35 Å	P41208	TRP848, LEU851, LEU855
C-terminal domain of human centrin 2 in complex with a repeat sequence of human Sfi 1	2K2I NMR	P41208	LEU651, LEU655, TRP658
Scherffelia dubia centrin in complex with smMLCK peptide	3KF9 2.60 Å	Q06827	TRP4, PHE8, VAL11
Human BCL-XL in complex with BAK peptide	1BXL* NMR	Q07817	VAL574, LEU578, ILE581
Human E3 ubiquitin-protein ligase MDM2 in complex with p53 tumor transactivation domain (fragment 17-125)	1YCR* 2.60 Å	Q00987	PHE19, TRP23, LEU26
Rabbit cardiac troponin C in complex with a fragment (residues 1-47) of cardiac troponin I	1A2X 2.30 Å	P02586	LEU17, MET21, ILE24

*known to be disrupted by terphenyl or its derivatives.

sequence similarities we performed sequence alignment using the CLUSTALW software [28]. Interacting residues at the protein-protein interface in terms of contact distances were found using the ContPro online freely available tool [29]. We identified the protein residues interacting with the three key residues of the alpha-helical peptide (occupying positions *i, i+3* and *i+7* or *i, i+4* and *i+7*) those relative positions are mimicked by terphenyl and its derivatives. The distance threshold was set to 5 Å for the side chain atoms.

In order to evaluate the protein surface properties, the bound peptide was removed for each complex. The surface characteristics of the entire protein and those of the peptide-binding cavity were analyzed. Using the approach of the fractal geometry we quantitatively described the surface roughness for the entire protein and

for the binding cavity, expressed by global surface fractal dimension (D_S) and local surface fractal dimension (D_L), respectively. In order to calculate the surface fractal dimension we used the method proposed by Lewis and Rees [30] based on the scaling law between the surface area (SA) and the radius of the rolling probe molecule (R) on the surface, i.e. SA is proportional to the radius to the power 2-Ds:

$$SA \sim R^{2-D_S} \tag{1}$$

The surface fractal dimension was determined from the slope of the double logarithmical plot of SA versus R. The surface area of the protein was computed using the on-line available software GETAREA [31]. Probe radii of 1, 1.2, 1.4, 1.6, 1.8 and 2 Å were used. For the

```
2OSG|P62149|CALM_CHICK    --FKEAFSLFDK-------------DGDGTITTKELGTVMRSLGQNPTE-     46
1ZUZ|P62158|CALM_HUMAN    --FKEAFSLFDK-------------DGDGTITTKELGTVMRSLGQNPTE-     46
2VAY|P62158|CALM_HUMAN    --FKEAFSLFDK-------------DGDGTITTKELGTVMRSLGQNPTE-     46
3DVE|P62158|CALM_HUMAN    --FKEAFSLFDK-------------DGDGTITTKELGTVMRSLGQNPTE-     46
1QTX                      --FKEAFSLFDK-------------DGDGTITTKELGTVMRSLGQNPTE-     46
2HQW|P62161|CALM_RAT      --FKEAFSLFDK-------------DGDGTITTKELGTVMRSLGQNPTE-     46
2GGM|P41208|CETN2_HUMAN   --IREAFDLFDA-------------DGTGTIDVKELKVAMRALGFEPKK-     67
2K2I|P41208|CETN2_HUMAN   --IREAFDLFDA-------------DGTGTIDVKELKVAMRALGFEPKK-     67
3KF9|Q06827|CATR_SCHDU    --IREAFDLFDT-------------DGSGTIDAKELKVAMRALGFEPKK-     62
1BXL|Q07817|B2CL1_HUMAN   INGNPSWHLADSPAVNGATGHSSSLDAREVIPMAAVKQALREAGDEFELR     99
1YCR|Q00987|MDM2_HUMAN    -------------------------LVRPKPLLLKLLKSVGAQKDT-     31
1A2X|P02586|TNNC2_RABIT   --FKAAFDMFDA-------------DGGGDISVKELGTVMRMLGQTPTK-     51
                                                            :       ::      *

2OSG|P62149|CALM_CHICK    ---------------------AELQDMINEVDADGNGTIDFPEFLTMMARK     76
1ZUZ|P62158|CALM_HUMAN    ---------------------AELQDMINEVDADGNGTIDFPEFLTMMARK     76
2VAY|P62158|CALM_HUMAN    ---------------------AELQDMINEVDADGNGTIDFPEFLTMMARK     76
3DVE|P62158|CALM_HUMAN    ---------------------AELQDMINEVDADGNGTIDFPEFLTMMARK     76
1QTX                      ---------------------AELQDMINEVDADGNGTIDFPEFLTMMARK     76
2HQW|P62161|CALM_RAT      ---------------------AELQDMINEVDADGNGTIDFPEFLTMMARK     76
2GGM|P41208|CETN2_HUMAN   ---------------------EEIKKMISEIDKEGTGKMNFGDFLTVMTQK     99
2K2I|P41208|CETN2_HUMAN   ---------------------EEIKKMISEIDKEGTGKMNFGDFLTVMTQK     99
3KF9|Q06827|CATR_SCHDU    ---------------------EEIKKMIADIDKDGSGTIDFEEFLQMMTAK     92
1BXL|Q07817|B2CL1_HUMAN   YRRAFSDLTSQLHITPGTAYQSFEQVVNELFRDGVNWGRIVAFFSFGGAL    149
1YCR|Q00987|MDM2_HUMAN    ----------------------YTMKEVLFYLGQYIMTKRLYDEKQQH     57
1A2X|P02586|TNNC2_RABIT   ---------------------EELDAIIEEVDEDGSGTIDFEEFLVMMVRQ     81
                                  :    ::                       :

2OSG|P62149|CALM_CHICK    MKDTD---SEEEIREAFRVFDKDGNGYISAAELRHVMTNLGEKLTDEEVD    122
1ZUZ|P62158|CALM_HUMAN    MKDTD---SEEEIREAFRVFDKDGNGYISAAELRHVMTNLGEKLTDEEVD    122
2VAY|P62158|CALM_HUMAN    MKDTD---SEEEIREAFRVFDKDGNGYISAAELRHVMTNLGEKLTDEEVD    122
3DVE|P62158|CALM_HUMAN    MKDTD---SEEEIREAFRVFDKDGNGYISAAELRHVMTNLGEKLTDEEVD    122
1QTX                      MKDTD---SEEEIREAFRVFDKDGNGYISAAELRHVMTNLGEKLTDEEVD    122
2HQW|P62161|CALM_RAT      MKDTD---SEEEIREAFRVFDKDGNGYISAAELRHVMTNLGEKLTDEEVD    122
2GGM|P41208|CETN2_HUMAN   MSEKD---TKEEILKAFKLFDDDETGKISFKNLKRVAKELGENLTDEELQ    146
2K2I|P41208|CETN2_HUMAN   MSEKD---TKEEILKAFKLFDDDETGKISFKNLKRVAKELGENLTDEELQ    146
3KF9|Q06827|CATR_SCHDU    MGERD---SREEIMKAFRLFDDDETGKISFKNLKRVAKELGENMTDEELQ    139
1BXL|Q07817|B2CL1_HUMAN   CVES----VDKEMQVLVSRIAAWMATYLNDHLEPWIQENGGWDTFVELYG    195
1YCR|Q00987|MDM2_HUMAN    IVYCS---------NDLLGDLFGVPSFSVKEHRKIYTMIYRNLVVVNQQ     97
1A2X|P02586|TNNC2_RABIT   MKEDAKGKSEEELAECFRIFDRNADGYIDAEELAEIFRASGEHVTDEEIE    131
                                  :.         :           .

2OSG|P62149|CALM_CHICK    EMIREADIDGDGQVNYEEFVQMMTAK-----------    149
1ZUZ|P62158|CALM_HUMAN    EMIREADIDGDGQVNYEEFVQMMTAK-----------    149
2VAY|P62158|CALM_HUMAN    EMIREADIDGDGQVNYEEFVQMMTAK-----------    149
3DVE|P62158|CALM_HUMAN    EMIREADIDGDGQVNYEEFVQMMTAK-----------    149
1QTX                      EMIREADIDGDGQVNYEEFVQMMTAK-----------    149
2HQW|P62161|CALM_RAT      EMIREADIDGDGQVNYEEFVQMMTAK-----------    149
2GGM|P41208|CETN2_HUMAN   EMIDEADRDGDGEVSEQEFLRIMKKTSLY--------    172
2K2I|P41208|CETN2_HUMAN   EMIDEADRDGDGEVSEQEFLRIMKKTSLY--------    172
3KF9|Q06827|CATR_SCHDU    EMIDEADRDGDGEVNEEEFFRIMKKTSLF--------    168
1BXL|Q07817|B2CL1_HUMAN   NNAAAESRKGQERFNRWFLTGMTVAGVVLLGSLFSRK    232
1YCR|Q00987|MDM2_HUMAN    ESSDSGTSVSE---NRCHLEGGSDQKDLV--------    123
1AX2|P02586|TNNC2_RABIT   SLMKDGDKNNDGRIDFDEFLKMMEGVQ----------    160
                                  .:            :
```

Figure 1 Sequence alignment of alpha-helix binding proteins. The amino acid residues interacting with alpha-helical peptides are presented in red.

Table 2 Sequence identity (in %) between the considered proteins (the binding area/entire protein)

Protein/ sequence identity	Human calmodulin	Human centrin 2	Scherffelia dubia centrin	Human BCL-X_2	Human E3 ubiquitin-protein ligase MDM2
Human centrin 2	54/50				
Scherffelia dubia centrin	56/55	90/74			
Human BCL-X_2	5/7	5/5	5/8		
Human E3 ubiquitin-protein ligase MDM2	5/4	5/10	7/6	9/5	
Rabbit cardiac troponin C	57/51	57/34	37/32	5/9	5/19

The binding area was defined here as all residues of the protein interacting with the helical peptide.

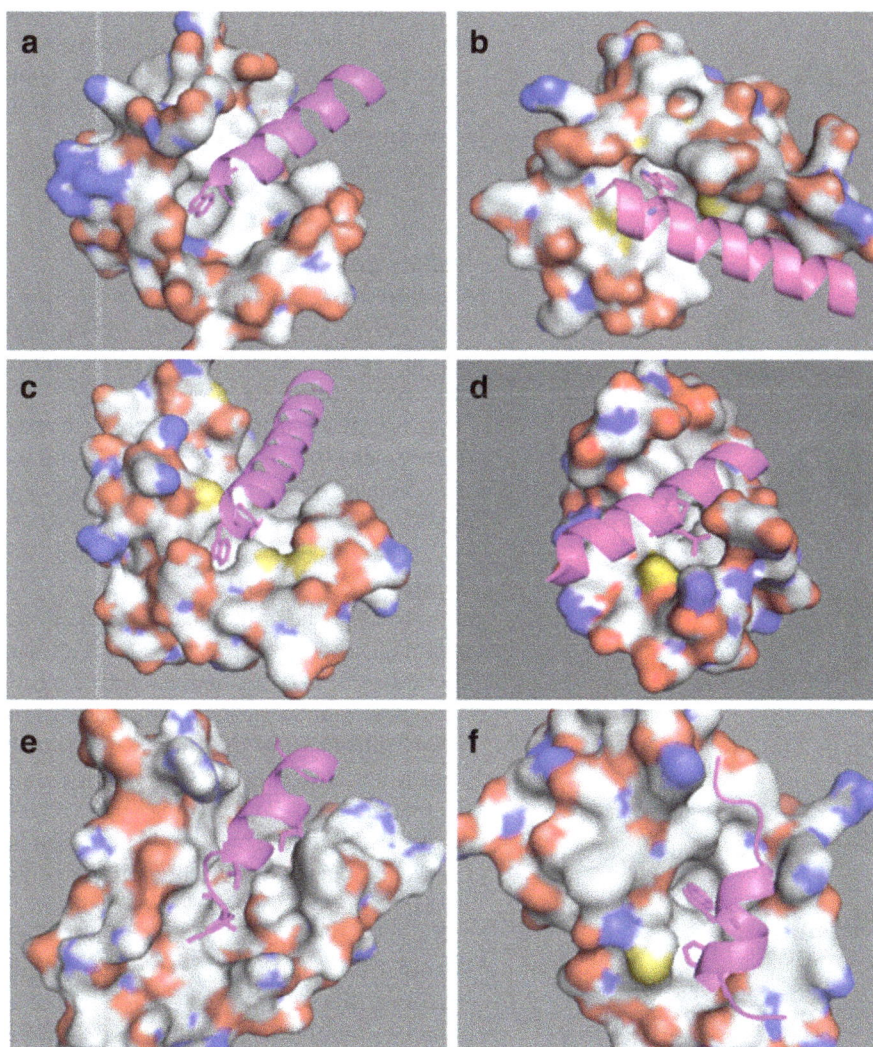

Figure 2 **3D structures of the complexes formed by:** (**a**) human centrin 2 and a 10 residue peptide of Xeroderma Pigmentosum group C protein, code entry 2GGM. (**b**) chicken calmodulin and smooth muscle myosin light chain kinase (smMLCK), code entry 2O5G. (**c**) scherffelia dubia centrin and smMLCK peptide, code entry 3KF9. (**d**) rabbit cardiac troponin C and a fragment of cardiac troponin I, code entry 1A2X. (**e**) human BCL-XL and BAK peptide, code entry 1BXL. (**f**) human E3 ubiquitin-protein ligase MDM2 and p53 tumor transactivation domain, code entry 1YCR. All proteins are shown as surface in atom color type (C and H-white, N – blue, O -red, S – yellow) and ligands are shown in magenta cartoon with hydrophobic interacting residues given as sticks.

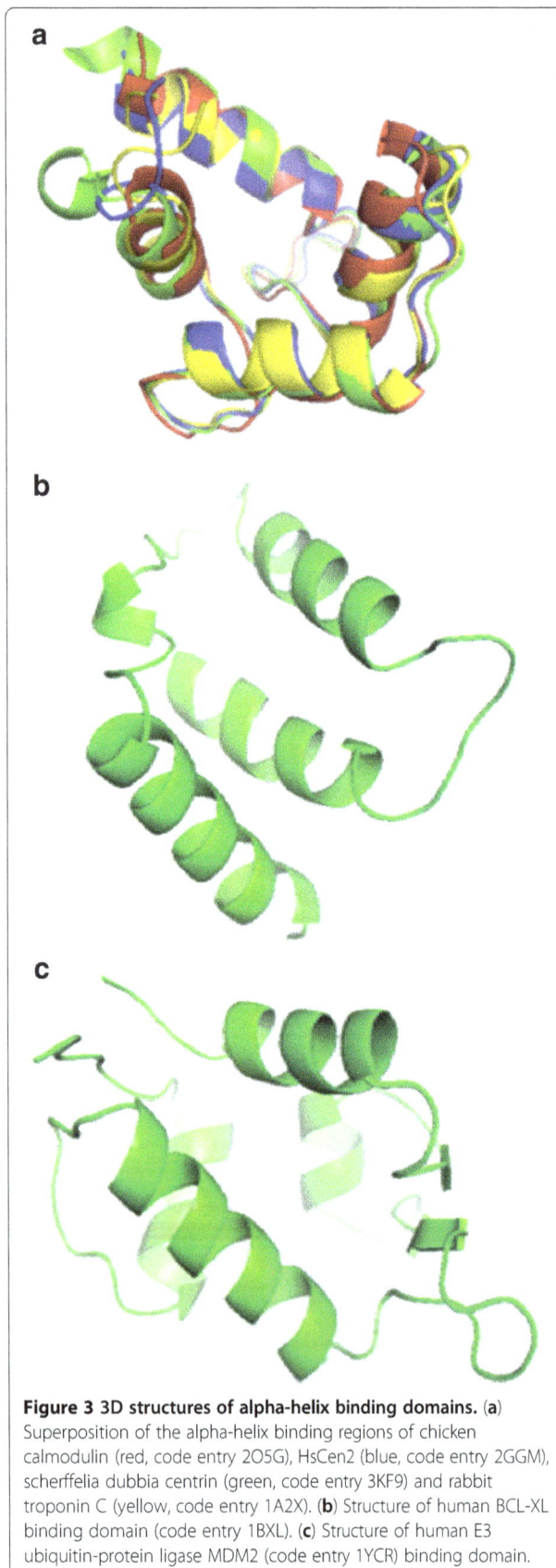

Figure 3 3D structures of alpha-helix binding domains. (a)
Superposition of the alpha-helix binding regions of chicken
calmodulin (red, code entry 2O5G), HsCen2 (blue, code entry 2GGM),
scherffelia dubbia centrin (green, code entry 3KF9) and rabbit
troponin C (yellow, code entry 1A2X). (b) Structure of human BCL-XL
binding domain (code entry 1BXL). (c) Structure of human E3
ubiquitin-protein ligase MDM2 (code entry 1YCR) binding domain.

proteins cavities, the same algorithm was employed
using the CASTp software [32]. Hydrophobicity and
local hydrophobic density for binding pockets were determined using Fpocket [33]. Pocket volumes were computed using CASTp [32].

Molecular docking of terphenyl 2 was performed into
the alpha-helical binding sites of calmodulin (code entry
2O5G) and troponin C (code entry 1A2X) using AutoDock
4.2 [34]. The input files preparation and docking analysis
were carried out using AutoDockTools. Grid maps were
centered in the alpha-helix binding site for both structures.
Grids sizes were 126 Å x 126 Å x 126 Å with a grid spacing of 0.33 Å for calmodulin and 126 Å x 126 Å x 126 Å
with a grid spacing of 0.28 Å for troponin C. Ligand conformational searching was performed using Lamarckian
genetic algorithm and all ligand torsion angles were flex-
ible. The following docking parameters were used: 250
Lamarckian genetic algorithm runs, a population size of
250, a maximum of 2 500 000 energy evaluations and a
maximum of 27000 generations.

Figures were prepared using PyMol [35] and CHIMERA
software [36].

Results and discussions
Sequence-based analysis
We analyze several proteins interacting with alpha-
helical peptides, some of them being known to bind also
terphenyl and/or its derivatives. To characterize and
compare their surface properties we examine the sequences and the three dimensional (3D) structures of
the complexes formed by the protein and the bound
peptide. The 3D structures are retrieved from the PDB
[37], the entry codes being presented in Table 1. Most of
the structures are crystallographic. Two NMR structures
are also used: the C-terminal domain of human centrin 2
in complex with the repeat sequence of human Sfi 1 and
the human BCL-XL in complex with the BAK peptide.

Multiple sequences alignment (Figure 1) shows low sequence identity for the most of the analyzed proteins
(shown in Table 2) both for the entire sequences and for
the binding areas. The binding areas included all residues
of the protein interacting with the alpha-helical peptide.
Chicken, human, E. coli and rat calmodulin have very
similar sequences (rat, chicken and human calmodulin are
100% identical; E coli has 98% identity with the others).
For BCL-XL and human ubiquitin carboxyl-terminal
hydrolase MDM2 only those fragments of sequences that
are present in the 3D structures are considered. There is a
high similarity only between the calmodulin, centrin 2 and
troponin C sequences.

Structure-based analysis
Figure 2 illustrates the complexes' structures of six alpha-
helix binding proteins. In all shown complexes, bulky

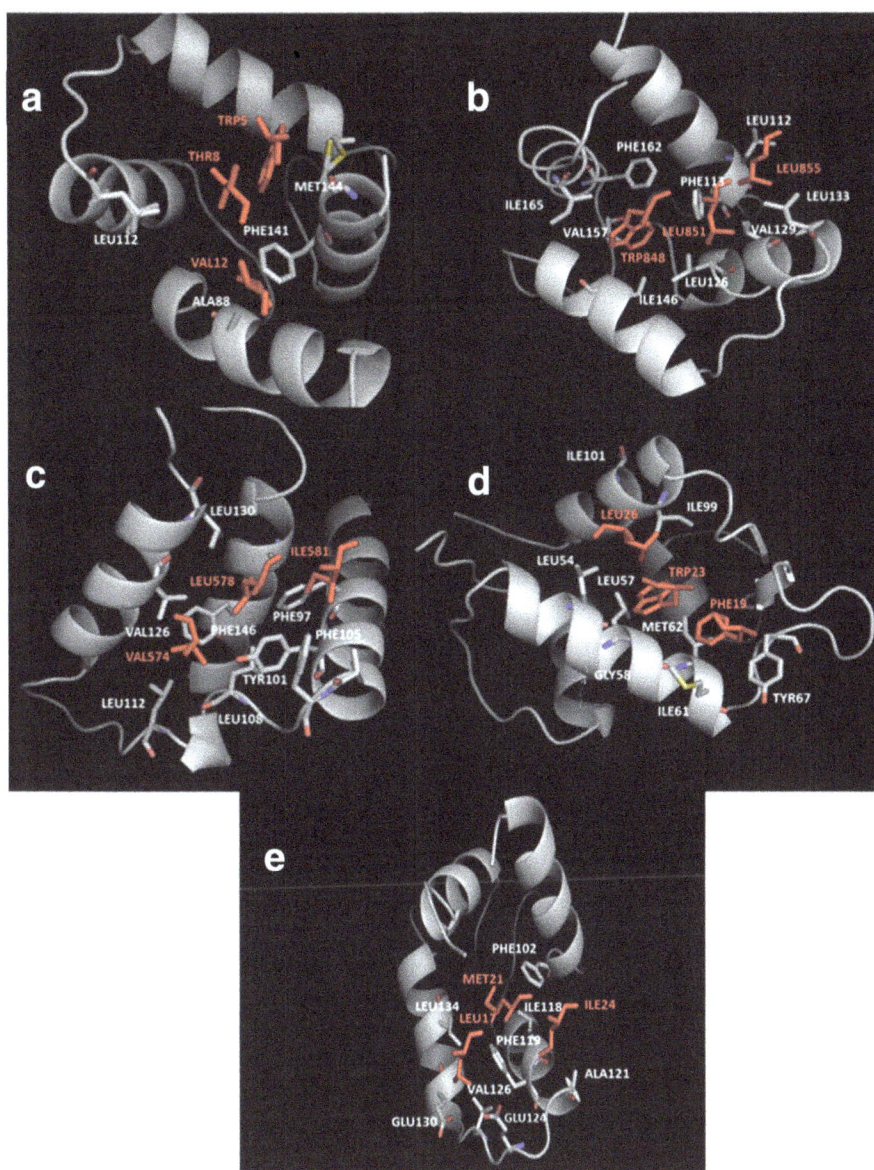

Figure 4 Illustration of the interacting residues (in sticks) of the protein (atom color type) and the bound peptide (red): (a) chicken calmodulin and smMLCK (code entry 2O5G), **(b)** human centrin 2 and the centrin binding region of XPC (code entry 2GGM), **(c)** human BCL-XL protein and BAK (code entry 1BXL), **(d)** human E3 ubiquitin- protein ligase MDM2 and p53 tumor transactivation domain (code entry 1YCR), **(e)** rabbit cardiac troponin C and cardiac troponin I (code entry 1A2X).

hydrophobic residues of the bound peptide anchor into the protein binding pocket. Following the sequence similarities we superimposed the alpha-helix binding regions structures of calmodulin, human centrin 2, scherffelia dubia centrin and rabbit troponin C (Figure 3a). Strong structural homology for binding regions is seen following the sequence similarity of these proteins. Figure 3b and 3c illustrate the binding pockets of BCL-XL and human E3 ubiquitin-protein ligase MDM2, respectively.

The interacting residues of the proteins and bound peptides, identified with ContPro [29], are shown in Figures 1 and 4 and Table 1. The results reveal that usually hydrophobic residues such as TRP, LEU, ILE, PHE, VAL, MET are involved in the interactions. The presence of hydrophobic residues suggests a favorable interaction with terphenyl-like molecules anchoring in the hydrophobic cavities. Most of the residues involved in the interactions between the proteins and alpha-helices are hydrophobic for both partners, as also observed in other studies [38]. We notice several key residues involved in the interaction of the same protein with different peptide partners. For example, in the case of calmodulin, PHE92, MET124, PHE141, MET144 and MET145 are involved in most of the peptides' interactions. These residues can thus be

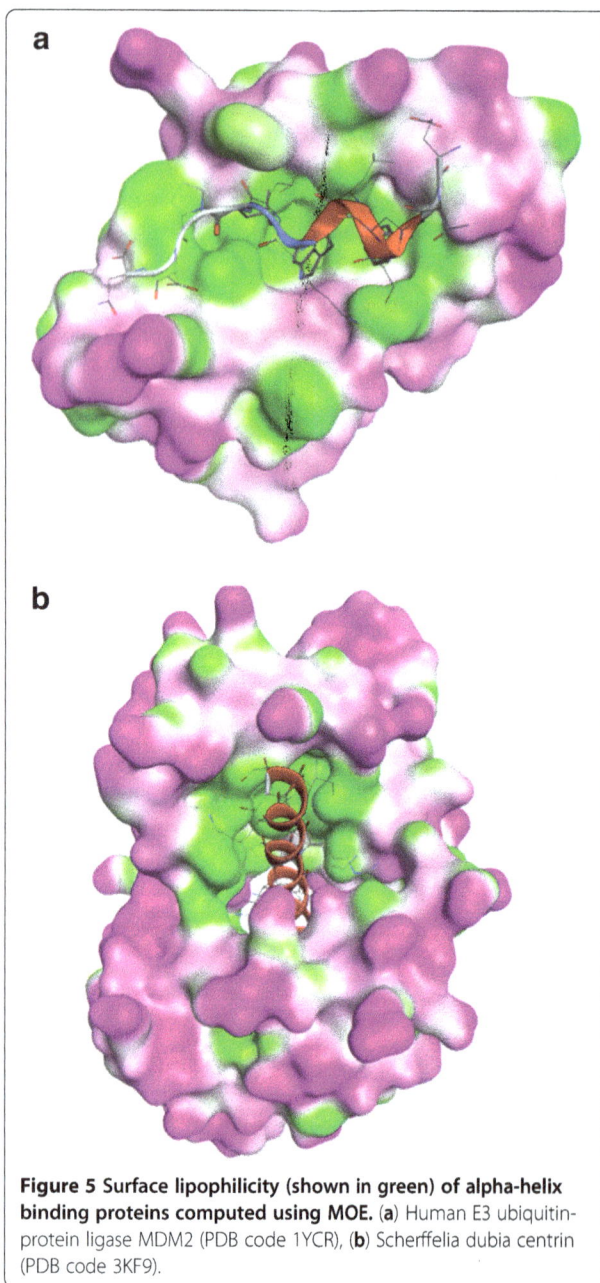

Figure 5 Surface lipophilicity (shown in green) of alpha-helix binding proteins computed using MOE. (a) Human E3 ubiquitin-protein ligase MDM2 (PDB code 1YCR), (b) Scherffelia dubia centrin (PDB code 3KF9).

transcriptase (p51/p66) and in cell-fusion processes, including the gp120-CD4 interaction and the gp41 six-helix bundle formation. They suggested that polarizability of MET allows it to assume roles of both hydrophobic and hydrophilic residues [40]. Further, its larger flexibility compared to other hydrophobic residues may facilitate the plasticity of hydrophobic binding pockets allowing to accommodate different ligands [27].

We used Fpocket [33] and CASTp [32] to calculate geometrical and physicochemical characteristics of the binding pockets taking into account the protein residues interacting with the alpha-helical peptides. The overall hydrophobic character of the binding pockets is again clearly identified. Yet, some specificity is also observed, several pockets show high hydrophobicity score but low local hydrophobic density, or vice versa, demonstrating that the hydrophobic patches are not always regularly distributed in the binding pockets. For example, 1YCR and 3KF9 have similar hydrophobicity scores but high and low calculated hydrophobic density, respectively. The differences of the hydrophobicity distribution are illustrated in Figure 5.

The volumes of the detected pockets in the peptide-binding regions computed with CASTp are given in Table 3. The average volume of the sub-cavities present at the PPI interfaces found by Fuller et al [41] was ~60 Å^3. Sonavane & Chakrabarti [42] found PPI pocket volumes to be up to ~330 Å^3. We found similar volumes to those reported in Bourgeas et al. [43]. Taking into account the various algorithms and different concepts for binding pocket definition, such differences for the computed volumes can be expected. Several small cavities are present in the binding region (seen in Figure 2 and Figure 5), as it has been previously observed for other targeted PPI interfaces [39]. For the proteins studied here, the presence of several small hydrophobic cavities in the alpha-helix binding region seems to be a typical surface feature guiding the anchoring of hydrophobic residues from the peptide side. Such characteristics can also facilitate targeting PPI mediated by alpha-helices by small molecules containing hydrophobic anchors (as terphenyl or other mimetics).

Further, we decided to explore the roughness of the alpha-helix binding sites. The methodology implemented to calculate the fractal surface dimensions, used for the roughness evaluation, is illustrated in Figure 6 for the global surface roughness of chicken calmodulin. The fractal global surface dimension and the fractal local surface dimension for the binding site of chicken calmodulin are calculated to be $D_S = 2.238$; ± 0.006 and $D_L = 2.616 \pm 0.072$, respectively. The global and local fractal dimensions for the other proteins are given in Table 4. Our results and other previously published data [44-47] suggest that the global fractal dimension of protein surface is

considered as key for the interaction with terphenyl and its derivatives, or other alpha-helix mimetics. We noticed the presence of MET residues in most of the alpha-helix binding pockets analyzed here. In a recent study, MET residues have not been identified to be a part of hot spot amino acids, in particular in alpha-helix mediated protein interfaces [39]. However, our analysis clearly indicates their presence in positions that are key for the interaction with the alpha-helical partner. Furthermore, Ma and Nussinov [40] have also concluded that the amino acids TRP, MET, and PHE are important for protein-protein interactions. They showed that TRP/MET/PHE residues play roles in the dimerization of the

Table 3 Geometrical and physicochemical characteristics of the identified pockets

Protein code PDB	Volume ($Å^3$)	Hydrophobicity score	Local hydrophobic density
Chicken calmodulin 2O5G	312.0	68.86	43.00
Human calmodulin 1ZUZ	203.0	68.86	42.00
Human calmodulin 2VAY	219.8	59.62	40.00
Human calmodulin 3DVE	226.4	61.00	39.32
E.coli calmodulin 1QTX	317.9	56.63	40.15
Rat calmodulin 2HQW	310.6	56.62	43.78
Human centrin 2 2GGM	147.9	41.47	32.00
Human centrin 2 2K2I	210.9	39.93	35.08
Scherffelia dubia centrin 3KF9	221.5	58.19	31.00
Human BCL-XL 1BXL	321.5	36.91	42.04
Human E3 ubiquitin-protein ligase MDM2 1YCR	201.9	51.18	55.20
Rabbit cardiac troponin C 1A2X	213.1	63.07	39.15

about 2. The local surface fractal dimensions for the binding cavities are computed to be larger than the global surface fractal dimensions for all studied proteins. This reflects the higher roughness of the binding site and its more complex shape and that can be considered as important for ligand binding. The most important differences between D_S and D_L are obtained for human

calmodulin (2VAY), centrin (3KF9, 2K2I), BCL-XL (1BXL), MDM2 (1YCR) and troponin C (1A2X). It has been experimentally demonstrated that human calmodulin [18], BCL-XL [19,20] and MDM2 [21,22] interact with terphenyl or its derivatives. Recently, we suggested

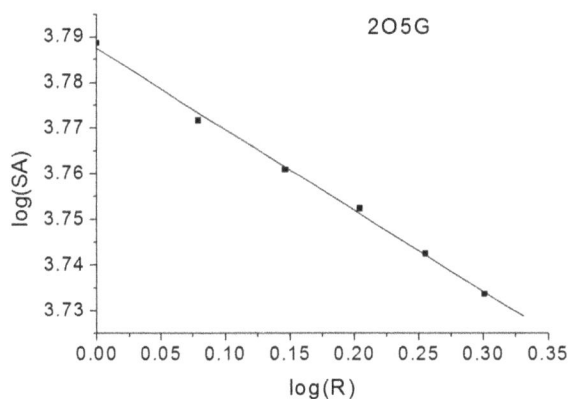

Figure 6 Double logarithmical plot of the surface area versus probe radii for chicken calmodulin (PDB code 2O5G).

Table 4 Global (D_S) and local (D_L) surface fractal dimensions of investigated proteins

Code PDB	D_S	D_L
2O5G	2.238 ± 0.006	2.616 ± 0.072
1ZUZ	2.181 ± 0.007	2.487 ± 0.058
2VAY	2.183 ± 0.006	2.757 ± 0.108
3DVE	2.217 ± 0.003	2.418 ± 0.040
1QTX	2.302 ± 0.002	2.494 ± 0.069
2HQW	2.172 ± 0.002	2.454 ± 0.082
2GGM	2.247 ± 0.004	2.373 ± 0.018
2K2I	2.167 ± 0.008	2.892 ± 0.124
3KF9	2.179 ± 0.006	2.892 ± 0.153
1BXL	2.230 ± 0.007	2.696 ± 0.225
1YCR	2.173 ± 0.014	2.708 ± 0.055
1A2X	2.177 ± 0.005	2.624 ± 0.032

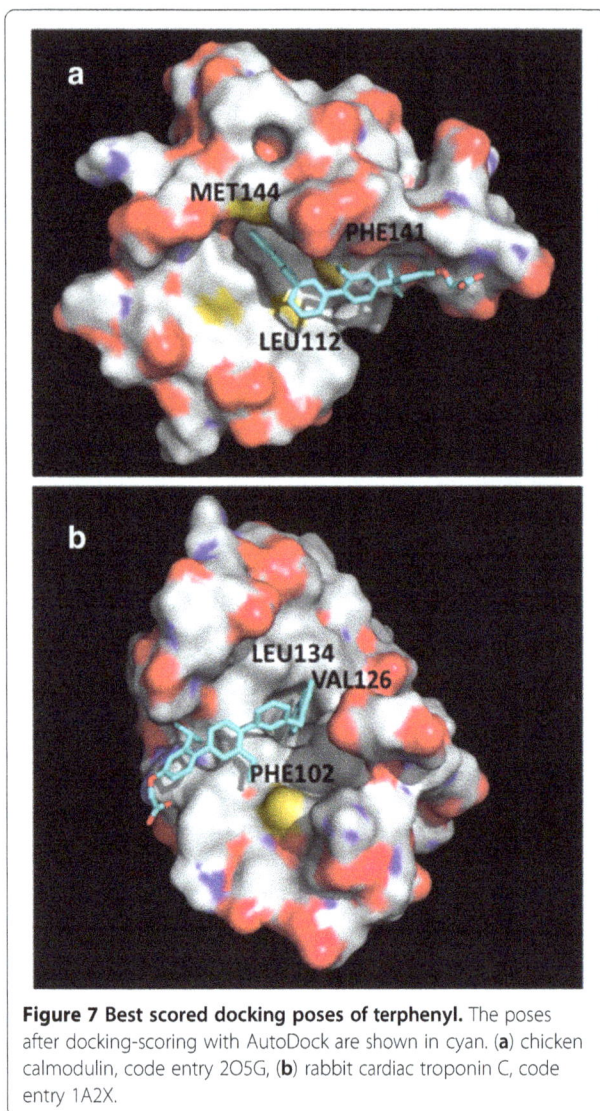

Figure 7 Best scored docking poses of terphenyl. The poses after docking-scoring with AutoDock are shown in cyan. (**a**) chicken calmodulin, code entry 2O5G, (**b**) rabbit cardiac troponin C, code entry 1A2X.

position of the bound alpha-helical peptides shown in Figure 2. The predicted interaction energies of -7.98 and -8.18 kcal/mol for terphenyl binding in calmodulin and troponin C, respectively, suggest favorable interactions with the two proteins.

In the light of the results obtained here, it is now interesting to discuss the physicochemical properties of known PPI modulators, such as terphenyl. In a previous work [10] we gathered a set of 66 PPI inhibitors among which some terphenyl derivatives and other inhibitors of alpha-helix mediated PPI were present. In that work we demonstrated the more hydrophobic character of these compounds but also their bigger size. Interestingly, we also showed the importance of a critical number of aromatic bonds and some specific molecular shapes (T-shaped, star-shaped, or L-shaped compounds), among which some correspond to terphenyl derivatives. The present work therefore confirms that such genuine properties on the ligand side seem to be cavity-driven, and that these small molecules must possess certain properties in order to efficiently modulate an alpha-helix mediated PPI and to mimic the native partner and its properties.

Conclusions

Modulating protein-protein interactions using small molecules based on surface recognition has been a field of increasing interest during the last decade. PPI interfaces are very complex and need to be analyzed in order to be efficiently targeted for drug discovery purposes. Designed compounds must bind with high affinity and selectivity to the target protein. The low sequence identity found between some of the analyzed proteins suggests that there are no sequence requirements for the ability of proteins to bind alpha-helical peptides and consequently small-molecule mimetics.

From the structural point of view, all investigated proteins show larger surface fractal dimensions for the peptide-binding pockets than the entire protein surface reflecting the higher complexity of the shape of the binding sites. Also, the presence of several hydrophobic patches at the protein surface seems to be an important property related to the ability of the protein to bind alpha-helical peptides and mimetics. Furthermore, we showed that hydrophobicity is not uniformly distributed across different alpha-helix binding pockets and that its distribution can be used to identify hydrophobic hot spots.

Many similarities between the binding sites studied here are observed and terphenyl or its derivatives binding to various alpha-helix binding proteins can be suggested. However, targeting various PPI complexes by similar small molecules can rise selectivity problems in the context of drug discovery or chemical biology

a possible binding of terphenyl 2, which mimics the relative positions of the side chains of residues TRP848, LEU851, LEU855 of the XPC peptide, into human centrin 2 following our energetic and conformational flexibility analysis performed for the alpha-helical peptide-binding pocket of centrin 2 [27]. The D_L value for the peptide-binding site of troponin C shows rougher surface than the entire protein, similarly to the above listed terphenyl-binding proteins.

Taking into consideration the sequence and structural homology of troponin C and calmodulin and other physicochemical similarities of the binding sites as discussed above, we decided to probe putative terphenyl binding into troponin C. We performed docking of terphenyl 2 into the peptide-binding sites of calmodulin and troponin C using AutoDock. The best scored docking poses are shown in Figure 7. The terphenyl orientations in the best scored poses correspond to the projects. Thus, the specificities found here for different binding sites, e.g. key residues, roughness and local hydrophobic density, can be further exploited to optimize terphenyl-like ligands in order to improve their selectivity.

Abbreviations

PPI: Protein-Protein interactions; smMLCK: smooth muscle myosin light chain kinase; CaM: Calmodulin; HsCen2: Human centrin 2; PDE: 3'-5'-cyclic nucleotide phosphodiesterase; XPC: Xeroderma pigmentosum group C.

Competing interests

The authors declare that they have no competing interests.

Authors' contributions

AI carried out the sequence alignment and binding pockets analysis. DC carried out the fractal calculations. AI and DC drafted the manuscript. VM carried out the volume calculations and docking analysis. OS participated in the protein-protein interface analysis and discussion writing. MAM designed and coordinated the study. All authors participated in manuscript writing and approved the final manuscript.

Acknowledgments

The financial support from the West University of Timisoara, the Inserm institute and the University Paris Diderot is greatly appreciated.

Author details

[1]Department of Biology and Chemistry, West University of Timisoara, 16 Pestalozzi, Timisoara 300115, Romania. [2]Advanced Environmental Researches Laboratory, 4 Oituz, Timisoara 300086, Romania. [3]Teacher Training Department, West University of Timisoara, 4 Blvd. V. ParvanTimisoara 300223, Romania. [4]Université Paris Diderot, Sorbonne Paris Cité, Molécules Thérapeutiques in silico, Inserm UMR-S 973, 35 rue Helene Brion, Paris 75013, France. [5]INSERM, U973, Paris F-75205, France.

References

1. Hunter T, Maniatis T, Califano A, Honig B, Zhang QC, Petrey D, Deng L, Qiang L, Shi Y, Thu CA, Bisikirska B, Lefebvre C, Accili D: **Structure-based prediction of protein-protein interactions on a genome-wide scale.** *Nature* 2012, **490**:556–660.
2. Stumpf MP, Thorne T, de Silva E, Stewart R, An HJ, Lappe M, Wiuf C: **Estimating the size of the human interactome.** *Proc Natl Acad Sci USA* 2008, **105**:6959–6964.
3. Stockwell BR: **Exploring biology with small organic molecules.** *Nature* 2004, **432**:846–854.
4. Wilson CG, Arkin MR: **Small-molecule inhibitors of IL-2/IL-2R: Lessons learned and applied.** *Curr Top Microbiol Immunol* 2011, **348**:25–29.
5. Villoutreix BO, Bastard K, Sperandio O, Fahraeus R, Poyet JL, Calvo F, Deprez B, Miteva MA: **In silico-in vitro screening of protein-protein interactions: towards the next generation of therapeutics.** *Curr Pharm Biotechnol* 2008, **9**:103–122.
6. Fry DC: **Protein-protein interactions as targets for small molecule drug discovery.** *Biopolymers* 2006, **84**:535–552.
7. Gautier B, Miteva MA, Goncalves V, Huguenot F, Coric P, Bouaziz S, Seijo B, Gaucher JF, Broutin I, Garbay C, Lesnard A, Rault S, Inguimbert N, Villoutreix BO, Vidal M: **Targeting the proangiogenic VEGF-VEGFR protein-protein interface with drug-like compounds by in silico and in vitro screening.** *Chem Biol* 2011, **18**(12):1631–1639.
8. Villoutreix BO, Laconde G, Lagorce D, Martineau P, Miteva MA, Dariavach P: **Tyrosine kinase syk non-enzymatic inhibitors and potential anti-allergic drug-like compounds discovered by virtual and in vitro screening.** *PLoS One* 2011, **6**(6):e21117.
9. Wells JA, McClendon CL: **Reaching for high-hanging fruit in drug discovery at protein-protein interfaces.** *Nature* 2007, **450**:1001–1009.
10. Sperandio O, Reynes CH, Camproux AC, Villoutreix BO: **Rationalizing the chemical space of protein-protein interaction inhibitors.** *Drug Discov Today* 2010, **15**:220–229.
11. Morelli X, Bourgeas R, Roche P: **Chemical and structural lessons from recent successes in protein-protein interaction inhibition (2P2I).** *Curr Opin Chem Biol* 2011, **15**:475–481.
12. Tripathi A, Kellogg GE: **A Novel and Efficient Tool for Locating and Characterizing Protein Cavities and Binding Sites.** *Proteins* 2010, **78**(4):825–842.
13. Grosdidier S, Fernández-Recio J: **Protein-protein Docking and Hot-spot Prediction for Drug Discovery.** *Curr Pharm Des* 2012, **18**(30):4607–4618.
14. Andersson CD, Chen BY, Linusson A: **Mapping of ligand-binding cavities in proteins.** *Proteins* 2010, **78**(6):1408–1422.
15. Koes D, Khoury K, Huang Y, Wang W, Bista M, Popowicz GM, Wolf S, Holak TA, Domling A, Camacho CJ: **Enabling Large-Scale Design, Synthesis and Validation of Small Molecule Protein-Protein Antagonists.** *PLoS One* 2012, **7**(3):e32839.
16. Petsko GA, Ringe D: *Protein structure and function.* London: New Science Press Ltd; 2004.
17. Bullock BN, Jochim AL, Arora PS: **Assessing helical protein interfaces for inhibitor Design.** *J Am Chem Soc* 2011, **133**(36):14220–14223.
18. Orner BP, Ernst JT, Hamilton AD: **Towards Proteomimetics: Terphenyl Derivatives as Structural and Functional Mimics of Extended Regions of an a-Helix.** *J Am Chem Soc* 2001, **123**(22):5382–5383.
19. Kutzki O, Park HS, Ernst JT, Orner BP, Yin H, Hamilton AD: **Development of a Potent Bcl-xL Antagonist Based on r-Helix Mimicry.** *J Am Chem Soc* 2002, **124**(40):11838–11839.
20. Yin H, Lee GI, Sedey KA, Kutzki O, Park HS, Orner BP, Ernst JT, Wang HG, Sebti SM, Hamilton AD: **Terphenyl-Based Bak BH3 alpha-helical proteomimetics as low-molecular-weight antagonists of Bcl-xL.** *J Am Chem Soc* 2005, **127**(29):10191–10196.
21. Yin H, Lee G, Park HS, Payne GA, Rodriguez JM, Sebti SM, Hamilton AD: **Terphenyl-Based Helical Mimetics That Disrupt the p53/HDM2 Interaction.** *Angew Chem* 2005, **117**(18):2764–2767.
22. Chen L, Yin H, Farooqi B, Sebti S, Hamilton AD, Chen J: **p53 alpha-Helix mimetics antagonize p53/MDM2 interaction and activate p53.** *Mol Canc Ther* 2005, **4**(6):1019–1025.
23. Che Y, Brooks BR, Marshall GR: **Protein recognition motifs: design of peptidomimetics of helix surfaces.** *Biopolymers* 2007, **86**(4):288–297.
24. Becerril J, Rodriguez JM, Wyrembak PN, Hamilton AD: **Inhibition of protein-protein interaction by peptide mimics.** In *Protein Surface Recognition: Approaches for Drug Discovery.* Edited by Giralt E, Peczuh M, Salvatella X. London: John Willey&Sons; 2011.
25. Fairlie DP, West ML, Wong AK: **Towards protein surface mimetics.** *Curr Med Chem* 1998, **5**(1):29–62.
26. Maity P, König B: **Synthesis and structure of 1,4-dipiperazino benzenes: chiral terphenyl-type peptide helix mimetics.** *Org Lett* 2008, **10**(7):1473–1476.
27. Isvoran A, Badel A, Craescu CT, Miron S, Miteva MA: **Exploring NMR ensembles of calcium binding proteins: Perspectives to design inhibitors of protein-protein interactions.** *BMC Struct Biol* 2011, **11**:24.
28. Thompson JD, Higgins DG, Gibson TJ: **CLUSTAL W: Improving the sensitivity of progressive multiple sequence alignment through sequence weighting, position specific gap penalties and weight matrix choice.** *Nucleic Acids Res* 1994, **22**:4673–4680.
29. Firoz A, Malik A, Afzal O, Jha V: **ContPro: A web tool for calculating amino acid contact distances in protein from 3D –structure at different distance threshold.** *Bioinformation* 2010, **5**(2):55–57.
30. Lewis M, Rees DC: **Fractal surfaces of proteins.** *Science* 1985, **230**:1163–1165.
31. Fraczkiewicz R, Braun W: **Exact and efficient analytical calculation of accesible surface areas and their gradients for macromolecules.** *J Compl Chem* 1998, **19**:319–333.
32. Dundas J, Ouyang Z, Tseng J, Binkowski A, Turpaz Y, Liang J: **CASTp: computed atlas of surface topography of proteins with structural and topographical mapping of functionally annotated resiudes.** *Nucleic Acid Res* 2006, **34**:W116–W118.
33. Guilleoux VL, Schmidtke P, Tuffery P: **Fpocket; An open source platform for ligand binding pocket detection.** *BMC Bioinforma* 2009, **10**:168.
34. Morris GM, Huey R, Lindstrom W, Sanner MF, Belew RK, Goodsell DS, Olson AJ: **AutoDock4 and AutoDockTools4: Automated docking with selective receptor flexibility.** *J Comput Chem* 2009, **30**(16):2785–2791.
35. DeLano WL: *The PyMol molecular graphics system.* San Carlos: DeLano Scientific; 2002.

36. Pettersen EF, Goddard TD, Huang CC, Couch GS, Greenblatt DM, Meng EC, Ferrin TE: **UCSF Chimera--a visualization system for exploratory research and analysis.** *J Comput Chem* 2004, **25**(13):1605–1612.

37. Berman HM, Westbrook J, Feng Z, Gilliland G, Bhat TN, Weissig H, Shindyalov IN, Bourne PE: **The Protein Data Bank.** *Nucleic Acids Res* 2000, **28**:235–242.

38. Moreira IS, Fernandes PA, Ramos MJ: **Hot spots—A review of the protein–protein interface determinant amino-acid residues.** *Proteins Struct Funct Bioinform* 2007, **68**(4):803–812.

39. Brooke N, Bullock A, Paramjit SA: **Assessing Helical Protein Interfaces for Inhibitor Design.** *J Am Chem Soc* 2011, **133**(36):14220–14223.

40. Ma B, Nussinov R: **Trp/Met/Phe Hot Spots in Protein-Protein Interactions: Potential Targets in Drug Design.** *Curr Top Med Chem* 2007, **7**:999–1005.

41. Fuller JC, Burgoyne NJ, Jackson RM: **Predicting druggable binding sites at the protein–protein interface.** *Drug Discov Today* 2009, **14**(3–4):155–161.

42. Sonavane S, Chakrabarti P: **Cavities and Atomic Packing in Protein Structures and Interfaces.** *PLoS Comput Biol* 2008, **4**:e100001188.

43. Bourgeas R, Basse MJ, Morelli X, Roche P: **Atomic Analysis of Protein-Protein Interfaces with Known Inhibitors: The 2P2I Database.** *PLoS One* 2010, **3**:e9598.

44. Goetze T, Brickmann J: **Self similarity of protein surfaces.** *Biophys J* 1992, **61**:109–118.

45. Pettit FK, Bowie JU: **Protein surface roughness and small molecular binding sites.** *J Mol Biol* 1999, **285**(4):1377–1382.

46. Stawiski EW, Baucom AE, Lohr SC, Gregoret LM: **Predicting protein function from structure: Unique structural features of proteases.** *Proc Natl Acad Sci* 2000, **97**:3954–3958.

47. Stawiski EW, Mandel-Goutfreund Y, Lowenthal AC, Gregoret LM: **Progress in predicting protein structure from sequence: unique features of O-glycosidases.** *Pacific Symp Biocomput* 2002, **7**:637–648.

19

Pharmaceutical quality of seven generic Levodopa/Benserazide products compared with original Madopar® / Prolopa®

Urs E Gasser[1], Anton Fischer[2], Jan P Timmermans[2] and Isabelle Arnet[3*]

Abstract

Background: By definition, a generic product is considered interchangeable with the innovator brand product. Controversy exists about interchangeability, and attention is predominantly directed to contaminants. In particular for chronic, degenerative conditions such as in Parkinson's disease (PD) generic substitution remains debated among physicians, patients and pharmacists. The objective of this study was to compare the pharmaceutical quality of seven generic levodopa/benserazide hydrochloride combination products marketed in Germany with the original product (Madopar® / Prolopa® 125, Roche, Switzerland) in order to evaluate the potential impact of Madopar® generics versus branded products for PD patients and clinicians.

Methods: Madopar® / Prolopa® 125 tablets and capsules were used as reference material. The generic products tested (all 100 mg/25 mg formulations) included four tablet and three capsule formulations. Colour, appearance of powder (capsules), disintegration and dissolution, mass of tablets and fill mass of capsules, content, identity and amounts of impurities were assessed along with standard physical and chemical laboratory tests developed and routinely practiced at Roche facilities. Results were compared to the original "shelf-life" specifications in use by Roche.

Results: Each of the seven generic products had one or two parameters outside the specifications. Deviations for the active ingredients ranged from +8.4% (benserazide) to −7.6% (levodopa) in two tablet formulations. Degradation products were measured in marked excess (+26.5%) in one capsule formulation. Disintegration time and dissolution for levodopa and benserazide hydrochloride at 30 min were within specifications for all seven generic samples analysed, however with some outliers.

Conclusions: Deviations for the active ingredients may go unnoticed by a new user of the generic product, but may entail clinical consequences when switching from original to generic during a long-term therapy. Degradation products may pose a safety concern. Our results should prompt caution when prescribing a generic of Madopar®/Prolopa®, and also invite to further investigations in view of a more comprehensive approach, both pharmaceutical and clinical.

Keywords: Parkinson's Disease, Levodopa, Benserazide hydrochloride, Pharmaceutical quality, Generics

Background

Parkinson's disease (PD) is a progressive neurodegenerative disorder affecting primarily dopaminergic neuronal systems. Typical manifestations include motor symptoms (bradykinesia, rigidity, tremor, gait and postural instability) and non-motor symptoms including cognitive and emotional dysfunction [1-3]. Levodopa or L-dopa is a naturally occurring amino acid (L-3,4-dihydroxyphenylalanine). It is a prodrug and the precursor of dopamine (DA), a neurotransmitter that is severely reduced in PD due to degeneration of neuronal cells [2,3]. Levodopa has been the standard medical therapy for PD since its discovery approximately 40 years ago [4] and is recognized as a classic example of a brain neurotransmitter substitution therapy. When given systemically, levodopa crosses the blood–brain barrier and is converted to DA by L-dopa decarboxylase (DDC) [5]. When administered orally, a high pre-systemic conversion to DA occurs in the gut by

* Correspondence: isabelle.arnet@unibas.ch
[3]Pharmaceutical Care Research Group, Department of Pharmaceutical Sciences, University of Basel, Klingelbergstr. 50, 4056, Basel, Switzerland
Full list of author information is available at the end of the article

the enzyme L-amino acid decarboxylase (AADC), reducing the systemic available dose of levodopa to 30% [6,7]. Levodopa is thus coadministered in a 4/1 ratio with an AADC inhibitor such as benserazide hydrochloride. This combination can triple the oral bioavailability of levodopa, and markedly reduces both the required levodopa therapeutic dose and the severity of dopamine-mediated gastrointestinal and cardiovascular side-effects [8]. Levodopa has a short half-life of 1.5 h, even when coadministered with an AADC inhibitor [9]. When administered with benserazide hydrochloride, the initial dose is 100 mg to 200 mg levodopa daily given as levodopa 50 mg/benserazide 25 mg up to 2 to 4 times a day. Treatment may start at levodopa 300 mg daily in advanced disease. The recommended maximum maintenance dose is 800 mg levodopa daily in multiple divided doses [9,10].

Levodopa is a white or almost white crystalline powder which darkens on exposure to air and light [10]. It is odourless, almost tasteless, slightly soluble in water and soluble in aqueous solutions of mineral acids and alkali carbonates [10]. Levodopa is purchased on the pharmaceutical market. Benserazide hydrochloride is a white or almost white crystalline powder, slightly soluble in ethanol, and soluble in water. Benserazide hydrochloride decomposes slowly in aqueous solution. It is synthetically produced by Roche.

Madopar®/Prolopa® 125 mg (levodopa 100 mg + benserazide hydrochloride 25 mg) exists as scored tablets and capsules for Parkinson's disease [9].

By definition, a generic product is considered interchangeable with the innovator brand product and needs to demonstrate the same qualitative and quantitative composition in active substances, the same pharmaceutical form and bioequivalence with the reference product after a single dose [11]. The different salts, esters, complexes or derivatives of an active substance are considered to be the same active substance, and thus different excipients, colour agents, flavours and preservatives are allowed. Generics may also differ in characteristics such as shape, size, colour, scoring configuration, and release mechanisms [12-16]. Controversy exists about interchangeability, mainly because of the questionable validity of the current criteria the evaluation is performed in a small, young and healthy population; no clinical efficacy data are required; short term study [17]. Thus, therapeutic equivalence is not necessarily guaranteed. However, attention is predominantly directed to contaminants that could cause adverse clinical events and ultimately fatal issues [5-7]. In clinical settings, health professionals are aware that patient response and susceptibility to levodopa vary widely, especially in advanced PD, and that levodopa blood levels correlate with the

emergence of many symptoms, including motor manifestations like dyskinesia and "off" periods. Thus, even small variations in levodopa availability and consequently subtle fluctuations in levodopa blood levels can trigger motor complications. Since generic formulations differ from the branded product mainly in their excipients, which may affect absorption and bioavailability [15], simple bioequivalence cannot suffice to ensure comparable clinical efficacy and safety, especially in PD.

Roche's standard operating procedures (SOPs) describe the qualitative and quantitative pharmaceutical tests for physical and chemical purity of the substance. They were accepted by regulatory authorities as part of the Madopar® registration documentation and form the basis of Mapopar®/Prolopa® specifications in the United States, European and British Pharmacopoeias. The current investigation compares the pharmaceutical quality of seven generic products with the specifications of the original Madopar® and raises questions about safety and interchangeability.

Methods
Samples of generic levodopa/benserazide hydrochloride products, all 100 mg/25 mg formulations, were purchased in 2011 as commercial goods in a community pharmacy in Germany and tested within their expiry dates.

Pharmaceutical quality tests
The tests were colour (tablets and capsules), colour and appearance of powder (capsules), mass of tablets and fill mass of capsules, disintegration and dissolution, content of active pharmaceutical ingredient (API), and the identity and amounts of impurities.

Colour
Tablet colour was assessed visually according to the standards described in the "Munsell Book of Color" (1996). Capsule colour was assessed by comparison to reference capsules. Madopar® specifications for colour are pale red for tablets and flesh-coloured opaque for the capsule body and powder-blue opaque for the capsule cap.

Mass of tablets
Twenty tablets were weighed and average mass was calculated. Madopar® specifications for average mass of tablets are 267–283 mg (275 mg ± 3%).

Fill mass of capsules
Twenty capsules were weighed, emptied, and the empty capsules weighed; the average weight of the capsule fill mass was derived from the difference. Madopar® specifications for capsule fill mass are 142.5-157.5 mg (150 mg ± 5%).

Disintegration time

Tablets and capsules were tested according to Ph. Eur. / USP (tablets: apparatus A without discs using water at 37°C; capsules: apparatus A using discs and 0.1 M HCl at 37°C). Madopar® specifications for disintegration time are not more than 15 min for tablets and not more than 30 min for capsules.

Dissolution

Dissolution was tested using the Ph. Eur. rotating basket apparatus and 0.1 N HCl at 37°C as the dissolution medium. Samples were measured by UV-HPLC at 220 nm. Madopar® shelf-life specifications for dissolution after 30 min are at least 75% for tablets and at least 80% for capsules.

Content of levodopa, benserazide hydrochloride, related substances and impurities

Madopar® specifications for content of active substances are levodopa 95.0-105.0 mg (100 mg ± 5%) and benserazide hydrochloride 27.1-29.9 mg (28.5 mg ± 5%) per unit. The content of active substances and degradation products was determined using HPLC. Benserazide is degradated by hydrolysis to Ro 04–1419, which can bind one molecule of benserazide to the dimer Ro 08–1580. The specifications for content of specific degradation products of benserazide hydrochloride are limited to 3.49%

(tablets) and 0.49% (capsules). The maximum permissible amount of other impurities is set at 1.04% (tablets) and 0.54% (capsules). The specifications for other impurities are no more than 0.54% (tablets) and 0.24% (capsules) for any individual impurity.

Results

Analysis was performed according to the standard physical and chemical laboratory tests developed and routinely practiced at Roche facilities.

Physical characteristics

The physical characteristics of the tested products are shown in Table 1. None of the generic tablets was cross-scored on both sides like the original product, but all had either a single break bar on both sides (Betapharm) or on one side only. The colours of all generic products were similar to Madopar®/Prolopa® except for one capsule formulation (Teva).

Mass, fill mass, disintegration time and dissolution rate

Mass exceeded the upper limits of the specifications in five of the seven generic products (Table 2), and by almost 200% for all three capsule formulations. Disintegration times (min - max: tablets 4.30 - 6.30 min; capsules 5.40 -16.10 min) were within specification. Dissolution values after 30 min complied with the specifications,

Table 1 Physical characteristics of Madopar®/Prolopa® and seven generic products

Brand name	Manufacturer	Colour	Appearance	
Tablets				
Madopar	Roche Pharmaceuticals	Pale red	Above: cross-scored	
			Below: cross-scored	
Levodopa/ Benserazid beta	Betapharm Arzneimittel GmbH	Pale red, speckled	Above: score line	
			Below: score line	
Levodopa/ Benserazid-CT	CT Arzneimittel GmbH	Pale red, speckled	Above: score line	
			Below: none	
dopadura B	MYLAN dura	Pale red, speckled	Above: score line	
			Below: none	
Levodopa/ Benserazid ratiopharm	ratiopharm GmbH	Pale red, strongly speckled	Above: score line	
			Below: none	
Capsules			**Appearance of the content**	**Colour of the content**
Madopar	Roche Pharmaceuticals	Body: flesh-coloured, opaque	Fine granular powder	Light beige
		Cap: powder-blue, opaque		
Levopar	HEXAL AG	Body: flesh-coloured, opaque	Fine granular powder	Brown
		Cap: powder-blue, opaque		
Levodopa comp. B STADA	STADApharm GmbH	Body: flesh-coloured, opaque	Fine granular powder	Almost white
		Cap: powder-blue, opaque		
Levobens-Teva	TEVA GmbH	Body: midnight blue, opaque	Fine granular powder	Almost white
		Cap: fluorescent-pink, opaque		

Table 2 Mass, content of active ingredients, and dissolution time of seven generic products compared to Madopar®/ Prolopa® specifications

Brand name	Mass (mg)	Levodopa (mg)	Benserazide hydrochloride (mg)	Dissolution after 30 min
Tablet specifications	267.0-283.0	95.0-105.0	27.1-29.9	>75%/ >75%
Levodopa/ Benserazid beta	265	92.4*	30.9*	99% / 99%
Levodopa/ Benserazid-CT	284*	98.2	27.8	101% / 97%
dopadura B	283	94.4*	26.9*	100% / 97%
Levodopa/ Benserazide ratiopharm	284*	95.5	28.8	101% / 98%
Capsule specifications	Fill mass (mg) 142.5-157.5	95.0-105.0	27.1-29.9	>80%/ >80%
Levopar	298.6*	98.3	27.5	80% / 84%
Levodopa comp. B STADA	299.0*	98.7	27.6	100% / 96%
Levobens-Teva	222.3*	99.5	28.3	89% / 86%

* Values marked with an asterisk indicate deviations from Roche specifications.

however, some single values were below specification (Levobens-Teva 16%, 25%; Levopar 68%, 49%, 72% 78%), indicating large variations in dissolution properties for single capsules.

Content of active substances, degradation products, and impurities

Content requirements for the active substances were unmet in two of the four tablet formulations, with content of levodopa below the limits, and content of benserazide hydrochloride below and above the limits (Table 2). All products contained impurities, exceeding the limits by 79% in one generic product (Table 3).

Discussion

Comparison of the pharmaceutical quality of Madopar®/ Prolopa® with seven generic products showed that at least one of the tested parameters fell outside Roche shelf-life specifications in all products tested and identified two areas of concern: Content of active substances and impurities. Since even small variations of levodopa availability and consequently subtle fluctuations in levodopa blood

levels can trigger motor complications, the observed out-of-specification values could suffice to unbalance symptom management, especially in stabilized patients. In switching to a new formulation, patients may face weeks of complex retitration and further visits to their neurologists. In 2010–11 the worldwide shortage of branded Sinemet (carbidopa-levodopa), followed by shortage of its generic formulation (all formulations and all dosages), revealed the distress of the Parkinson community through the testimony of thousands of patients forced to switch to generics [18]. Patients uniformly reported a negative experience and several clinical issues, e.g. slower onset of effect, faster waning of effect, dose adjustment to compensate for the decreased medication effect, symptom exacerbation (e.g. dyskinesia), and side effects such as poorer sleep quality and increased impulsivity. No patient reported a preference for the generic version. Replacement medication was perceived as less effective, probably due to patients receiving differing generics at each renewal, thus getting fluctuations in blood levels with every new product.

The development of a branded formulation requires the assessment of pharmacokinetic parameters in healthy

Table 3 Identity and amounts of related substances and impurities in seven generic products compared to Madopar®/ Prolopa® specifications

Degradation product	Ro 04-1419	Ro 08-1580	Ro 04-1419 + Ro 08-1580	Others each	Others total
Tablets Upper limits (%)	1.54	2.49	3.49	0.54	1.04
Levodopa/ Benserazid beta	0.35	0.47	0.83	0.19, 0.09	0.28
Levodopa/ Benserazid-CT	0.28	0.48	0.75	0.09, 0.08	0.17
Levodopa/ Benserazide ratiopharm	0.25	0.37	0.62	0.16, 0.05	0.21
dopadura B	0.26	0.34	0.60	0.12	0.12
Capsules Upper limits (%)	0.54	0.54	0.49	0.24	0.54
Levopar	0.12	0.34	0.46	0.10	0.10
Levodopa comp. B STADA	0.16	0.32	0.49	0.11, 0.11	0.11
Levobens-Teva	0.36	0.25	0.62*	0.10, 0.12, 0.10	0.33

*Values marked with an asterisk indicate deviations from Roche specifications.

subjects, and a clinical study program to proof efficacy, safety and tolerability in the target patient population. Market authorisation for generic equivalents, however, requires only the documentation of bioequivalence with branded counterparts in healthy subjects, using one lot of branded product, and without accounting for country to country differences [19,20]. Some small studies [21,22] suggested that the generic formulation of carbidopa-levodopa given in a single dose to PD patients was bioequivalent to brand Sinemet. However, the same authors report clinical worsening with marked motor fluctuations in a long-term open-label study following conversion to generic carbidopa-levodopa [21]. Approval by the authorities is based on the assumption that demonstrating bioequivalence in pharmacokinetic studies in healthy volunteers suffices to demonstrate similar tolerability and efficacy in patients. Differences in the excipients used for generic formulations and the presence of impurities which may affect both the absorption and bioavailability of active ingredients in patients create a potential risk of "relative therapeutic in-equivalence" [15]. Furthermore, the intra-individual peculiarity of PD patients, such as slow absorption of the first orally administered dose of medication in the morning due to low gastric motility [23] makes the variability of blood concentrations from generic drugs unpredictable. Furthermore, PD patients often use multiple drugs e.g., dopamine agonists, monoamine oxydase inhibitors, anticholinergics, and psychotropics. Since issues regarding drug-drug interactions are not addressed by bioequivalence studies, potential risks cannot be excluded [1,23]. Unpredictable blood concentrations also expose patients to a higher risk of concentration-dependent drug-drug interactions. In addition, unknown excipients and impurities may trigger allergic reactions or even intolerance [24,25]. Score lines are a further area of concern. Madopar®/Prolopa® is cross-scored for easy splitting, since many patients commonly split their tablets to adjust their doses. Easy splitting of the medication for optimal individual dosing is a critical patient-care requirement. Without score lines, or with only one score line on one side, as in three of the test generic tablets, tablet splitting usually requires the use of a sharp blade, which is a clear safety issue for a person with PD.

Conclusions

In conclusion, these results demonstrate areas of concern in the pharmaceutical quality of generic products, such as the content of active substances, and the composition and amount of impurities. The potential risks of "relative therapeutic in-equivalence," drug-drug interactions, and allergic reactions or intolerance should prompt caution when prescribing a generic product of

Madopar®/Prolopa®, in particular in highly susceptible PD patients with co-morbidities requiring comedication. We recommend considering the substitution of Parkinson's medication as a change in medication, requiring guidance and supervision by the patient's physician. Any generic can be used to initiate first treatment. It will be effective and less expensive than the branded product, but will need a similar process of titration until symptom control is achieved. The challenge for patient, prescribing physician and pharmacist will be to ensure that the same generic formulation is dispensed at each refill. Switching back and forth between brand and generic, or even between generics, is a recipe for problems that may cancel out the savings achieved with the cheaper drug. Ultimately, it is the responsibility of the physician-patient-pharmacist triad to arrive at the best choice for the best patient outcome.

Abbreviations
AADC: L-amino acid decarboxylase; API: Active pharmaceutical ingredient; DA: Dopamine; DDC: L-Dopa decarboxylase; HCl: Hydrochloride; L-dopa: Levodopa; PD: Parkinson's Disease.

Competing interests
FA and JPT are employees at Roche. UA and IA received consultant fees.

Authors' contributions
FA and JPT conceived and designed the study, and collected the data. UA and IA analysed and interpretated the data. All authors were involved in drafting and revising the manuscript critically for intellectual content and gave final approval of the version to be published.

Author's information
UA is an independent senior scientist working for different companies as a consultant. IA is a researcher at the University of Basel specialised in adherence to medication and in guidelines developement for community pharmacies. She is a lecturer and member of several pharmacy and pharmacology societies.

Author details
[1]ClinResearch Ltd, Aesch, Switzerland. [2]F. Hoffmann-La Roche Ltd, Basel, Switzerland. [3]Pharmaceutical Care Research Group, Department of Pharmaceutical Sciences, University of Basel, Klingelbergstr. 50, 4056, Basel, Switzerland.

References
1. Schapira AHV, Olanow CE, eds: *Principles of treatment in Parkinson's disease.* Philadelphia, PA: Elsevier Health Sciences; 2005.
2. Fahn S, Sulzer D: **Neurodegeneration and neuroprotection in Parkinson disease.** *NeuroRx* 2004, 1:139–154.
3. Sulzer D: **Multiple hit hypotheses for dopamine neuron loss in Parkinson's disease.** *Trends Neurosci* 2007, 30(5):244–250.
4. Yahr MD, Duvoisin RC, Schear MJ, Barrett RE, Hoehn MM: **Treatment of Parkinsonism with levodopa.** *Arch Neurol* 1969, 4:343–354.
5. Hauser RA, Zesiewicz TA: **Advances in the pharmacologic management of early Parkinson disease.** *Neurologist* 2007, 13(3):126–132.
6. Jankovic J, Stacy M: **Medical management of levodopa-associated motor complications in patients with Parkinson's disease.** *CNS Drugs* 2007, 21(8):677–692.
7. Esposito E, Cuzzocrea S: **New therapeutic strategy for Parkinson's and Alzheimer's disease.** *Curr Med Chem* 2010, 17(25):2764–2774.
8. Contin M, Martinelli P: **Pharmacokinetics of levodopa.** *J Neurol* 2010, 257(Suppl 2):S253–S261.

9.   Swiss Summary of product characteristics of Madopar®/ Prolopa®. www.
     swissmedicinfo.ch>Madopar.
10. Reynolds JEF (Ed): *Martindale - the Extra Pharmacopoeia.* 30th edition.
     London: The Pharmaceutical Press; 1993.
11. EU/1/98/071/001-006 - Type II Variation EMEA/H/C/00154/II/0045: Widening
     of dissolution specification Q-value at shelf-life from 75% to 65%. 2007.
     www.ema.europa.eu/docs/en_GB/document_library/Scientific_guideline/
     2010/01/WC500070039.pdf.
12. Duh MS, Cahill KE, Paradis PE, Cremieux PY, Greenberg PE: The economic
     implications of generic substitution of antiepileptic drugs: a review of
     recent evidence. *Expert Opin Pharmacother* 2009, 10(14):2317e28.
13. Berg MJ, Gross RA, Haskins LS, Zingaro WM, Tomaszewski KJ: Generic
     substitution in the treatment of epilepsy: patient and physician
     perceptions. *Epilepsy Behav* 2008, 13(4):693e9.
14. Andermann F, Duh MS, Gosselin A, Paradis PE: Compulsory generic switching
     of antiepileptic drugs: high switchback rates to branded compounds
     compared with other drug classes. *Epilepsia* 2007, 8(3):464–469.
15. Go C, Rosales RL, Schmidt P, Lyons KE, Pahwa R, Okun MS: A generic versus
     branded pharmacotherapy in Parkinson's disease: Does it matter? A
     review. *Parkinsonism Relat Disords* 2011, 17:308–312.
16. Ferner RE, Lenney W, Marriott JF: Controversy over generic substitution.
     BMJ 2010, 340:c2548.
17. Borgheini G: The bioequivalence and therapeutic efficacy of generic
     versus brand-name psychoactive drugs. *Clin Ther* 2003, 25(6):1578–1592.
18. National Parkinson Foundation: Lessons from the 2011 Sinemet shortage-
     The National Parkinson Foundation's Helpline speaks. 2012. Available
     from: www.parkinson.org [March 15, 2013] www.parkinson.org/
     NationalParkinsonFoundation/files/ae/aea8377b-cf22-46d0-bdc6-
     3922290efb60pdf.
19. Meredith P: Bioequivalence and other unresolved issues in generic drug
     substitution. *Clin Ther* 2003, 5(11):2875e90.
20. US Food and Drug Administration: Guidance for industry: Bioavailability
     and bioequivalence studies for orally administered drug products -
     general consideration. [July 18, 2010]. 2010. Available from: www.fda.
     gov/cder/guidance/4964dft.pdf.
21. Pahwa R, Marjama J, McGuire D, Lyons K, Zwiebel F, Silverstein P, *et al*:
     Pharmacokinetic comparison of Sinemet and Atamet (generic
     carbidopa/levodopa): a single-dose study. *Mov Disord* 1996, 11:427–430.
22. Chaná P, Fierro A, Reyes-Parada M, Sáez-Briones P: Pharmacokinetic
     comparison of Sinemet and Grifoparkin (levodopa/carbidopa 250/
     25 mg) in Parkinson s disease: a single dose study [Article in Spanish].
     Rev Med Chil 2003, 131:623–631.
23. Fernandez N, Garcia JJ, Diez MJ, Sahagun AM, Gonzalez A, Diez R, *et al*:
     Effects of slowed gastrointestinal motility on levodopa
     pharmacokinetics. *Auton Neurosci* 2010, 156(1–2):67e72.
24. Sims-McCallum RP: Adverse reaction caused by excipients in
     mercaptopurine tablets. *Ann Pharmacother* 2007, 41(9):1548.
25. Hebron BS, Hebron HJ: Aspirin sensitivity: acetylsalicylate or excipients.
     Intern Med 2009, 39(8):546–549.

20

Effects of packaging and storage conditions on the quality of amoxicillin-clavulanic acid – an analysis of Cambodian samples

Mohiuddin Hussain Khan[1,2*], Kirara Hatanaka[1,3], Tey Sovannarith[4], Nam Nivanna[4], Lidia Cecilia Cadena Casas[1,5], Naoko Yoshida[1], Hirohito Tsuboi[1], Tsuyoshi Tanimoto[6] and Kazuko Kimura[1]

Abstract

Background: The use of substandard and degraded medicines is a major public health problem in developing countries such as Cambodia. A collaborative study was conducted to evaluate the quality of amoxicillin–clavulanic acid preparations under tropical conditions in a developing country.

Methods: Amoxicillin-clavulanic acid tablets were obtained from outlets in Cambodia. Packaging condition, printed information, and other sources of information were examined. The samples were tested for quantity, content uniformity, and dissolution. Authenticity was verified with manufacturers and regulatory authorities.

Results: A total of 59 samples were collected from 48 medicine outlets. Most (93.2%) of the samples were of foreign origin. Using predetermined acceptance criteria, 12 samples (20.3%) were non-compliant. Eight (13.6%), 10 (16.9%), and 20 (33.9%) samples failed quantity, content uniformity, and dissolution tests, respectively. Samples that violated our observational acceptance criteria were significantly more likely to fail the quality tests (Fisher's exact test, p < 0.05).

Conclusions: Improper packaging and storage conditions may reduce the quality of amoxicillin–clavulanic acid preparations at community pharmacies. Strict quality control measures are urgently needed to maintain the quality of amoxicillin–clavulanic acid in tropical countries.

Keywords: Medicine quality, Tropical country, Public health, Packaging condition, Substandard medicine, Developing country

Background

Medicine plays an important role in maintaining health, preventing disease and saving lives. However, ineffective medicines pose great risks to individuals and even threaten lives in emergencies [1,2]. Ineffectiveness takes several forms, such as medicines containing less than the stated dose of the active ingredient or containing unstated or harmful substance(s). Similarly, fake or counterfeit medicines and medicines that have been degraded or adulterated due to improper storage and handling may be ineffective [3,4]. Hence, the health ministries of many countries, especially developing nations, struggle to prevent the circulation of substandard and counterfeit medicines [5-10].

A combination of amoxicillin and clavulanic acid was introduced in the United Kingdom in 1981 as Augmentin and eventually became the treatment of choice for many infections [11,12]. Amoxicillin–clavulanic acid is available in a variety of doses: 250/125 mg (2:1), 500/125 mg (4:1), 875/125 mg (7:1), 1000/125 mg (8:1), and 2000/125 mg (16:1). In combined preparations, 125 mg of clavulanic acid is sufficient to inhibit β-lactamase–producing organisms. Amoxicillin–clavulanic acid also has proven more effective for the eradication of *H. pylori* than conventional monotherapies [13,14]. However, insufficient doses and inappropriate use of such potent antibiotics may lead to the development of resistance [15].

---

* Correspondence: mohiuddin_khn@yahoo.com
[1]Drug Management & Policy, Kanazawa University, Kakuma-machi, Kanazawa, Ishikawa 920-1192, Japan
[2]Médecins Sans Frontières, 14 Sayat-Nova street, Vanadzor, Lori, Armenia
Full list of author information is available at the end of the article

Several studies have reported the presence of substandard and counterfeit medicines in Cambodian pharmaceutical markets, with prevalences ranging from 4% to 90% [5,7]. Several of these studies suggest that antibiotics are deliberately counterfeited in some cases but unintentionally degraded in others [7,16]. The improper storage and handling of medicines in tropical countries may cause the unintentional degradation of medicines [17]. Based on previous studies in Cambodia, the Cambodian Ministry of Health (MoH), and Kanazawa University decided to conduct a collaborative study of the quality of amoxicillin–clavulanic acid in the private pharmaceutical market under tropical conditions in a developing country [7,9].

Methods
Selection of medication and study area
Combination tablets of amoxicillin–clavulanic acid were selected from the essential medicine list of Cambodia in consultation with the country's MoH. Of the various formulations of amoxicillin-clavulanic acid, only tablets appear on the essential medicine list of Cambodia. Because this study did not involve human subjects, ethical clearance was not sought. However, a memorandum of understanding was signed by the Cambodian MoH before commencement. Equal numbers of samples were collected from urban and rural areas. Seven districts of the capital (Phnom Penh) were selected to represent urban areas, and three provinces (Kandal, Takeo, and Kampong Speu) were selected to represent rural areas. The locations were selected after taking into account population density, the number of outlets, and budgetary limitations. The selections were made in consultation with the Department of Drugs and Food and the National Health Product Quality Control Center.

Collection of samples
Sampling was conducted in July-August 2009 by two teams. Each team consisted of three members: a researcher, a locally recruited supervisor and an assistant. All members of the sampling teams were provided with training beforehand and instructed to pose as typical customers. Stratified random sampling was used to collect samples from four types of private drug outlet (Pharmacy, Depot-A, Depot-B and nonlicensed outlets). A sampling form was completed for each sample after payment. Each sample was then labeled with a code number and stored at 20-25°C until analysis.

Sample analysis
Observational analysis
Primary and secondary packaging and printed labels were carefully observed with the naked eye at the Department of Drug Management and Policy, Kanazawa University, Japan. Samples were classified into five types according

to package type and the presence of desiccants (e.g., silica gel):

Type A: Press-through packaging (PTP) of aluminum-aluminum materials in cardboard boxes.
Type B: Type A tablets wrapped in transparent plastic with silica gel.
Type C: Type A tablets wrapped in aluminum with silica gel.
Type D: Similar to Type C, but with PTP made of an aluminum-plastic composite.
Type E: Strip packaging (SP) in cardboard boxes without silica gel.

Samples having any of the following packaging defects were considered unacceptable: 1) PTP/SP packaging with peeling of the cover; 2) missing tablet(s); 3) PTP/SP without any clear pocket breaks.

Authenticity
A database of manufacturer addresses was prepared using labels, online searches, e-mail and telephone communication. Portions of all samples were sent to the manufacturer with a request for authentication. Furthermore, the medical regulatory authorities (MRAs) of the manufacturers' countries were queried on the legitimacy of the manufacturers and their products. Taking into consideration the WHO definition of counterfeit medicines, all information was then cross-checked to arrive at a final determination on the authenticity of the samples and their manufacturers [9,18].

Chemical analysis
Dosage and uniformity tests were conducted on 10 tablets according to the United States Pharmacopoeia (USP 30) by high-performance liquid chromatography. A Shim-pack CLC-ODS (M) 15 cm column (Shimadzu, Kyoto, Japan) was used. Dissolution tests were conducted on 6 tablets for each sample using an NTR-VS6P dissolution tester (Toyama, Osaka, Japan) according to USP 30. For quantity tests, tablets were expected to contain 90-120% of the labeled dose. The maximum value accepted in the content uniformity test was 15.0. For dissolution tests, $\geq 85\%$ of the labeled dose of amoxicillin, and $\geq 80\%$ of the labeled dose of clavulanic acid was expected to dissolve in 30 minutes, respectively [19,20].

A stability test was conducted on amoxicillin/clavulanic acid at 37°C with 100% relative humidity (RH). We used one control sample with no visible defect, one with torn wrapping but no strip defect, and one in which the strips were deliberately perforated. In all three samples, amoxicillin and clavulanic acid contents were measured at 0, 24, 48, 72, and 96 hours. These times were based on an exploratory experiment: significant degradation of amoxicillin was observed within 24 hours under tropical conditions (37°C, 100% RH) (unpublished report).

Statistical analysis

Data analysis was performed using SPSS version 17.0.0 (SPSS Inc., Chicago). When appropriate, Fisher's exact test and the Bonferroni multiple t-test were used to test the significance of differences in categorical and quantitative variables, respectively. Statistical significance was evaluated at the 5% level.

Results

Medicine outlets

A total of 59 samples were collected from 48 outlets in Phnom Penh and surrounding provinces. Of these samples, 26 (44.1%) were collected from Phnom Penh, and the rest from the provinces. Forty-eight (81.4%) of the samples were from licensed outlets (31 (52.5%) Pharmacy, 4 (6.8%) Depot A and 13 (22%) Depot B); the rest (11/18.6%) were from unlicensed outlets. At least one pharmacist was found to be present in 14 of the pharmacies. Air conditioning was present in only one pharmacy. A Cambodian registration number was found on 93.2% of the samples. No sample was past the expiration date.

Package condition

According to the printed information, most of the samples (55, 93.2%) were imported. Only four (6.8%) samples were manufactured domestically. Fourteen (23.73%) of the samples were branded, and the rest (45, 76.27%) were generic. Fifty-seven (96.6%) of the samples were of 500 mg/125 mg strength, and the rest were 875 mg/125 mg. The labels on 16 samples recommended storage below 25°C; most others simply recommended avoidance of humid conditions. On one product, storage below 15°C was recommended.

On observation of all samples, 32 (54.2%) from six manufacturers were categorized as type A, six (10.2%) from one manufacturer as type B, 2 (3.4%) from one manufacturer as type C, eight (13.6%) from four manufacturers

as type D and 11 (18.6%) from four manufacturers as type E (Table 1). We found 12 (20.3%) samples with defective packaging. Two samples had the plastic covers peeled off the strips, one had a strip with missing tablets, and nine had an unclear scored line of package break for individual tablets (Table 1). There was a significant association between the presence of instructions on humidity and the pass rate in the observational test (p < 0.05). No significant association was found between the results of the observational test and any of the following parameters: sampling location, shop category, registered or unregistered store, country of origin, branded/generic product or condition of packaging (intact or sealed and unsealed or open).

Authenticity

Requests were sent asking 15 manufacturers to authenticate 57 products. One manufacturer could not be contacted. Six manufacturers responded for 28 (49.1%) of the samples. All of these samples were described as authentic. Only three of 11 MRAs replied to our requests for verification of the legitimacy of manufacturers and samples.

Quality analysis

Of 59 samples, eight (13.6%), 10 (16.9%), and 20 (33.9%) failed the dose, content uniformity and dissolution tests, respectively. No significant relationship was observed between failure rate and area of collection, shop category, registration status, origin, branded/generic product type, intactness of packaging (i.e., sealed or opened) or response to authenticity investigation. However, failure rates in the quality tests were significantly associated with the outcome of observational analysis (Fisher's exact test, p < 0.05; Table 2).

Interestingly, clavulanic acid accounted for most failures in the quantity and content uniformity tests (87.5% and 70% of failures, respectively), whereas amoxicillin accounted for most failures (80%) in the dissolution tests. Most of the samples (7 of 8 and 9 of 10, respectively) that failed the quantity and uniformity tests, as well as all (20)

Table 1 Results of observational tests

Type	No. of manufacturers	No. of samples	No. of samples with packaging defects*			No. of total failed samples	(%)
			a	b	c		
A	6	32	2	0	4	6	18.8
B	1	6	0	0	3	3	50.0
C	1	2	0	0	0	0	0.0
D	4	8	0	0	0	0	0.0
E	4	11	0	1	2	3	27.3
Total	16	59	2	1	9	12	20.3

* Identified packaging defects:
a = PTP/SP packaging with peeling of the outer plastic or aluminum cover.
b = missing tablet(s) in intact PTP or SP.
c = PTP/SP without clear pocket breaks.

Table 2 Comparison of quality tests with observation

		Quantity test (n = 59)		Fisher's exact test	Content uniformity (n = 59)		Fisher's exact test	Dissolution test (n = 59)		Fisher's exact test	Failed ≥ 1 test (n = 59)		Fisher's exact test
		Passed	Failed		Passed	Failed		Passed	Failed		Passed	Failed	
Condition of packaging	No defects	46	1	p < 0.05	44	3	p < 0.05	35	12	p < 0.05	33	14	p < 0.05
	Defects	5	7		5	7		4	8		2	10	

samples that failed the dissolution tests, were generic. The results of the stability test suggest that both amoxicillin and clavulanic acid decompose significantly within one day (Bonferroni's multiple t-test, P < 0.05, Figure 1).

Discussion

Medicine outlets

Public medical services in Cambodia still struggle with a lack of medical staff in hospitals, and there are other problems such as long waiting times and high costs [21]. The sale of antibiotics without a prescription for the treatment of mild symptoms is very common at pharmacies and clinics [22]. Seeking health care in the private sector as a first choice is widely observed in many developing countries [23]. Our study found a prescription regulation warning on the packaging of less than half (40.7%) of the samples. The inappropriate use of antibiotics without prescription may promote resistance to even the newest and most effective antibiotics [24]. Sample collection was conducted in July-August, when average daytime temperatures were 30-40°C with high humidity. Although there were recommended storage conditions in the package inserts of several samples, air conditioning was found in only one pharmacy out of 54 outlets.

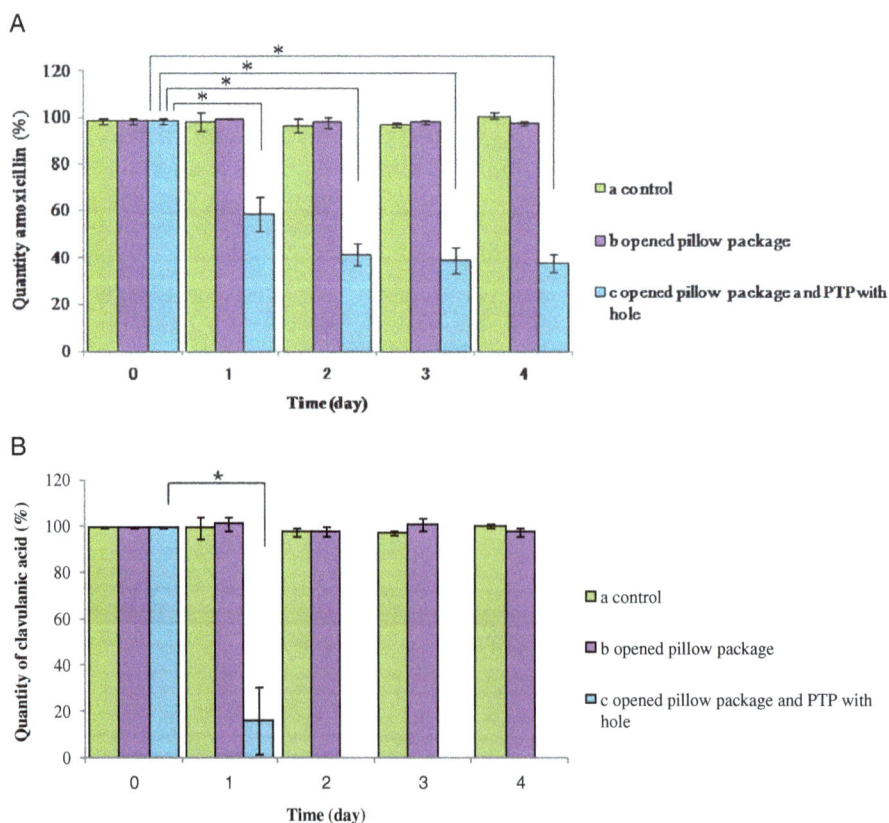

Figure 1 Changes in concentrations of amoxicillin and clavulanic acid (n = 3) in each packaging condition during storage. Each value represents the mean ± SD of three experiments. *Significant difference (p < 0.01) compared to baseline using Bonferroni's multiple t-test. **A.** Changes in the concentration of amoxicillin in tablets (n=3) with each packaging condition during storage (**A**). Each value represents the mean ± SD of three experiments. *Significant difference (p<0.01) compared to baseline using Bonferroni's multiple t-test. **B.** Changes in the concentration of clavulanic acid in tablets (n=3) with each packaging condition during storage (**B**). Each value represents the mean ± SD of three experiments. *Significant difference (p<0.01) compared to baseline using Bonferroni's multiple t-test.

Medicines that are rapidly degraded in adverse environments should not be supplied by outlets that cannot comply with storage requirements [25,26].

Condition of packaging

Pharmaceutical packaging is an important part of the overall manufacturing and distribution process. Good packaging can ensure the quality and effectiveness of its contents [27]. Several of the samples in this study had no clear-cut break lines between tablets; thus, adjacent tablets may be exposed to air when a tablet is torn from a strip. Two samples that failed the observational test due to peeling of the outer plastic or aluminum cover might have been affected by improper handling during distribution. One sample that failed due to missing tablets in intact PTP and 9 samples that failed due to indistinct pocket breaks may have resulted from poor manufacturing practices. Ten of these samples also failed one of the quality tests. Hence, these 10 samples are not counterfeit but rather degraded authentic products. Strict adherence to good manufacturing, distribution, and pharmacy practices may improve the quality of medicines for end users [27].

Authenticity

This study received few responses from MRAs and manufacturers, which may be due to the methodology used in the authenticity investigation. This issue is a low priority for manufacturers and MRAs [7]. Failed samples were attributed to degradation; no counterfeit products were identified. Nevertheless, cooperation from all stakeholders is crucial to safeguard medicine quality, especially from counterfeits [7,28].

Quality analysis

Samples that failed the content uniformity test usually came from open packages/containers during sampling (Fisher's exact test, p = 0.057). Moreover, samples that failed the quality test were significantly more likely to fail the observational test of this study (p < 0.05, Table 2). This outcome indicates that appropriate storage conditions and packaging may help prevent deterioration in the quality and bio-availability of medicines. Some previous studies also reported damaged packaging as a prominent characteristic of counterfeit and substandard medicines [15,29].

Clavulanic acid is volatile and unstable when exposed to high temperatures and high pH [30]. In addition, clavulanic acid is hygroscopic; therefore, 30% RH or less is desirable for storage [31,32]. The harmful effects of experimentally introduced packaging defects on amoxicillin–clavulanic acid revealed here were in accord with recent studies: clavulanic acid was the main factor in the degradation of mixtures [33-35]. Our results show that several samples failed the quantity and content uniformity tests because of low clavulanic acid contents. Degradation of clavulanic acid may occur during manufacturing, in distribution, or in storage at the pharmacy. Packaging practices and materials have been reported to contribute to the degradation of medicines in several studies [19,36]. Improvement and standardization of packaging, as well as strict compliance with good distribution and pharmacy practices, may help to maintain the quality of medicines for the end user.

Most of the samples that failed the quality tests in this study were generic. The circulation of substandard generic amoxicillin-clavulanic acid was reported in two recent studies in other countries [37,38]. Some reports suggest that different coatings and additives with similar active ingredients are used to make medicines bio-available [39]. Therefore, the low dissolution rate of amoxicillin observed in this study might be due to the additives used in generic formulations. There is evidence that poor-quality medicines commonly fail dissolution tests, which is in accord with our findings [40].

Limitation

We did not measure potassium content; this omission could be considered a limitation of this study. This decision was made because of the low number of tablets in each samples and limited resource. Analysis of potassium might provide important clues as to whether the degradation of clavulanic acid occurred in the supply chain or at the manufacturer. One objective of this study is to check quality authenticity and pharmacopoeial quality within the framework of limited collected samples and resource and quickly report these values for necessary measures, even in cases of incomplete investigation of the cause and source of such medicines. Another limitation of this study was the absence of liquid formulations such as syrups and suspensions due to our selection criteria. Further study is required to evaluate these commonly used products.

Conclusion

This study shows that the condition of packaging is an important factor in maintaining the quality of amoxicillin–clavulanic acid products. To ensure quality, manufacturers must comply with GMP requirements. Distributors and service providers also need to be very stringent in adhering to quality assurance and standard operating procedures. It may not be possible to completely eliminate antibiotic resistance; however, through the improved management and rational use of antibiotics, we may be able to delay the process.

Competing interests
The authors declare that they have no competing interests.

Authors' contributions

MHK, KH, TS, NN, TT and KK participated in design, fieldwork and documentation; MHK, KH, TS, NN, LCCC, NY, HT and KK participated in data analysis; MHK, KH, TS, NN, NY, HT, TT and KK participated in the interpretation of results. MHK wrote the first draft. All authors participated in a critical review of the manuscript and approved the submitted version. Additionally, all authors have read and approved the final manuscript.

Acknowledgments

We gratefully acknowledge the cooperation of the Department of Drugs and Food (DDF), Ministry of Health, Cambodia, and the manufacturers and MRAs of the samples. This study received grant support from the Japan Pharmaceutical Manufacturers Association (JPMA). Additionally, MHK was supported by a Monbukagakusho scholarship and Takeda Science Foundation fellowship, and LCCC was supported by Japan International Cooperation Agency (JICA).

Author details

[1]Drug Management & Policy, Kanazawa University, Kakuma-machi, Kanazawa, Ishikawa 920-1192, Japan. [2]Médecins Sans Frontières, 14 Sayat-Nova street, Vanadzor, Lori, Armenia. [3]Department of Pharmacy, Saiseikai-Nakatu Hospital, Shibata, Osaka 530-0012, Japan. [4]National Health Product Quality Control Center, Ministry of Health, Phnom Penh, Cambodia. [5]Becton Dickinson de México, S.A.de C.V. Km 37.5 – Aut. México-Qro. Parque Industrial Cuamatla, Cuautitlán Izcalli., Edo. De México, CP 54730, México. [6]Department of Analytical Sciences, Faculty of Pharmaceutical Sciences, Doshisha Women's College, Kyoto, Japan.

References

1. Hanif M, Mobarak MR, Ronan A, Rahman D, Donovan JJJ, Bennish ML: **Fatal renal failure caused by diethylene glycol in paracetamol elixir: the Bangladesh epidemic.** *Br Med J* 1995, **311**:88–91.

2. Keoluangkhot V, Green M, Nyadong L, Fernandez F, Mayxay M, Newton P: **Impaired clinical response in a patient with uncomplicated falciparum malaria who received poor-quality and underdosed intramuscular artemether.** *Am J Trop Med Hyg* 2008, **78**:552–555.

3. Amin AA, Kokwaro GO: **Antimalarial drug quality in Africa.** *J Clin Pharm Ther* 2007, **32**:429–440.

4. Gaudiano M, Di Maggio A, Cocchieri E, Antoniella E, Bertocchi P, Alimonti S, Valvo L: **Medicines informal market in Congo Burundi and Angola: counterfeit and sub-standard antimalarials.** *Malar J* 2007, **6**:22.

5. Lon CT, Tsuyuoka R, Phanouvong S, Nivanna N, Socheat D, Sokhan C, Blum N, Christophel EM, Smine A: **Counterfeit and substandard antimalarial drugs in Cambodia.** *Trans R Soc Trop Med Hyg* 2006, **100**:1019–1024.

6. MOH: *2nd Study Report on Counterfeit and Substandard Drugs in Cambodia 2004.* Cambodia: Phnom Penh: Ministry of Health; 2004.

7. Khan MH, Okumura J, Sovannarith T, Nivanna N, Nagai H, Taga M, Yoshida N, Akazawa M, Tanimoto T, Kimura K: **Counterfeit Medicines in Cambodia—Possible Causes.** *Pharm Res* 2011, **28**:484–489.

8. Khan MH, Akazawa M, Dararath E, Kiet HB, Sovannarith T, Nivanna N, Yoshida N, Kimura K: **Perceptions and practices of pharmaceutical wholesalers surrounding counterfeit medicines in a developing country: a baseline survey.** *BMC Health Serv Res* 2011, **11**:306.

9. Khan MH, Okumura J, Sovannarith T, Nivanna N, Akazawa M, Kimura K: **Prevalence of counterfeit anti-helminthic medicines: a cross-sectional survey in Cambodia.** *Trop Med Int Health* 2010, **15**:639–644.

10. Khan MH, Tanimoto T, Nakanishi Y, Yoshida N, Tsuboi H, Kimura K: **Public health concerns for anti-obesity medicines imported for personal use through the internet: a cross-sectional study.** *BMJ Open* 2012, **2**.

11. Berry V, Hoover J, Singley C, Woodnutt G: **Comparative Bacteriological Efficacy of Pharmacokinetically Enhanced Amoxicillin-Clavulanate against Streptococcus pneumoniae with Elevated Amoxicillin MICs and Haemophilus influenzae.** *Antimicrob Agents Chemother* 2005, **49**:908–915.

12. White AR, Kaye C, Poupard J, Pypstra R, Woodnutt G, Wynne B: **Augmentin®(amoxicillin/clavulanate) in the treatment of community-acquired respiratory tract infection: a review of the continuing development of an innovative antimicrobial agent.** *J Antimicrob Chemother* 2004, **53**:i3–i20.

13. Abbas Z, Yakoob J, Abid S, Jafri W, Islam M, Azam Z, Hilal I: **Furazolidone, co-amoxiclav, colloidal bismuth subcitrate, and esomeprazole for patients who failed to eradicate helicobacter pylori with triple therapy.** *Dig Dis Sci* 2009, **54**:1953–1957.

14. Ojetti V, Migneco A, Zocco MA, Nista EC, Gasbarrini G, Gasbarrini A: **Beta-lactamase inhibitor enhances Helicobacter pylori eradication rate.** *J Intern Med* 2004, **255**:125–129.

15. Kelesidis T, Kelesidis I, Rafailidis PI, Falagas ME: **Counterfeit or substandard antimicrobial drugs: a review of the scientific evidence.** *J Antimicrob Chemother* 2007, **60**:214–236.

16. Newton PN, Green MD, Ferndez FM: **Impact of poor-quality medicines in the developing world.** *Trends Pharmacol Sci* 2010, **31**:99–101.

17. Shakoor O, Taylor R, Behrens R: **Assessment of the incidence of substandard drugs in developing countries.** *Trop Med Int Health* 1997, **2**:839–845.

18. WHO: *Counterfeit Drugs: Guidelines for the development of measures to combat counterfeit drugs pp. 60.* Geneva, Switzerland: World Health Organization; 1999:60.

19. Nagaraju R, Kaza R: **Stability evaluation of amoxicillin and potassium clavulanate tablets USP by accelerated studies.** *Turkish Journal of Pharmaceutical Science* 2008, **5**:201–214.

20. USP: *The United States Pharmacopeia (USP 30/NF 25).* 12601 Twinbrook Parkway, Rockville, MD 20852: The United States Pharmacopeial Convention; 2007.

21. Chhea C, Warren N, Manderson L: **Health worker effectiveness and retention in rural Cambodia.** *Rural Remote Heal* 2010, **10**:1391.

22. Yanagisawa S, Mey V, Wakai S: **Comparison of health-seeking behaviour between poor and better-off people after health sector reform in Cambodia.** *Public Health* 2004, **118**:21–30.

23. Ahmed SM, Hossain MA, Chowdhury MR: **Informal sector providers in Bangladesh: how equipped are they to provide rational health care?** *Health Policy Plan* 2009, **24**:467–478.

24. Kunin CM: **Resistance to Antimicrobial Drugs - A Worldwide Calamity.** *Ann Intern Med* 1993, **118**:557–561.

25. MOH: *Good Pharmacy Practice (GPP) in Cambodia.* Phnom Penh. Cambodia: Department of Drugs and Food, Ministry of Health; 2006.

26. Pharmaceutical Compounding Expert Committee: *Pharmaceutical compounding. In: United States Pharmacopeia 34/National Formulary 29.* Rockville, Md: United States Pharmacopeial Convention; 2011.

27. WHO: *Technical Report Series 957: WHO Expert Committee on Specifications for Pharmaceutical Preparations (annex 5).* Geneva, Switzerland: World Health Organization; 2010.

28. Newton PN, Fernández FM, Plançon A, Mildenhall DC, Green MD, Ziyong L, Christophel EM, Phanouvong S, Howells S, McIntosh E, et al: **A Collaborative Epidemiological Investigation into the Criminal Fake Artesunate Trade in South East Asia.** *PLoS Med* 2008, **5**:e32.

29. Abounassif MA, Abdel-Moety EM, Mohamed ME, Gad-Kariem E-RA: **Liquid chromatographic determination of amoxycillin and clavulanic acid in pharmaceutical preparations.** *J Pharm Biomed Anal* 1991, **9**:731–735.

30. Abu Reid I, El-Samani S, Hag Omer A, Khalil N, Mahgoub K, Everitt G, Grundstrom K, Lindgren B, Stjernstrom N: **Stability of drugs in tropics. A study in Sudan.** *Int Pharm J* 1990, **4**:6–10.

31. Lee YB, Kim DJ, Ahn CH, Scholtz EC: *Pharmaceutical formulation of clavulanic acid.* USA: Rexahn Pharmaceuticals, Inc.; 2009.

32. Ramsey MG, Rickman JT: *Pharmaceutical Formulations. (GLXOSMITHKLINE ed., vol. US 2005/0136117A1.* Ramsey et al.: USA; 2005.

33. Jerzsele Á, Nagy G: **The stability of amoxicillin trihydrate and potassium clavulanate combination in aqueous solutions.** *Acta Vet Hung* 2009, **57**:485–493.

34. Risha P, Shewiyo D, Msami A, Masuki G, Vergote G, Vervaet C, Remon J: **In vitro evaluation of the quality of essential drugs on the Tanzanian market.** *Trop Med Int Health* 2002, **7**:701–707.

35. Caudron J-M, Ford N, Henkens M, Mac C, Kiddle-Monroe R, Pinel J: **Substandard medicines in resource-poor settings: a problem that can no longer be ignored.** *Trop Med Int Health* 2008, **13**:1062–1072.

36. Yamazaki N, Taya K, Shimokawa K-i, Ishii F: **The most appropriate storage method in unit-dose package and correlation between color change and decomposition rate of aspirin tablets.** *Int J Pharm* 2010, **396**:105–110.

37. Olanrewaju OJ, Paul AC, Olusola AM: **Quality assessment of amoxicillin-clavulanate potassium tablets in Lagos, Nigeria.** *Journal of Chemical and Paharmaceutical Research* 2012, **4**:5032–5038.

38. Al Ameri MN, Nayuni N, Anil Kumar KG, Perrett D, Tucker A, Johnston A: The differences between the branded and generic medicines using solid dosage forms: In-vitro dissolution testing. *Results in Pharma Sciences* 2011, **2**:1–8.
39. Markman BEO, Rosa PCP, Koschtschak MRW: Assessment of the quality of simvastatin capsules from compounding pharmacies. *Rev Saude Publica* 2010, **44**:1055–1062.
40. Kayumba PC, Risha PG, Shewiyo D, Msami A, Masuki G, Ameye D, Vergote G, Ntawukuliryayo JD, Remon JP, Vervaet C: The quality of essential antimicrobial and antimalarial drugs marketed in Rwanda and Tanzania: influence of tropical storage conditions on in vitro dissolution. *J Clin Pharm Ther* 2004, **29**:331–338.

21

Dipyrithione induces cell-cycle arrest and apoptosis in four cancer cell lines *in vitro* and inhibits tumor growth in a mouse model

Yumei Fan[1], Caizhi Liu[1], Yongmao Huang[2], Jie Zhang[1], Linlin Cai[1], Shengnan Wang[1], Yongze Zhang[1], Xianglin Duan[1*] and Zhimin Yin[3*]

Abstract

Background: Dipyrithione (PTS2) is widely used as a bactericide and fungicide. Here, we investigated whether PTS2 has broad-spectrum antitumor activity by studying its cytotoxicity and proapoptotic effects in four cancer cell lines.

Methods: We used MTT assays and trypan blue staining to test the viability of cancer cell lines. Hoechst 33258 and DAPI staining were used to observe cell apoptosis. Cell-cycle percentages were analyzed by flow cytometry. Apoptosis was assayed using caspase-3 and poly (ADP-ribose) polymerase (PARP) combined with Western blotting. Student's *t*-test was used for statistical analysis.

Results: PTS2 inhibited proliferation in four cancer cell lines in a dose-dependent manner. Treated cells showed shrinkage, irregular fragments, condensed and dispersed blue fluorescent particles compared with control cells. PTS2 induced cycle-arrest and death. Cleavage of caspase-9, caspase-3, and PARP were detected in PTS2-treated cells. Antitumor activity of PTS2 was more effective against widely used cancer drugs and its precursor.

Conclusions: PTS2 appears to have novel cytotoxicity and potent broad-spectrum antitumor activity, which suggests its potential as the basis of an anticancer drug.

Keywords: PTS2, Anti-tumor activity, Chemotherapy

Background

Apoptosis is a cellular progression characterized by a series of tightly regulated molecular processes leading to cell death [1]. There are two independent apoptosis pathways: the death receptor pathway and the mitochondria pathway [2], both of which converge on a family of cysteine aspartases called caspases, whose activity drives the biochemical events leading to cellular disassembly and death. Novel second mitochondria-derived activator of caspases (Smac) mimetic compounds sensitize human leukemia cell lines to conventional chemotherapies that induce death receptor-mediated apoptosis [3,4]. During apoptosis, cytochrome *c*, a component of the mitochondrial electron transfer chain, releases from mitochondria to the cytosol, and binds to Apaf-1, a cytosolic protein, forming the Apaf-1/cytochrome *c* complex, which then oligomerizes and forms apoptosomes by recruiting multiple procaspase-9 molecules, and then cleaving and activating downstream apoptosis effectors such as caspase-3, and PARP [5]. As malignancies grow, cancer cells evolve around mechanisms that limit cell proliferation, such as apoptosis and replicative senescence. Successful cancer therapies may trigger tumor-selective apoptosis [6].

Pyrithione (2-pyridinethiol-1-oxide, PT) has been used as a bactericide and fungicide for more than 50 years [7]. PT derivatives, such as zinc PT and sodium PT, are widely used as cosmetic preservatives and as anti-dandruff agents in shampoos. Zinc PT can reportedly induce apoptosis because of its role as a zinc-ionophore [8,9]. Compounds containing -SH group are quickly oxidized to generate disulfide. For PT, such self-oxidation would result in the formation of the dimer, 2,2'-dithiobispyridine-1,1'-dioxide

---

* Correspondence: xlduan0311@163.com; yinzhimin@njnu.edu.cn
[1]The Key Lab of Animal Physiology, College of Life Science, Hebei Normal University, Hebei Province, Shijiazhuang 050024, China
[3]Jiangsu Province Key Laboratory of Molecular and Medical Biotechnology, College of Life Science, Nanjing Normal University, Nanjing 210046, China
Full list of author information is available at the end of the article

(dipyrithione, PTS2; Figure 1), which also possesses anti-bacterial and anti-fungal activity. Our previous study demonstrated the cytotoxicity and effect of PTS2 in HeLa cells [4], and PTS2 inhibited inflammatory responses induced by lipopolysaccharides (LPS) in RAW264.7 cells, thus protecting mice against endotoxic shock by exerting anti-inflammatory effects through decreased formation of chemokine IP-10/CXCL10 and reduced acute oleic acid-induced lung injury [10-12].

Here we reported novel toxicity, including inhibited proliferation and induced apoptosis, of PTS2 in four cancer cell lines. Our results indicated that PTS2 has broad-spectrum antitumor activity, suggesting its potential as the basis of an anticancer drug.

Methods

Cell culture

MDA-MB-231 (human breast cancer cell line), KB (nasopharyngeal carcinoma cell line), U937 (human monoblast leukemia cell line), and K562 (human leukemia cell line) were purchased from the CBCAS (Cell Bank of the Chinese Academic of Sciences, Shanghai, China). Cells were maintained in RPMI1640 (GIBCO), supplemented with 10% (v/v) fetal bovine serum (HyClone), sodium bicarbonate, 100 µg/ml streptomycin and 100 U/ml penicillin (HyClone) at 37°C, in a humidified 5% CO_2 atmosphere.

Antibodies and reagents

PTS2 and PT were purchased from J&K Chemical LTD. Adriamycin (ADM) was purchased from Hisun (Zhejiang Hisun Pharceutical Co., LTD). Cisplatin (DDP) was purchased from QiLu (QiLu Pharmaceutical Co., LTD.). MTT, Hoechst33258, DAPI and propidium iodide (PI) were from Sigma (Sigma Chemical Co., St Louis, MO). Antibodies to caspase-3, PARP, CyclinD1, CyclinE1 and caspase-9 were purchased from Cell Signaling Technology (Beverly, MA). Antibodies to p21 were purchased from Santa Cruz Biotechnology (Santa Cruz, CA). All chemicals and drugs were prepared in PBS immediately before use.

Western blotting

Western blotting was performed as described previously [13]. Cells were washed twice with ice-cold PBS (pH 7.4)

and lysed in a lysis buffer containing 50 mM Tris–HCl (pH 8.0), 150 mM NaCl, 0.5 mM dithiothreitol, 1 mM EDTA, 1% NP-40, 10% (v/v) glycerol, 50 µg/ml phenylmethylsulfonyl fluoride, 2 µg/ml aprotinin, 1 µg/ml leupeptin, 1 µg/ml pepstatin and 1 mM Na_3VO_4. After incubation on ice for 20 min, lysates were centrifuged at 15,000× g for 10 min at 4°C and the supernatant was transferred to a clean microfuge tube. Equal amounts of the soluble protein were denatured in SDS, electrophoresed on SDS-polyacrylamide gel, and transferred to a PVDF membrane. Horseradish peroxidase (HRP)-conjugated goat anti-rabbit IgG antibodies were used against respective primary antibodies. Proteins were visualized using Lumi-Light Western Blotting Substrate (Roche Molecular Biochemicals). The total density of the protein bands was calculated using the Scion Image software program (Scion Corp., Frederick, MD).

Cell proliferation assay

Cells were seeded into 96-well plates at 5×10^3 cells per well 24 h before treatment. After treatment with different drugs, cell proliferation was determined using MTT (3-(4,5 dimethylthiazol-2-yl)-2,5-diphenyltetrazolium bromide) assay. Briefly, 15 µl (5 mg/ml) MTT solution was added to each well, and incubated at 37°C for 4 h, after which the MTT solution was removed and 200 µl of dimethylsulfoxide (DMSO) added to dissolve the crystals. Absorbance of each well was measured at 570 nm using an ELx 800 Universal Microplate Reader (Bio-Tek, Inc.) according to manufacturer's instructions.

Trypan blue assay

Cells were seeded in 6-well culture plates. After 24 h, culture medium containing 2.5 µg/ml of PTS2 was added to the wells. Cells were harvested at indicated times and washed with PBS, followed by centrifugation at 2500 g for 5 min. The cell pellet was then resuspended in 1 ml of fresh culture medium; 10 µl of the cell suspension was stained with an equal volume of trypan blue (Sigma, Germany) and incubated for 2 min at 37°C. The total number of viable cells was estimated using a hemocytometer chamber.

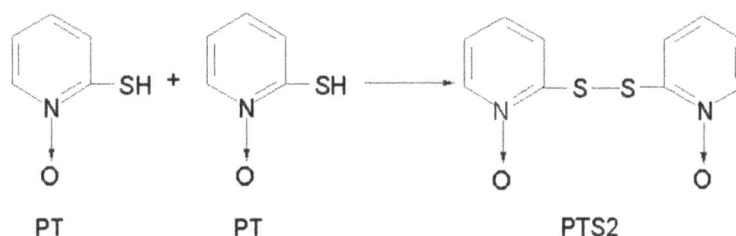

Figure 1 Chemical structure of PTS2.

Hoechst33258 Staining

A staining solution of Hoechst33258 was prepared immediately before use. After drug treatment, cells were collected and fixed in acetic acid/methanol (1:3) solution for 5 min at 4°C, washed 3 times with PBS, and then incubated with Hoechst33258 (50 ng /ml) for 5 min and washed 3 times with PBS. Cells were then assessed for Hoechst fluorescence in a Nikon Optiphot fluorescence microscope (magnification: ×400).

DAPI staining

Cells for 4′-6-diamidino-2-phenylindole (DAPI) staining underwent the same PTS2 treatment as those stained with Hoechst33258. Collected cells were fixed with acetic acid/methanol (1:3) solution for 10 min at room temperature and then incubated in DAPI (1 µg/ml) for 5 min. After being washed 3 times with PBS, cells were examined using a Nikon Optiphot fluorescence microscope (magnification: ×400).

Cell cycle analysis

Cell cycle distribution was analyzed by flow cytometry. Control and treated cells were harvested, washed twice with PBS, and fixed in 70% ethanol overnight at –20°C. Fixed cells were washed twice with PBS, incubated with 1 ml of PBS containing 50 µg/ml propidium iodide, 100 µg/ml RNase A and 0.1% Triton X-100 for 30 min at 37°C. Stained cells were analyzed using a FAScan laser flow cytometer (Becton Dickinson) and ModFit LT cell cycle analysis software (Verity Software).

Apoptosis assay

Apoptosis was determined using Annexin V-FITC/ PI double staining. After treatment, floating and adherent cells were collected, washed twice with PBS (pH 7.4), resuspended in 150 µl of Annexin-binding buffer and incubated with 0.4 µl of Annexin V-FITC. After 20 min incubation in the dark at room temperature, 150 µl of Annexin-binding buffer with 3 µl of PI (50 µg/ml) was added just before flow cytometry. Data were analyzed by flow cytometry using the FACSCalibur and Cell Quest software (Becton Dickinson).

Animals and solid tumor models

All experiments followed the recommendations of the Chinese Experimental Animals Administration Legislation, as approved by the Science and Technology Department of Jiangsu Province. Male ICR mice (6 weeks old, 18–20 g) purchased from Shanghai Laboratory Animal Center, Chinese Academy Sciences, were kept in groups of five animals per cage in a temperature-controlled room at 20 ± 2°C. They were fed a standard pellet diet and water *ad libitum*. As described in [4], two groups of 40 animals each were transplanted subcutaneously with hepatoma 22 (H22) tumor cells (5×10^6 cells/ml) in 0.2 ml PBS into their right groins. At 24 h after tumor inoculation, each set of 40 mice was randomly divided into 4 groups (10 mice per group) and injected intraperitoneally with PTS2 (0.25 or 2.5 mg/kg/day), DDP (25 mg/kg/day) or 0.2 ml 0.9% saline for a further 10 days. On day 11, all the animals were killed, and the tumors were dissected and weighed. Tumor growth inhibition was calculated using the formula:% inhibition = $100 \times ([C – T]/C)$, where C is the average tumor weight of the control group and T is the average tumor weight of each treated group.

Statistics

Statistical analysis used SPSS 12.0 (SPSS, Chicago, IL, USA). Results are expressed as means ± S.D. Differences between means were determined by one-way ANOVA, followed by Student–Newman–Keuls tests for multiple comparisons and Student's *t* test for other data. $P < 0.05$ was considered statistically significant.

Results

PTS2 decreases cancer cell viability

To assess effects of PTS2 on cancer cell growth or proliferation, 4 cancer cell lines, including KB, 231, U937 and K562, were assayed using MTT. After 36 h treatment with various concentrations of PTS2, cell viability was determined for all 4 cell lines. PTS2 (0.25–5 µg/ml) was found to decrease cell viability in a dose-dependent manner (Figure 2A). The effect of PTS2 on cell proliferation was also examined. Results showed that PTS2 significantly decreased cell numbers in all 4 cancer cell lines compared with controls, as assessed using trypan blue (Figure 2B). These data indicate that PTS2 can decrease cell viability or proliferation within a suitable concentration range.

PTS2 induces cell cycle arrest in cancer cells

Cell proliferation is well correlated to regulation of cell cycle progression. A common mechanism for chemotherapeutic drugs is blocking passage through the G_1 phase of the cell cycle [14]. We therefore investigated whether PTS2 can cause G_1 cell cycle arrest in treated cancer cells (Figure 3). Cells exposed to PTS2 at 2.5 µg/ml for 24 h showed a marked increase in the percentage in G_1 phase, and concomitant decreases in S phase and G_2 phase populations, compared with vehicle-treated controls (Figure 3A).

As p21$^{WAF1/Cip1}$ (p21) inhibits the cell cycle through its interaction with cyclin–CDK complexes [15], and is induced by p53 in response to DNA damage resulting in CDK inhibition and G_1 growth arrest [16]. We further tested the effect of PTS2 on endogenous p53, p21, CyclinD1 and CyclinE1 expression in the four cancer cell lines. After cells were treated with PTS2 (2.5 µg/ml) for

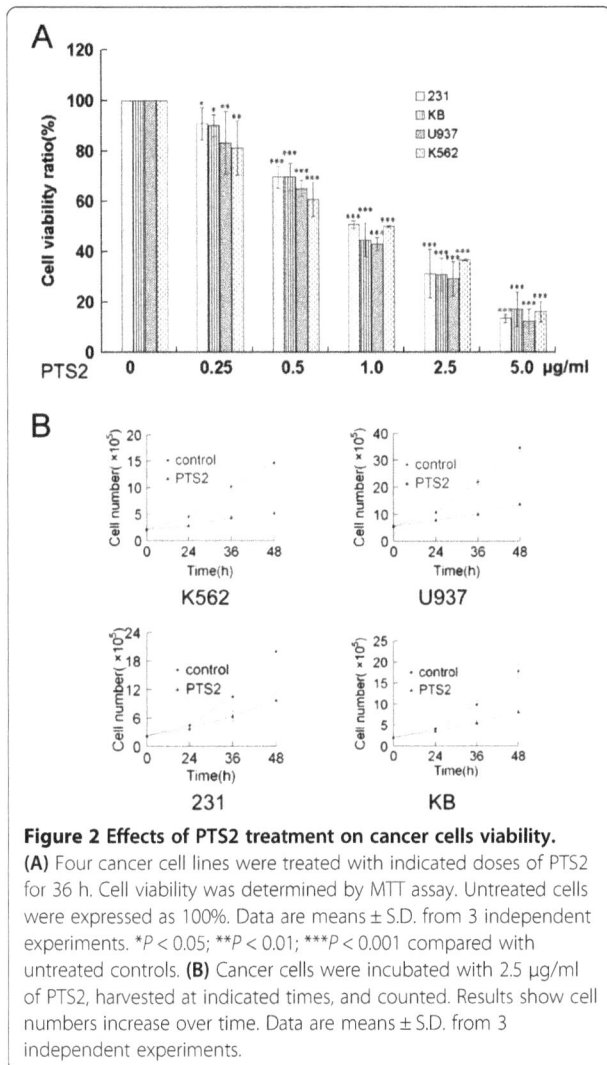

Figure 2 Effects of PTS2 treatment on cancer cells viability.
(A) Four cancer cell lines were treated with indicated doses of PTS2 for 36 h. Cell viability was determined by MTT assay. Untreated cells were expressed as 100%. Data are means ± S.D. from 3 independent experiments. *$P < 0.05$; **$P < 0.01$; ***$P < 0.001$ compared with untreated controls. **(B)** Cancer cells were incubated with 2.5 µg/ml of PTS2, harvested at indicated times, and counted. Results show cell numbers increase over time. Data are means ± S.D. from 3 independent experiments.

24 h, PTS2 induced p21 accumulation in all cells as shown by Western blot (Figure 3B). CyclinD1 and CyclinE1 expressions were downregulated. These results were in accordance with the cell cycle experiment and previous reports [17,18], and suggest that PTS2-induced G_1 arrest in cancer cells could be mediated via modulation of p53, p21, CyclinD1 and CyclinE1 levels.

PTS2 induces cancer cell apoptosis
Morphology alteration and chromatin condensation are two indicators of cell apoptosis. To verify whether the growth inhibitory effect of PTS2 was due to apoptosis, KB, 231, U937 and K562 cells were treated with PTS2 at 2.5 µg/ml for 36 h, and then observed under a light microscope or under a fluorescence microscope after Hoechst33258 and DAPI staining. We found the PTS2-treated cells were shrunken, with irregular fragments and apoptotic bodies, in contrast to control cells (Figure 4A). The typical apoptosis appearance, including condensed

and dispersed or fragmented blue fluorescent particles was observed in PTS2-treated cells compared with control cells (Figure 4B, C), which suggests that PTS2 induces apoptosis in these types of cancer cells obviously.

PTS2 induced cleavage of caspase-9, caspase-3 and PARP
Caspase family members, including caspase-9 and caspase-3, as well as downstream substrates such as PARP, are crucial mediators of the apoptotic process. To see whether PTS2-induced cell death involved activation of caspases and PARP, we analyzed cleavage of caspase-9, caspase-3 and PARP in PTS2-treated cancer cells. Cells were incubated with 2.5 µg/ml of PTS2 for 36 h. As expected, Western blot results showed that caspase-9, caspase-3 and PARP were cleaved (Figure 5). Activation of caspases and PARP thereby confirmed apoptosis. This suggests that cleavage of caspase-9, caspase-3 and PARP are involved in PTS2-induced cancer cell apoptosis.

PTS2 is more effective to induce cancer cell apoptosis against DDP, ADM or PT
Adriamycin (ADM) and cisplatin (DDP) are widely used cancer drugs. To further evaluate the efficacy of PTS2 in decreasing cancer cell viability, we compared its effects on KB cells to those of ADM and DDP. KB cells were exposed to 2.5 µg/ml of PTS2, ADM or DDP and assayed with MTT. At 3–36 h after treatment, PTS2 also showed faster results than did ADM or DDP (Figure 6A). In the dose range of 0.25–5.0 µg/ml, PTS2 was more effective in inhibiting cell viability than was ADM or DDP, although PT, the precursor of PTS2, exerted no obvious effect (Figure 6B). Flow cytometry analysis showed 2.5 µg/ml of PTS2 to be more effective in killing KB cell than PT and DDP (Figure 6C). These results strongly suggest that PTS2 can induce cancer cell death at least as efficiently as current anti-tumor drugs.

PTS2 inhibits tumor growth
To see effects of PTS2 on murine solid tumors, hepatoma 22 (H22) cells (5×10^6 cells/ml) were transplanted subcutaneously into the right groins of mice; 24 h after tumor implantation, the mice were injected intraperitoneally with PTS2, DDP or saline and observed for 10 days. PTS2 at 2.5 mg/kg/day reduced the weight of H22 tumors; DDP had a similar effect at 25 mg/kg/day (Figure 7A). The tumor growth inhibition rate of PTS2 (2.5 mg/kg/day) was more effective than DDP (25 mg/kg/day) (Figure 7B). Moreover, the body weight increase of the PTS2-treated mice was greater than that of the DDP-treated mice (data not shown).

Discussion
PTS2, a compound related to pyridinethione, has been used as a bactericide, pesticide and fungicide for a long

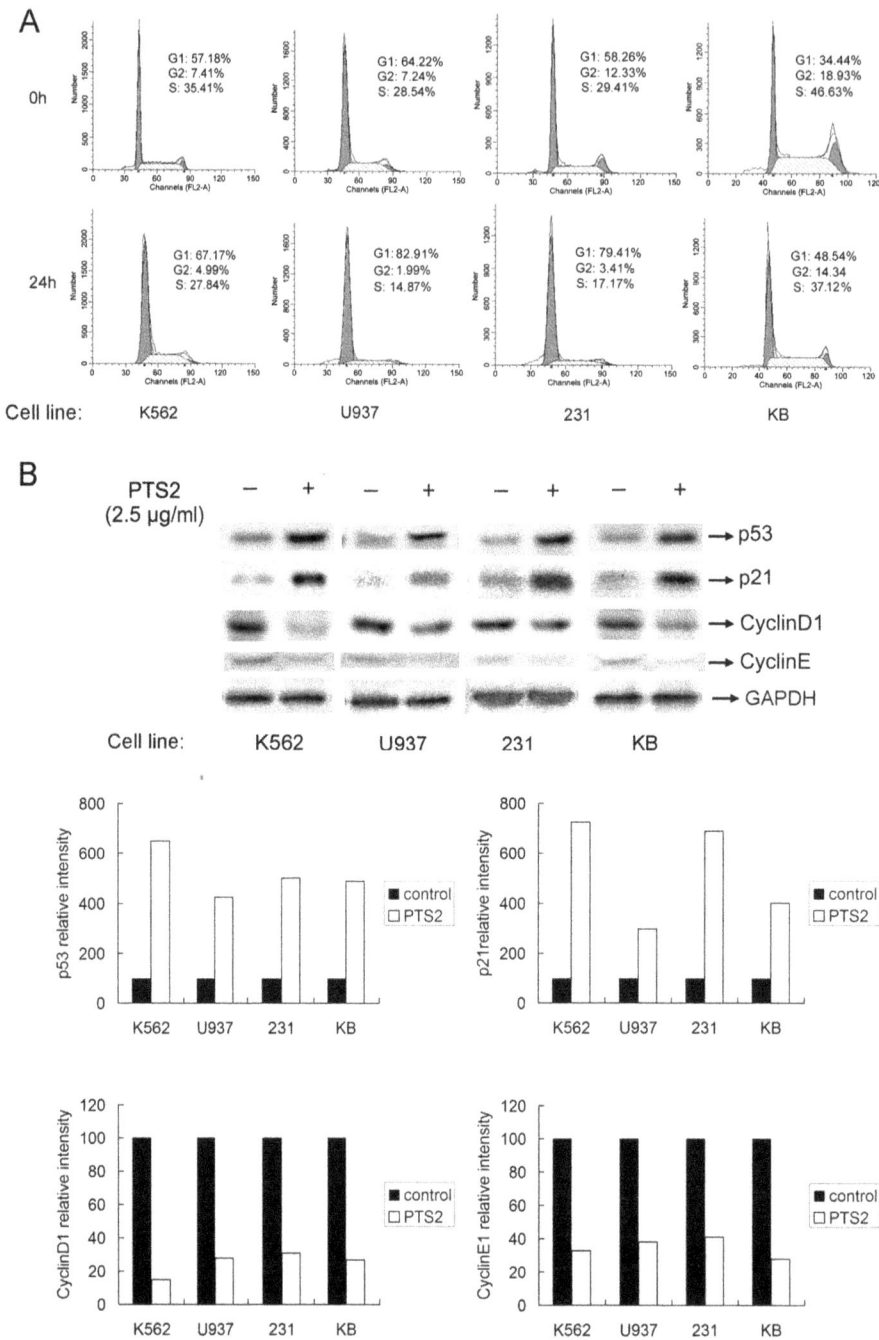

Figure 3 PTS2 induces cell cycle arrest in cancer cells. (A) Cancer cells were incubated with PTS2 (2.5 µg/ml) for 24 h, harvested and stained with propidium iodide (PI). Nuclei fluorescence was measured. Percentages of cells in each cell cycle phase are also shown. Results are representative of 3 independent experiments. **(B)** Cells were incubated with PTS2 (2.5 µg/ml) for 24 h, and then harvested. Western blot was performed using antibodies to p53, p21, CyclinD1, CyclinE1 and GAPDH. Results represent three independent experiments.

time. Our previous report showed that PTS2 exerted cytotoxicity on HeLa cells and reduced the weight of S180 and H22 tumors [4]. The goal of the present study was to explore the cytotoxicity of PTS2 in other cancer cell lines and assess its potential broad-spectrum antitumor activity. We found PTS2 induced cell death in four cancer cell lines *in vitro*, and decreased viability in these cell lines in a dose-dependent manner (Figure 2). At a dose of 2.5 µg/ml, PTS2 induced apoptosis in various cancer cell lines, as detected by morphological and fluorescence analysis (Figure 4), thus raising the possibility that capsaicin might be a potential chemopreventive or therapeutic agent.

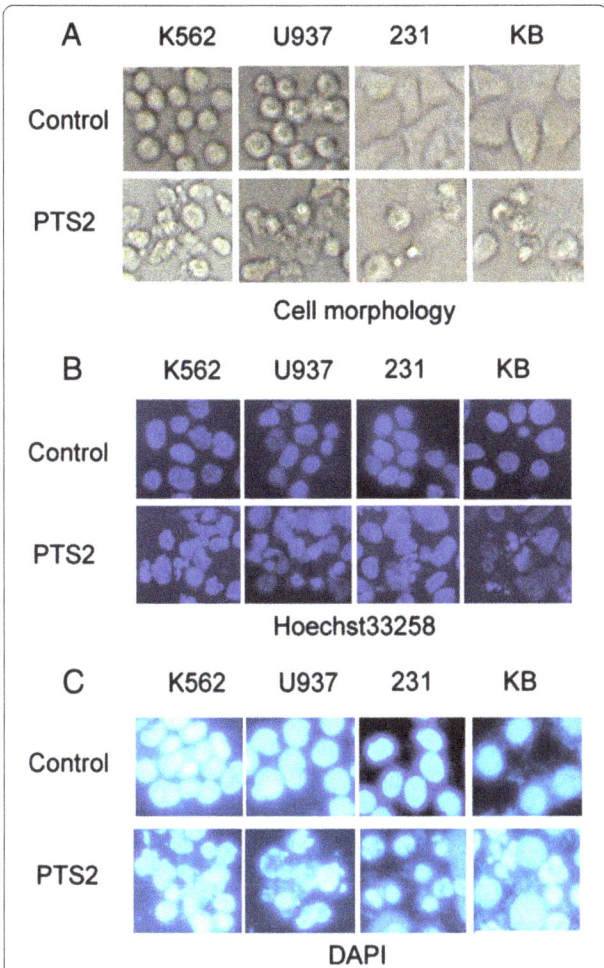

Figure 4 Treatment with PTS2 induces apoptosis in cancer cells. All 4 cancer cell lines were treated with PTS2 (2.5 μg/ml) for 36 h, along with untreated controls. Apoptotic nuclear fragmentation bodies, condensed and dispersed or fragmented particle were stained with blue fluorescence by Hoechst33258 (50 ng/ml) **(B)** and DAPI (1 μg/ml) **(C)**. Cell morphology **(A)** was observed in cells treated with PTS2 compared with control cells, using fluorescence microscopy (magnification: × 400).

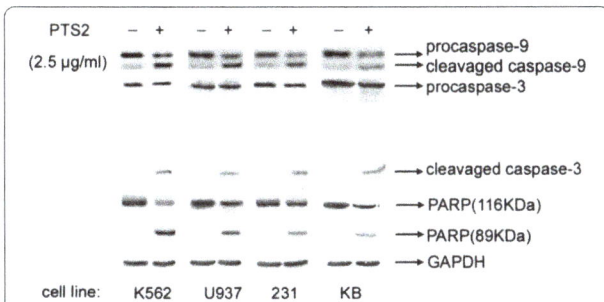

Figure 5 Effects of PTS2 treatment on caspase-9, caspase-3 and PARP. Cancer cells were treated with 2.5 μg/ml of PTS2 for 36 h, and then harvested. Western blot was used to determine proteolytic cleavage of caspase-9, caspase-3 and PARP. GAPDH was used as internal control. Results represent 3 independent experiments.

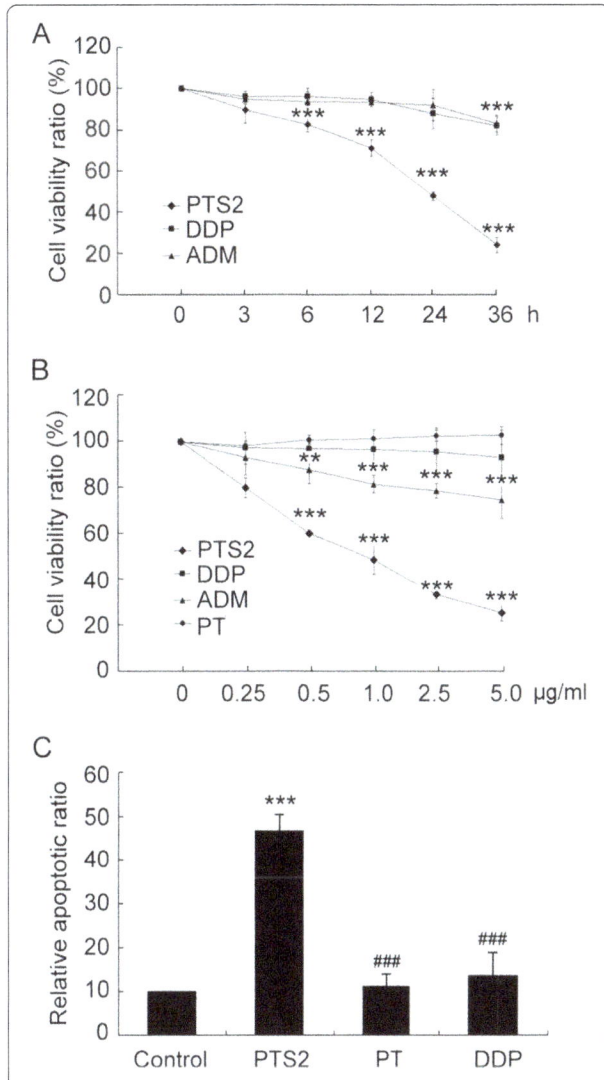

Figure 6 Comparison of effects of PTS2, PT, DDP and ADM on KB cell viability. (A) PTS2, PT, DDP and ADM (2.5 μg/ml) were added to KB cells, and assayed using MTT to determine cell viability after incubation for the indicated times. **(B)** In KB cells exposed to the indicated amounts of PTS2, PT, DDP and ADM for 36 h, cell viability was assayed using MTT. Data are means ± S.D. from 3 independent experiments. $**P < 0.01$; $***P < 0.001$ compared with untreated controls. **(C)** KB cells were treated with 2.5 μg/ml of PTS2, PT, and DDP for 36 h, stained with Annexin V/PI, and examined with flow cytometry. Data are means ± S.D. $***P < 0.001$, compared with viability of untreated cells. $###P < 0.001$, compared with viability of PTS2-treated cells. Results are representative of 3 independent experiments.

Many chemotherapeutic agents reportedly suppress cancer cell growth through disruption of cell cycle progression [19]. Upon cellular stress or DNA damage, these mechanisms induce cells to undergo either cell-cycle arrest, activation of repair systems, or apoptotic induction. In our present study, we showed that PTS2 evidently interferes with the cell cycle in vitro (Figure 3), arresting cells at G_1 phase, and thus leading them to

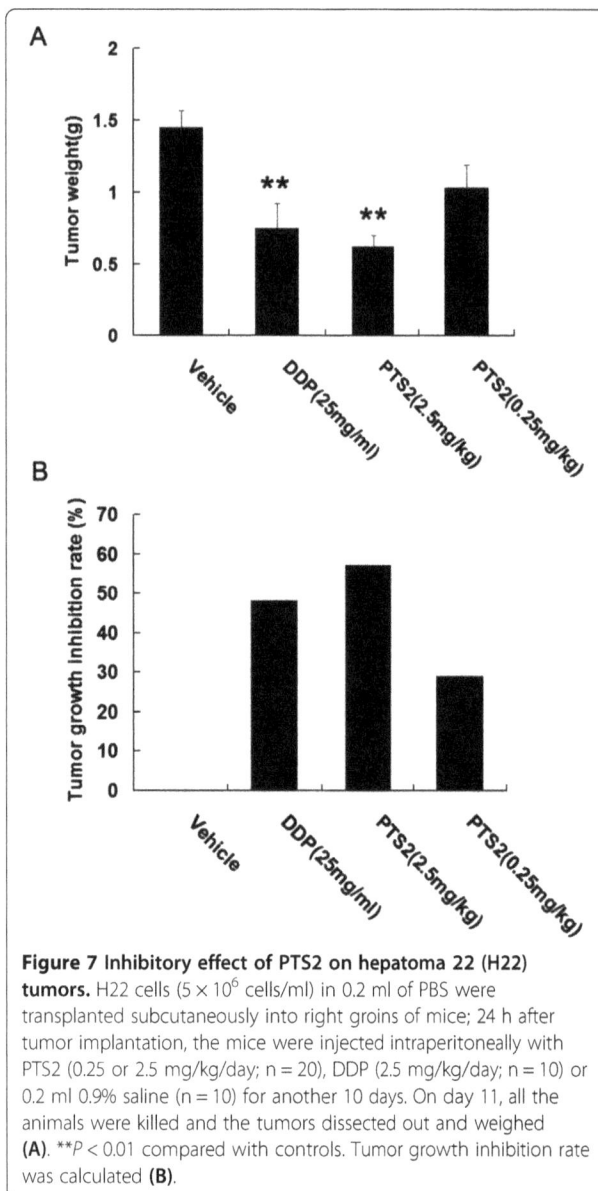

Figure 7 Inhibitory effect of PTS2 on hepatoma 22 (H22) tumors. H22 cells (5×10^6 cells/ml) in 0.2 ml of PBS were transplanted subcutaneously into right groins of mice; 24 h after tumor implantation, the mice were injected intraperitoneally with PTS2 (0.25 or 2.5 mg/kg/day; n = 20), DDP (2.5 mg/kg/day; n = 10) or 0.2 ml 0.9% saline (n = 10) for another 10 days. On day 11, all the animals were killed and the tumors dissected out and weighed **(A)**. **P < 0.01 compared with controls. Tumor growth inhibition rate was calculated **(B)**.

apoptosis. Presently, the molecular mechanisms of PTS2-induced cell cycle arrest in cancer cells require further investigation. Cells treated with PTS2 appear morphologically damaged and decreased in number (Figure 4). PTS2's apparent induction of G_1 arrest and subsequent apoptosis suggest that it could be the basis of an anticancer therapy. PTS2 can also induce p53, p21 accumulation and CyclinD1 and CyclinE1 downregulation in the four tested cancer cell lines (Figure 3B).

Caspase family members, including caspases 3 and 9, are crucial effectors of apoptosis, and are cleaved during apoptosis [19,20]. PARP is a substrate of caspase-3; its cleavage can indicate caspase activation in response to apoptotic stimulus [21,22], and generation of cleaved caspase-3 and PARP as markers for apoptosis [23]. In

analyzing the mechanism of PTS2-induced apoptosis, we found PTS2 treatment induced cleavage of caspase-9, caspase-3 and PARP in cancer cells (Figure 5), which implies that activation of caspase-9, caspase-3 and PARP is involved in PTS2-induced cell death.

Such specific knowledge of PTS2's anticancer effects is of great benefit in antitumor therapeutic strategy. PTS2 showed both dose and time advantages in inducing cancer cell death over adriamycin (an amino-glycosidic anthracycline antibiotic) and cisplatin (a platinum compound), which suggests PTS2's potential as an anticancer drug (Figure 6). Although both PT and its derivative, PTS2, have antifungal activities [24], PT showed no obvious anticancer activity in this study.

Conclusions

Here, we report novel toxicity of PTS2 on various cancers, and show PTS2 to inhibit proliferation of four cancer cell lines and induce apoptosis involving activation of caspase-9, caspase-3 and PARP. These results suggest that PTS2 has broad-spectrum antitumor activity and could be the basis of an anticancer drug.

Competing interests
The authors declare that they have no competing interests.

Authors' contributions
YF, CL and SW carried out the experimental studies. YF and YZ drafted and completed the manuscript. YH performed the statistical analysis. JZ and LC cultured cells. ZY proofread the manuscript. XD and ZY refined the manuscript. FY and XD conceived of and designed the study. All authors read and approved the final manuscript.

Acknowledgements
We thank Professor Lan Luo for critically reading the manuscript. This work was supported by grants from the National Natural Science Foundation of China (31000632), Natural Science Foundation of Hebei Province (C2010000409) and Educational Commission of Hebei Province (2008129). No competing financial interests exist for any of the authors.

Author details
[1]The Key Lab of Animal Physiology, College of Life Science, Hebei Normal University, Hebei Province, Shijiazhuang 050024, China. [2]Laboratory of Medical Biotechnology, Hebei Chemical and Pharmaceutical College, Hebei Province, Shijiazhuang 050026, China. [3]Jiangsu Province Key Laboratory of Molecular and Medical Biotechnology, College of Life Science, Nanjing Normal University, Nanjing 210046, China.

References
1. Jang TH, Lee SJ, Woo CH, Lee KJ, Jeon JH, Lee DS, Choi K, Kim IG, Kim YW, Lee TJ, Park HH: **Inhibition of genotoxic stress induced apoptosis by novel TAT-fused peptides targeting PIDDosome.** *Biochem Pharmacol* 2012, **83**:218–227.
2. Sun R, Zhang Y, Lv Q, Liu B, Jin M, Zhang W, He Q, Deng M, Liu X, Li G, Li Y, Zhou G, Xie P, Xie X, Hu J, Duan Z: **Toll-like receptor 3 (TLR3) induces apoptosis via death receptors and mitochondria by up-regulating the transactivating p63 isoform alpha (TAP63alpha).** *J Biol Chem* 2011, **286**:15918–15928.
3. Servida F, Lecis D, Scavullo C, Drago C, Seneci P, Carlo-Stella C, Manzoni L, Polli E, Lambertenghi Deliliers G, Delia D, Onida F: **Novel second mitochondria-derived activator of caspases (Smac) mimetic compounds sensitize human leukemic cell lines to conventional chemotherapeutic**

drug-induced and death receptor-mediated apoptosis. *Invest New Drugs* 2011, **29**:1264–1275.

4. Fan Y, Chen H, Qiao B, Luo L, Ma H, Li H, Jiang J, Niu D, Yin Z: **Opposing effects of ERK and p38 MAP kinases on HeLa cell apoptosis induced by dipyrithione.** *Mol Cells* 2007, **23**:30–38.

5. Garrido C, Galluzzi L, Brunet M, Puig PE, Didelot C, Kroemer G: **Mechanisms of cytochrome c release from mitochondria.** *Cell Death Differ* 2006, **13**:1423–1433.

6. Rinner B, Li ZX, Haas H, Siegl V, Sturm S, Stuppner H, Pfragner R: **Antiproliferative and pro-apoptotic effects of Uncaria tomentosa in human medullary thyroid carcinoma cells.** *Anticancer Res* 2009, **29**:4519–4528.

7. Doose CA, Szaleniec M, Behrend P, Muller A, Jastorff B: **Chromatographic behavior of pyrithiones.** *J Chromatogr A* 2004, **1052**:103–110.

8. Mann JJ, Fraker PJ: **Zinc pyrithione induces apoptosis and increases expression of Bim.** *Apoptosis* 2005, **10**:369–379.

9. Kondoh M, Tasaki E, Takiguchi M, Higashimoto M, Watanabe Y, Sato M: **Activation of caspase-3 in HL-60 cells treated with pyrithione and zinc.** *Biol Pharm Bull* 2005, **28**:757–759.

10. Huang H, Pan Y, Ye Y, Gao M, Yin Z, Luo L: **Dipyrithione attenuates oleic acid-induced acute lung injury.** *Pulm Pharmacol Ther* 2011, **24**:74–80.

11. Liu Z, Fan Y, Wang Y, Han C, Pan Y, Huang H, Ye Y, Luo L, Yin Z: **Dipyrithione inhibits lipopolysaccharide-induced iNOS and COX-2 up-regulation in macrophages and protects against endotoxic shock in mice.** *FEBS Lett* 2008, **582**:1643–1650.

12. Han C, Fu J, Liu Z, Huang H, Luo L, Yin Z: **Dipyrithione inhibits IFN-gamma-induced JAK/STAT1 signaling pathway activation and IP-10/CXCL10 expression in RAW264.7 cells.** *Inflamm Res* 2010, **59**:809–816.

13. Fan Y, Wu D, Jin L, Yin Z: **Human glutamylcysteine synthetase protects HEK293 cells against UV-induced cell death through inhibition of c-Jun NH2-terminal kinase.** *Cell Biol Int* 2005, **29**:695–702.

14. Morishita D, Takami M, Yoshikawa S, Katayama R, Sato S, Kukimoto-Niino M, Umehara T, Shirouzu M, Sekimizu K, Yokoyama S, Fujita N: **Cell-permeable carboxyl-terminal p27(Kip1) peptide exhibits anti-tumor activity by inhibiting Pim-1 kinase.** *J Biol Chem* 2011, **286**:2681–2688.

15. Kiraly R, Demeny M, Fesus L: **Protein transamidation by transglutaminase 2 in cells: a disputed Ca2 + –dependent action of a multifunctional protein.** *FEBS J* 2011, **278**:4717–4739.

16. Dulic V, Kaufmann WK, Wilson SJ, Tlsty TD, Lees E, Harper JW, Elledge SJ, Reed SI: **p53-dependent inhibition of cyclin-dependent kinase activities in human fibroblasts during radiation-induced G1 arrest.** *Cell* 1994, **76**:1013–1023.

17. Singh N, Nambiar D, Kale RK, Singh RP: **Usnic acid inhibits growth and induces cell cycle arrest and apoptosis in human lung carcinoma A549 cells.** *Nutr Cancer* 2013, **65**(Suppl 1):36–43.

18. Gulappa T, Reddy RS, Suman S, Nyakeriga AM, Damodaran C: **Molecular interplay between cdk4 and p21 dictates G0/G1 cell cycle arrest in prostate cancer cells.** *Cancer Lett* 2013, **337**:177–183.

19. Lin CH, Lu WC, Wang CW, Chan YC, Chen MK: **Capsaicin induces cell cycle arrest and apoptosis in human KB cancer cells.** *BMC Complement Altern Med* 2013, **13**:46.

20. Walsh JG, Cullen SP, Sheridan C, Luthi AU, Gerner C, Martin SJ: **Executioner caspase-3 and caspase-7 are functionally distinct proteases.** *Proc Natl Acad Sci U S A* 2008, **105**:12815–12819.

21. Shao L, Guo X, Plate M, Li T, Wang Y, Ma D, Han W: **CMTM5-v1 induces apoptosis in cervical carcinoma cells.** *Biochem Biophys Res Commun* 2009, **379**:866–871.

22. Rodriguez-Hernandez A, Brea-Calvo G, Fernandez-Ayala DJ, Cordero M, Navas P, Sanchez-Alcazar JA: **Nuclear caspase-3 and caspase-7 activation, and poly(ADP-ribose) polymerase cleavage are early events in camptothecin-induced apoptosis.** *Apoptosis* 2006, **11**:131–139.

23. Yang C, Choy E, Hornicek FJ, Wood KB, Schwab JH, Liu X, Mankin H, Duan Z: **Histone deacetylase inhibitor PCI-24781 enhances chemotherapy-induced apoptosis in multidrug-resistant sarcoma cell lines.** *Anticancer Res* 2011, **31**:1115–1123.

24. Malhotra GG, Zatz JL: **Investigation of nail permeation enhancement by chemical modification using water as a probe.** *J Pharm Sci* 2002, **91**:312–323.

22

Lean body mass: the development and validation of prediction equations in healthy adults

Solomon Yu[1,2,3,6]*, Thavarajah Visvanathan[4], John Field[3], Leigh C Ward[5], Ian Chapman[3], Robert Adams[6], Gary Wittert[3] and Renuka Visvanathan[1,2,3,6]

Abstract

Background: There is a loss of lean body mass (LBM) with increasing age. A low LBM has been associated with increased adverse effects from prescribed medications such as chemotherapy. Accurate assessment of LBM may allow for more accurate drug prescribing. The aims of this study were to develop new prediction equations (PEs) for LBM with anthropometric and biochemical variables from a development cohort and then validate the best performing PEs in validation cohorts.

Methods: PEs were developed in a cohort of 188 healthy subjects and then validated in a convenience cohort of 52 healthy subjects. The best performing anthropometric PE was then compared to published anthropometric PEs in an older (age $\geq$ 50 years) cohort of 2287 people. Best subset regression analysis was used to derive PEs. Correlation, Bland-Altman and Sheiner & Beal methods were used to validate and compare the PEs against dual X-ray absorptiometry (DXA)-derived LBM.

Results: The PE which included biochemistry variables performed only marginally better than the anthropometric PE. The anthropometric PE on average over-estimated LBM by 0.74 kg in the combined cohort. Across gender (male vs. female), body mass index (< 22, 22-< 27, 27-< 30 and $\geq$30 kg/m^2) and age groups (50–64, 65–79 and $\geq$80 years), the maximum mean over-estimation of the anthropometric PE was 1.36 kg.

Conclusions: A new anthropometric PE has been developed that offers an alternative for clinicians when access to DXA is limited. Further research is required to determine the clinical utility and if it will improve the safety of medication use.

Keywords: Lean body mass, Weight, Older people, Drugs

Background

With increasing age, there is a decline in lean body mass (LBM) and very often an increase in adiposity [1]. The decline in LBM may also be accompanied by a reduction in physical function and when a pathological threshold is reached, the person is said to have sarcopenia [2]. In recent times, sarcopenia has been recognized as an independent predictor of drug related adverse outcomes in the oncology setting where muscle wasting can be common [3,4]. Drug-related adverse effects are defined as medical events related to the use of medication which may result in disability, hospital admissions or death [5]. In patients with cancer, the use of LBM might be superior to body surface area (BSA) [6]. For example, in a prospective study of colon cancer patients treated with 5-fluorouracil (5-FU), the incidence of dose limiting toxicity was examined with respect to conventional dosing of 5-FU/m^2 of BSA versus 5-FU/kg of LBM. LBM was a better predictor of toxicity (p = 0.011) but not BSA [6]. Similar findings have been reported in other studies [7,8]. In anaesthesia, propofol pharmacokinetic parameters scaled linearly to LBM is also said to provide for improved dosing in adults [9]. Therefore, accurate measurement of LBM may have clinical application in improving drug prescribing safety and efficacy, especially in older people where loss of lean mass is common.

* Correspondence: solomon.yu@adelaide.edu.au
[1]Aged and Extended Care Services, Level 8B Main Building, The Queen Elizabeth Hospital, Central Adelaide Local Health Network, 21 Woodville Road, 5011 Woodville South, SA, Australia
[2]Adelaide Geriatrics Training and Research with Aged Care (G-TRAC) Center, School of Medicine, University of Adelaide, South Australia, Australia
Full list of author information is available at the end of the article

A major impediment to the routine clinical use of LBM is the reliance on relatively inaccessible or expensive methods of body composition measurements. Computed tomography (CT), magnetic resonance imaging and dual absorptiometry x-ray (DXA) are used to assess LBM but these methods may be difficult to access in clinical practice (e.g. frail or rural patients) [10]. Although the bioelectrical impedance analysis (BIA) method is portable, it still requires the purchase of special equipment and it's accuracy is also dependent on many other factors such as state of hydration, food intake and exercise [11].

Total body weight consists of fat mass and fat free mass. Fat free mass (FFM) consists of bone, muscle, vital organs and extracellular fluid. LBM differs from FFM in that lipid in cellular membranes are included in LBM but this accounts for only a small fraction of total body weight (up to 3% in men and 5% in women) [12]. In the literature, bone mass has at times been included in LBM and at other times not included [4,13].

Anthropometric-based prediction equations (PEs) have been examined as an alternative in measuring LBM in settings where access to these accurate methods is limited. In a very recent study of older (≥70 years) Australian men, FFM as estimated by three PEs were compared to FFM as estimated by DXA (FFM_{DXA}) [14]. The three PEs were the Heitmann, Janmahasatian and Deurenberg equations as shown below:

Heitmann equation [15]:

$$Body\ fat\ (kg)_{male} = (0.988 \times BMI)$$
$$+ (0.242 \times weight)$$
$$+ (0.094 \times age) - 30.180$$

$$Body\ fat\ (kg)_{female} = (0.988 \times BMI)$$
$$+ (0.344 \times weight)$$
$$+ (0.094 \times age) - 30.180.$$

Janmahasatian equation [12] :

$$FFM\ (kg)_{female} = (9270 \times weight)$$
$$/ (8780 + (244 \times BMI))$$

$$FFM\ (kg)_{male} = (9270 \times weight)$$
$$/ (6680 + (216 \times BMI))$$

Deurenberg equation [16]:

$$Body\ fat(\%) = (1.2 \times BMI)$$
$$+ (0.23 \times Age) - (10.8 \times Sex) - 5.4$$

Male = 1, Female = 0

For two of the PEs (Heitmann and Deurenberg equations), FFM was calculated by subtracting fat mass from total body mass. In defining the FFM and LBM, the authors in that study proposed that FFM and LBM could be used interchangeably. Mitchell et al. reported that

FFM as estimated by Deurenberg equation had the smallest mean difference and overestimated FFM_{DXA} for overweight men but underestimated FFM_{DXA} for all other body mass index (BMI) subgroups [14]. The Heitmann and Janmahasatian equations, on the other hand, overestimated FFM_{DXA} across various BMI categories [14].

The addition of biochemistry variables might improve the performance of prediction equations but few studies have examined this. Creatine Kinase (CK) is found predominantly in skeletal muscle and serum levels were associated with the lean muscle mass [17]. There has only been one study evaluating the relationship between LBM and plasma creatine kinase activity (CK) and a weak and partial correlation ($r < 0.262$) between log CK and LBM was reported [18]. Serum albumin has also been reported to reflect protein reserve and lower albumin levels have been shown to be associated with loss of lean mass [19].

Therefore, the aims of this study were to develop and validate PEs for LBM with anthropometric and biochemistry variables against DXA.

Methods

The Central Northern Adelaide Health Service Ethics of Human Research Committee approved this study. All participants provided written informed consent.

Study cohorts

Four study cohorts were investigated in this study: a) the Cytokine, Adiposity, Sarcopenia and Ageing (CASA) cohort; b) the validation cohort (VC); c) the North West Adelaide Health Study (NWAHS) cohort and d) the Florey Adelaide Male Ageing Study (FAMAS) cohort. CASA was used to derive the PEs for LBM which included anthropometric and biochemistry variables. The selected LBM PEs were then validated in a second independent cohort, the VC (n = 52). As sarcopenia is more prevalent in older populations, validation of the best performing PE and other published FFM PEs (Heitmann, Janmahasatian and Deurenberg equations) were then undertaken in the larger population representative NWAHS and FAMAS cohorts (n = 2287, age ≥ 50 years).

CASA

195 population representative healthy subjects (age 18 to 83 years) were recruited from the western suburbs of Adelaide [20]. The inclusion criteria were: being aged 18 and above, able to comply with study protocol and weight stable over the last 3 months. We excluded those with a serious medical illness, an acute illness in the pass 3 months or in the 2 weeks following blood sampling, an inability to stop medications for 3 days prior to blood sampling, being in receipt of vaccinations and pregnancy. In undertaking the analysis, data from 7 subjects were excluded due to haemolysed or insufficient blood samples.

VC

This was a convenience sample of 52 healthy subjects (age 22 – 83 years) recruited through advertisement for another study [21]. Subjects with known medical illness including gastrointestinal disease or symptoms, significant respiratory, renal or cardiac disease and who were pregnant were excluded from this study.

NWAHS

This is a longitudinal study of community dwelling adults aged eighteen years and older. The population which is a representative biomedical cohort of predominantly of mixed European descent has been described in detail previously [22]. DXA scans were offered to NWAHS participants who were aged ≥ 50 years at follow up (median time = 4 years). Participants with complete anthropometric and DXA measurements at follow up (2004–06) aged ≥50 were included in this analysis (n = 1575).

FAMAS

This male only cohort has also been described in detail elsewhere [23]. The recruitment process was very similar to that used for the NWAHS and so the men in FAMAS were comparable with men in the same age groups from the NWAHS study and of mixed European descent [24]. DXA measurements at baseline (2002–2005) were obtained on 700 participants aged 50 years and over.

Measurements

Anthropometry

Height (m) was measured without shoes using a wall-mounted SECA stadiometer to the nearest 0.1 cm. Weight (kg) was measured wearing light clothing to the nearest 0.1 kg (A&D FV platform scales 0.5 – 150 kg). Body mass index (BMI, weight/height^2) was calculated. The healthy BMI for older people is said to be between 22–27 kg/m^2 [25]. Caucasians with BMI > 30 kg/m^2 were classified as obese [26].

Dual Energy X-ray Absorptiometry (DXA)

DXA analysis in all cohorts measured 3 compartments of the total body composition; fat mass, LBM and bone mineral content. For the purpose of this study, LBM refers to soft tissues and muscle mass, but excludes fat and bone mass. CASA: A Lunar PRODIGY whole-body scanner (GE Medical Systems, Madison, WI), in conjunction with Encore 2002 software, was used to estimate LBM. The majority of subjects underwent DXA within 2 hours of attending the morning clinic when blood sampling occurred. VC: A Norland densitometer XR36 (Norland Medical Systems, Fort Atkinson, Wisconsin, USA), in conjunction with Illuminatus 4.2.4a software, was used to estimate LBM. The DXA was performed on a separate study

day but within 2 weeks of blood sampling and given that the subjects were healthy, it is unlikely that there would have been significant change in body composition within that time frame. To account for differences between machines, LBM data from the VC had a correction factor applied to convert the data to Lunar equivalent [27]. NWAHS and FAMAS: The fan-beam Lunar PRODIGY (GE Medical Systems, Madison, WI) in conjunction with Encore 2002 software and a pencil-beam DPX + (GE Medical Systems, Madison, WI) in conjunction with LUNAR software version 4.7e were used. Cross-calibration analysis had been undertaken and no differences between these 2 densitometers were reported [28].

Blood analyses

For both the CASA and VC cohorts, a venous sample was obtained from each participant after an overnight fast. Both cohorts were asked to refrain from smoking, consuming alcohol or vigorous exercise in the 24 hours before the clinic appointment. Last regular medications were taken the day before and the morning dose was held until after venous sampling. For CASA, the blood was placed in ethylenediaminetetraacetic acid (EDTA) tubes and transported immediately to the Institute for Medical and Veterinary Sciences Laboratories (IMVS) in South Australia for analysis. The blood was centrifuged at 5000 rpm for 7 minutes and analyzed immediately at 37°C. For the VC, samples that had been centrifuged and stored at –70°C were transferred to be processed by the IMVS using the same methodology. The measured co-efficients of variation (CV) were: alanine transferase (ALT, 1.98%), aspartate transaminase (AST, 2.8%),albumin (2.8%), creatinine (3%), lactate dehydrogenase (LDH, 2.2%), creatinine kinase (CK, 2.2%) and high sensitivity C-reactive protein (hsCRP, 1.4%). A Beckman Coulter AU 2700 was used to perform the blood analysis and the methods, reagents and calibration were as per manufacturer instructions.

Statistical analysis

Demographic characteristics in both groups were expressed as mean ± standard deviation (SD). Independent samples t test was used to compare means between the two cohorts. Differences between methods of LBM measurements in the same cohort were examined by paired t test. PEs for LBM were developed from CASA where the independent variable was DXA derived LBM. The initial 10 independent variables were gender, age, weight, height, body mass index, albumin, AST, LDH, CK and hsCRP. The best PEs (as assessed by adjusted R^2: the proportion of the variance of the dependent variable accounted for by the independent variables, and adjusted for the number of independent variables) were developed considering up to 6 equations with n predictors.

For each n, the PE for validation was selected by considering the adjusted R^2 value and likely clinical utility. In the VC, LBM was calculated from the developed prediction equations (LBM_{PE}) and compared with DXA derived LBM (LBM_{DXA}).

The anthropometric PE was also compared to other known PEs [12,15,16] in the NWAHS and FAMAS cohorts.

To assess the accuracy and predictive performance of the prediction equations against LBM_{DXA}, a regression analysis as proposed by Lin [29] was undertaken and the concordance correlation coefficient (ρ_c) was derived. ρ_c measures how much the data deviates from the line of identity representing congruence between the methods. It is a product of Pearson correlation (ρ) and bias correction factor (C_b): $\rho_c = \rho \ C_b$ [30].

In addition, to assess the level of agreement between the two methods, Bland-Altman analysis was performed to obtain the 95% limits of agreement [31]. Furthermore, the goodness of fit with root mean square error (RMSE) and bias (mean error [ME]) was also determined. RMSE and ME were calculated according to the method of Sheiner and Beal [32]. When the 95% confidence interval of the ME includes 0 (i.e. no error), it indicates that the model is not biased. In this study, mean difference was taken to be the same as ME. This gives an estimation of R^2 and the standard error of the estimate [SEE]. SPSS 11.5 for Windows software (SPSS, Inc., Chicago, IL) and the R statistical language (R Foundation for Statistical Computing, Vienna, Austria) were used for the analyses. $P < 0.05$ was considered statistically significant.

Results

The CASA and VC cohorts were similar in age (CASA mean [SD] 49.2 [17.0] vs. VC 50.6 [15.7] years), but younger than the NWAHS (64.7 [9.84] years) and FAMAS (62.3 [8.2] years) cohorts. The BMI (23.7 [2.3] vs. 26.7 [5.2] kg/m^2) and CK (93.3 [54.7] vs. 114.3 [66.0] U/L), were significantly lower in the VC compared to the CASA. LDH (194.4 [37.8] vs. 175.0 [37.4] U/L) and albumin (40.4 [2.5] vs. 39.1 [3.1] g/L) were significantly higher in the VC compared to the CASA. No significant differences between the two cohorts were noted for hsCRP or LBM. The BMI of subjects in the NWAHS and FAMAS studies were higher at 28.2 [4.8] and 28.6 [4.6] kg/m^2 respectively.

Based on adjusted R^2 and potential clinical utility, the following PEs were selected for further validation in the VC:

Table 1 compares LBM_{PE1-4} to LBM_{DXA} in the VC. LBM predicted by all PEs was highly correlated with LBM_{DXA}. Concordance correlations, a measure of the degree to which the data lie on the line of identity, were all around 0.9 and similar to the Pearsons correlation coefficient. All PEs over-estimated LBM_{DXA}, ranging from 1.9% for PE_1 to 4.1% for PE_4. The limits of agreement were similar for all PEs, approximately ± 15%. With increasing number of variables, there were reducing RMSE and mean error indicating improving precision and reducing bias. Because of the costs involved with blood investigations and the marginal benefits, only the anthropometric PE_1 was selected for further comparison in the combined NWAHS and FAMAS cohorts (Tables 2, 3 and 4). Furthermore, biochemistry was not readily available from those cohorts.

Table 2 compares the performance of various PEs including PE_1 against LBM_{DXA} in the total combined NWAHS and FAMAS cohorts as well as in the two gender groups, men and women. All PEs over-estimated the LBM_{DXA} in the total group. PE_1 demonstrated a lower mean error and RMSE score than the Heitmann and Janmahasatian equations in the total population, men and women cohorts. The Deurenberg equation performed the best in the total population with the lowest mean error and RMSE. However, when reviewed within gender groups, PE_1 performed better than the Deurenberg equation in women where both equations over-estimated LBM. In men, the Deurenberg equation under-estimated LBM whilst all other equations over-estimated LBM.

Table 3 compares the performance of the various PEs across age groups (60–64, 65–79, ≥80). PE_1 consistently over-estimated LBM_{DXA} across the age groups but performed better (lowest ME, RMSE values and higher concordance correlation coefficient) than the Janmahasatian and Heitmann equations. The Deurenberg equation did not perform as well as PE_1 in the 50- < 65 years age group and the ≥ 80 years age group and over-estimated LBM in the 50- < 65 years age group but under-estimated LBM in the other two age groups.

Table 4 compares the performance of the various PEs across various BMI groups. Once again, PE_1 has the smallest ME and RMSE compared with the Janmahasatian and Heitmann equations across all the BMI groups analyzed but all of these consistently over-estimated LBM_{DXA} across the various BMI groups. PE_1, in comparison with the Deurenberg equation has a lower ME and RMSE in the obese BMI (>30 kg/m^2) and underweight BMI

$LBM_{PE1} = 22.93 + 0.68(weight) - 1.14(BMI) - 0.01(age) + 9.94(if\ male)\ SEE = 3.61, R^2 = 90.7$
$LBM_{PE2} = 22.06 + 0.67(weight) - 1.11(BMI) + 9.76(if\ male) + 0.01(CK)\ SEE = 3.56, R^2 = 91.0$
$LBM_{PE3} = 21.19 + 0.67(weight) - 1.04(BMI) + 9.51(if\ male) - 0.56(CRP) + 0.01(CK)\ SEE = 3.47, R^2 = 91.4$
$LBM_{PE4} = 23.17 + 0.64(weight) - 0.91(BMI) + 9.45(if\ male) + 0.02(CK) - 0.58(CRP) - 0.02(LDH)\ SEE = 3.38, R^2 = 91.9$

Table 1 Validation of PE LBM in healthy adults from the Cytokine, Adiposity, Sarcopenia and Ageing (CASA) study cohort (n = 195) against DXA derived LBM in the validation cohort (n = 52)

	Mean (SD), kg	Mean error (95%CI), kg	P-value for mean error	R	ρ_c (95% CI) [C_b]	95% limits of agreement	RMSE (95% CI), kg
Total (n = 52)							
LBM$_{DXA}$	46.2 (9.49)						
LBM$_{PE1}$	48.1 (8.93)	1.88 (0.79, 2.97)	0.001	0.911*	0.891 (0.820, 0.935) [0.977]	−9.72, 5.96 (−20.7 to 12.6%)	4.32 (2.84, 5.80)
LBM$_{PE2}$	47.9 (8.95)	1.69 (0.62, 2.75)	0.003	0.915*	0.899 (0.832, 0.940) [0.982]	−9.20, 5.83 (−19.9 to 12.6%)	4.15 (2.70, 5.60)
LBM$_{PE3}$	47.7 (9.13)	1.50 (0.44 ,2.57)	0.006	0.917*	0.904 (0.840, 0.943) [0.986]	−8.99, 5.98 (−19.5 to 13.0%)	4.07 (2.63, 5.51)
LBM$_{PE4}$	47.1 (8.96)	0.86 (−0.22, 1.94)	0.114	0.914*	0.908 (0.846, 0.946) [0.994]	−8.44, 6.72 (−18.3 to 14.6%)	3.93 (2.51, 5.35)

*P-value <0.001, R = correlation, SD = Standard Deviation.
RMSE = root mean squared prediction error, CI = confidence interval, R = Pearson Correlation Coefficient, C_b = Bias Correction Factor, ρ_c = Concordance Correlation Coefficient.

(< 22 kg/m^2) groups. Interestingly, the Deurenberg equation has less bias and better precision than PE$_1$ in predicting LBM$_{DXA}$ in the 22-27 kg/m^2 BMI group. The Deurenberg equation overestimated LBM$_{DXA}$ except in the underweight and obese categories.

Discussion

In this study, prediction equations for LBM were developed and validated. It was hypothesized that the addition of biochemistry variables would result in an improvement in the performance of the PEs and this was seen.

However, the improvement was marginal and insufficient to justify the additional costs.

A significant finding from this study wasthe development of a new anthropometric PE (PE$_1$) for LBM: $LBM = 22.932326 + 0.684668\ (weight)\ -1.137156\ (BMI)\ -0.009213\ (age) + 9.940015\ (if\ male)$. The close approximation to LBM$_{DXA}$ generated by this equation was reflected by its small bias (ME = 0.74 kg) and precision (RMSE = 3.73 kg). It overestimated LBM$_{DXA}$ across gender, age and BMI groups. This PE may be useful in care settings where access to DXA may be limited, providing clinicians a

Table 2 Performance of the CASA (LBM$_{PE1}$) and previously published FFM prediction equations in the NWAHS and FAMAS cohorts (age 50 years and over) in the combined cohort and by gender

	Mean (SD), kg	Mean error (95%CI), kg	P-value for mean error	R	ρ_c (95% CI) [C_b]	95% limits of agreement	RMSE (95% CI), kg
Total (n = 2287)							
LBM$_{DXA}$	50.62 (10.8)						
Heitmann equation	54.30 (10.7)	3.68 (3.53, 3.83)	<0.001	0.940*	0.888 (0.880, 0.896) [0.945]	−3.77, 11.1	5.24 (4.97, 5.51)
Janmahasatian equation	54.23 (11.0)	3.61 (3.46, 3.76)	<0.001	0.943*	0.884 (0.884, 0.899) [0.946]	−3.78, 11.0	5.17 (4.90, 5.44)
Deurenberg equation	50.64 (10.1)	0.02 (−0.14, 0.19)	0.777	0.931*	0.928 (0.923, 0.934) [0.998]	−7.89, 7.93	3.95 (3.70, 4.20)
LBM$_{PE1}$	51.36 (10.6)	0.74 (0.59, 0.89)	<0.001	0.942*	0.939 (0.934, 0.944) [0.998]	−6.58, 8.06	3.73 (2.48, 4.98)
Men (n = 1436)							
LBM$_{DXA}$	57.09 (7.50)						
Heitmann equation	60.56 (7.80)	3.46 (3.25. 3.67)	<0.001	0.863*	0.782 (0.764, 0.800) [0.906]	−11.5, 4.57	5.30 (4.93, 5.67)
Janmahasatian equation	61.18 (6.80)	4.09 (3.89, 4.29)	<0.001	0.852*	0.728 (0.707, 0.747) [0.853]	−12.0, 3.82	5.69 (5.32, 6.06)
Deurenberg equation	56.76 (6.80)	- 0.34 (−0.55, -0.12)	0.002	0.838*	0.834 (0.818, 0.848) [0.995]	−7.92, 8.60	4.14 (3.85, 4.43)
LBM$_{PE1}$	58.22 (6.11)	1.12 (0.92, 1.33)	<0.001	0.851*	0.822 (0.806, 0.837) [0.851]	−6.78, 9.02	4.11 (3.80, 4.42)
Women (n = 851)							
LBM$_{DXA}$	39.70 (5.30)						
Heitmann equation	43.74 (5.55)	4.04 (3.83, 4.26)	<0.001	0.833*	0.651 (0.620, 0.680) [0.782]	−10.3, 2.26	5.12 (4.75, 5.49)
Janmahasatian equation	42.50 (5.39)	2.81 (2.60, 3.01)	<0.001	0.837*	0.722 (0.693, 0.749) [0.872]	−8.91, 3.29	4.14 (3.83, 4.45)
Deurenberg equation	40.32 (4.90)	0.63 (0.39, 0.87)	<0.001	0.759*	0.751 (0.721, 0.779) [0.990]	−7.75, 6.49	3.61 (3.29, 3.93)
LBM$_{PE1}$	39.78 (5.11)	0.08 (−0.12, 0.28)	0.433	0.835*	0.835 (0.813, 0.854) [0.999]	−5.91, 6.07	2.99 (2.74, 3.24)

Mean Error = DXA-PE; LBM, Lean Body Mass; DXA, Dual X-ray absorptiometry; RMSE, Root Mean Square Error; CI, Confidence interval; SD, Standard Deviation; R, Pearson Correlation; C_b = Bias Correction Factor; ρ_c = Concordance Correlation Coefficient; *p-value <0.001.

Table 3 Performance of the CASA (LBM$_{PE1}$) and previously published FFM prediction equations in the NWAHS and FAMAS cohorts (age 50 years and over) across various age groupings

	Mean (SD), kg	Mean error (95%CI), kg	P-value for mean error	R	ρ_c (95% CI) [C$_b$]	95% limits of agreement	RMSE (95% CI), kg
Age 50–64, years (n = 1265)							
LBM$_{DXA}$	52.27 (11.2)						
Heitmann equation	56.47 (10.8)	4.20 (3.99, 4.40)	<0.001	0.944*	0.879 (0.868, 0.890) [0.932]	−11.6, 3.23	5.60 (5.26, 5.95)
Janmahasatian equation	55.62 (11.2)	3.35 (3.15, 3.55)	<0.001	0.948*	0.907 (0.897, 0.915) [0.956]	−10.6, 3.85	4.92 (4.61, 5.23)
Deurenberg equation	53.15 (10.0)	0.87 (0.66, 1.09)	<0.001	0.938*	0.929 (0.921, 0.936) [0.990]	−8.72, 6.98	4.02 (3.73, 4.31)
LBM$_{PE1}$	52.77 (10.7)	0.50 (0.30, 0.70)	<0.001	0.948*	0.946 (0.939, 0.951) [0.998]	−6.68, 7.68	3.62 (3.36, 3.88)
Age 65–79, years (n = 882)							
LBM$_{DXA}$	49.09 (9.91)						
Heitmann equation	52.23 (10.0)	3.14 (2.90, 3.38)	<0.001	0.933*	0.887 (0.873, 0.899) [0.951]	−10.5, 4.18	4.82 (4.35, 5.29)
Janmahasatian equation	53.03 (10.5)	3.93 (3.69, 4.18)	<0.001	0.933*	0.862 (0.846, 0.876) [0.925]	−11.5, 3.66	5.46 (4.97, 5.95)
Deurenberg equation	48.19 (9.14)	−0.90 (−1.15, -0.65)	<0.001	0.924*	0.916 (0.905, 0.926) [0.993]	−6.70, 8.50	3.90 (3.45, 4.35)
LBM$_{PE1}$	50.20 (10.2)	0.98 (0.73, 1.22)	<0.001	0.929*	0.925 (0.915, 0.934) [0.995]	−6.57, 8.53	3.90 (3.48, 4.32)
Age ≥80, years (n = 140)							
LBM$_{DXA}$	44.48 (8.64)						
Heitmann equation	46.71 (9.20)	2.23 (1.60, 2.85)	<0.001	0.929*	0.902 (0.868, 0.928) [0.969]	−9.05, 4.59	4.06 (3.20, 4.92)
Janmahasatian equation	48.46 (10.1)	3.97 (3.29, 4.66)	<0.001	0.936*	0.850 (0.806, 0.883) [0.906]	−11.4, 3.46	5.43 (4.31, 6.55)
Deurenberg equation	42.46 (8.41)	−2.03 (−2.58, -1.48)	<0.001	0.937*	0.911 (0.880, 0.934) [0.971]	−3.97, 8.03	3.61 (2.85, 4.37)
LBM$_{PE1}$	45.84 (9.81)	1.36 (0.80, 1.93)	<0.001	0.941*	0.923 (0.897, 0.943) [0.981]	−5.39, 8.11	3.63 (2.90, 4.36)

Mean Error = DXA-PE; LBM, Lean Body Mass; DXA, Dual X-ray absorptiometry; RMSE, Root Mean Square Error; CI, Confidence interval; SD, Standard Deviation; R, Pearson Correlation; C$_b$ = Bias Correction Factor; ρ_c = Concordance Correlation Coefficient; *p-value <0.001.

practical alternative to assess LBM. Furthermore, it also provides a bedside option in hospitals for ill and frail patients where transport for DXA assessment may be difficult. Whilst BIA may be simple technique to be used at the beside, BIA may be affected by clinical factors such as ascites, hydration status, food intake and exercise and cannot be used in older people with pacemakers [11]. Skin fold measurements may be a cheaper option but the accuracy is operator dependent and the loss of subcutaneous tissue in older people may also affect accuracy [33].

Interestingly, the Deurenberg equation appeared to have less bias with a ME of 0.02 kg but similar precision with a RMSE of 3.95 when compared to the newly developed PE. However, across gender, age and BMI groups, it at times over-estimated and at other times underestimated the LBM$_{DXA}$ [14]. The newly developed PE$_1$ appeared to have better precision (smaller RMSE) and less bias (lower ME) than the Deurenberg equation only in women and in obese older individuals. In clinical settings where the dose normalization to LBM is required, an overestimation of LBM could potentially lead to higher incidence of dose limiting toxicity. Sarcopenia was an important predictor of toxicity in women with metastatic cancer and colon cancer receiving

chemotherapy [4,6]. It was suggested that chemotherapy dose normalization to LBM may reduce the excess toxicity in women. PE$_1$ in our study potentially offers a more accurate estimation of LBM over Deurenberg equation in women and obese individuals and may have clinical utility in this two patient population groups.

This study had several limitations. Only 6% of the study population was under-weight with a BMI < 22 kg/m^2 and therefore, it remains important to validate this newly developed PE in an under-weight population where sarcopenia is likely to be common. Furthermore, only Caucasians were studied and therefore generalizing these results to other ethnic communities is not possible and ethnic specific PEs will need to be developed. Different DXA machines were used in the CASA and VC cohort studies. This may have affected the results as even in the same person, reported measurements of the same tissue mass can be different with different DXA machines [34]. The researchers adjusted for the difference between the machines in the validation aspects of this study but clearly, it would have been preferable to use the same DXA machine in both cohorts. The use of other anthropometry measurements such as calf or arm circumference may improve the performance of prediction equations and needs to be explored in future studies.

Table 4 Performance of the CASA (LBM$_{PE1}$) and previously published FFM prediction equations in the NWAHS and FAMAS cohorts (age 50 years and over) across various body mass index groupings

	Mean (SD), kg	Mean error (95%CI), kg	P-value for mean error	R	ρ_c (95% CI) [C$_b$]	95% limits of agreement	RMSE (95% CI), kg
BMI < 22 kg/m^2 (n = 135)							
LBM$_{DXA}$	42.45 (8.85)						
Heitmann equation	44.85 (7.65)	2.40 (1.85, 2.96)	<0.001	0.932*	0.885 (0.847, 0.914) [0.949]	−4.12, 8.92	4.04 (3.21, 4.87)
Janmahasatian equation	43.72 (9.26)	1.27 (0.77, 1.77)	<0.001	0.946*	0.937 (0.914, 0.955) [0.989]	−4.65, 7.19	3.21 (2.55, 3.87)
Deurenberg equation	41.26 (8.04)	−1.18 (−1.77, -0.60)	<0.001	0.921*	0.909 (0.876, 0.933) [0.986]	−8.04, 5.68	3.62 (2.86, 4.36)
LBM$_{PE1}$	43.52 (9.04)	1.08 (0.57, 1.59)	<0.001	0.944*	0.937 (0.913, 0.955) [0.993]	−4.92, 7.08	3.18 (2.53, 3.83)
BMI 22- < 27 kg/m^2 (n = 847)							
LBM$_{DXA}$	47.45 (9.18)						
Heitmann equation	50.67 (8.67)	3.22 (2.99, 3.44)	<0.001	0.933*	0.874 (0.860, 0.888) [0.938]	−3.42, 9.86	4.62 (4.26,4.98)
Janmahasatian equation	50.81 (9.71)	3.36 (3.13, 3.59)	<0.001	0.937*	0.880 (0.866, 0.893) [0.939]	−3.41, 10.1	4.77 (4.39, 5.15)
Deurenberg equation	47.91 (8.68)	0.45 (0.22, 0.68)	0.001	0.928*	0.925 (0.915, 0.934) [0.997]	−6.42, 7.32	3.46 (3.16, 3.76)
LBM$_{PE1}$	48.64 (9.45)	1.19 (0.96, 1.41)	<0.001	0.938*	0.930 (0.920, 0.938) [0.992]	−5.41, 7.79	3.51 (3.20, 3.82)
BMI 27- < 30 kg/m^2 (n = 596)							
LBM$_{DXA}$	52.00 (9.83)						
Heitmann equation	55.65 (9.48)	3.65 (3.36, 3.95)	<0.001	0.929*	0.867 (0.847, 0.883) [0.933]	−3.65, 10.9	5.16 (4.69, 5.63)
Janmahasatian equation	56.11 (9.75)	4.12 (3.83, 4.41)	<0.001	0.932*	0.857 (0.837, 0.874) [0.919]	−3.08, 11.3	5.47 (4.97, 5.97)
Deurenberg equation	52.58 (9.23)	0.59 (0.30, 0.88)	<0.001	0.928*	0.925 (0.912, 0.935) [0.996]	−6.72, 7.90	3.70 (3.35, 4.05)
LBM$_{PE1}$	52.80 (9.69)	0.81 (0.52, 1.09)	<0.001	0.933*	0.929 (0.918, 0.939) [0.997]	−6.37, 7.99	3.67 (3.31, 4.03)
BMI ≥30 kg/m^2 (n = 709)							
LBM$_{DXA}$	54.80 (11.7)						
Heitmann equation	59.30 (11.7)	4.50 (4.19, 4.80)	<0.001	0.937*	0.867 (0.847, 0.883) [0.933]	−3.80, 12.8	6.12 (5.53, 6.71)
Janmahasatian equation	58.93 (11.0)	4.13 (3.83, 4.43)	<0.001	0.937*	0.857 (0.837, 0.974) [0.919]	−4.02, 12.3	5.80 (5.22, 6.38)
Deurenberg equation	54.07 (10.6)	−0.74 (−1.08, -0.39)	<0.001	0.917*	0.925 (0.912, 0.935) [0.996]	−10.0, 8.55	4.70 (4.14, 5.26)
LBM$_{PE1}$	54.88 (11.3)	0.08 (−0.23, 0.38)	0.628	0.936*	0.929 (0.918, 0.939) [0.997]	−8.15, 8.31	4.11 (3.61, 4.61)

Mean Error = DXA-PE; LBM, Lean Body Mass; DXA, Dual X-ray absorptiometry; RMSE, Root Mean Square Error; CI, Confidence interval; SD, Standard Deviation; R, Pearson Correlation; C$_b$ = Bias Correction Factor; ρ_c = Concordance Correlation Coefficient.
*p-value <0.001.

Conclusions

This study describes the development of a new prediction equation for LBM as estimated by DXA. This new PE consistently over-estimates across gender, age and BMI groups. There remains a need to confirm these findings in older and leaner cohorts, cohorts with diseases (e.g. renal failure), as well as other cohorts with varying ethnicity. The anthropometric PE is an alternative when access to DXA is difficult and this might occur with home bound frail older people as well as people residing in rural areas. The availability of simple and accuratemethods to estimate LBM might be the necessary catalyst required to support better prescribing to limit toxicity in the oncology setting.

Competing interests

TV, JF, JCW, IC, RA and GW have no conflicts of interest; SY received scholarship from University of Adelaide, Faculty of Health Sciences, Divisional Scholarship to support his PhD studies; RV received research grants from: i) University of Adelaide, Faculty of Health Sciences, Establishment Grant; ii) University of Adelaide, Faculty of Health Sciences, Early Career Grant; iii) Vincent Fairfax Family Foundation Research Fellowship through the Royal Australasian College of Physicians; iv) Bernie Lewis Foundation Grant through the Hospital Research Foundation; RVis a member of the Nestle Nutrition Australia Malnutrition In The Elderly Board and receives a honorarium for this activity. She has previously also been a member of Mini Nutritional Assessment (MNA) International Group to refine the MNA and more recently attended the International Consensus Meeting On Protein Intake In The Elderly and both meetings were undertaken independently but supported by an educational grant from Nestle Pty Ltd. She has no other relationships or activities that could appear to have influenced the submitted work. LCW has provided consultancy services to ImpediMed Ltd. The authors declare that they have no competing interests.

Authors' contributions
RV, TV, RA and SY contributed to the initial study design. SY contributed to the data collection, data entry and statistical analysis. JF undertook the statistical analysis required to develop the PEs. LW performed the LBM data correction to adjust differences between dual x-ray absorptiometry machines in this study. All authors contributed to the interpretation of the analysis and preparation of this manuscript. All authors read and approved the final manuscript.

Acknowledgements
We acknowledge the support from the Department of Endocrinology, Queen Elizabeth Hospital for their support with regards to undertaking the required DXA assessments. The Florey Adelaide Males Study is funded by the National Health and Medical Research Council Project grant #627227, and research support has previously been provide by the Florey Foundation, South Australian Health Department, and Premiers Science Research Fund.

Author details
[1]Aged and Extended Care Services, Level 8B Main Building, The Queen Elizabeth Hospital, Central Adelaide Local Health Network, 21 Woodville Road, 5011 Woodville South, SA, Australia. [2]Adelaide Geriatrics Training and Research with Aged Care (G-TRAC) Center, School of Medicine, University of Adelaide, South Australia, Australia. [3]Discipline of Medicine, School of Medicine, Faculty of Health Science, University of Adelaide, Adelaide, SA, Australia. [4]Department of Anaesthesia, The Queen Elizabeth Hospital, Central Adelaide Local Health Network, South Australia, Australia. [5]School of Chemistry and Molecular Biosciences, The University of Queensland, Brisbane, QLD, Australia. [6]The Health Observatory, Discipline of Medicine, School of Medicine, Faculty of Health Science, University of Adelaide, Adelaide, South Australia, Australia.

References
1. Visvanathan R, Chapman I: **Preventing sarcopaenia in older people.** *Maturitas* 2010, **66**(4):383–388.
2. Cruz-Jentoft AJ, Baeyens JP, Bauer JM, Boirie Y, Cederholm T, Landi F, Martin FC, Michel JP, Rolland Y, Schneider SM, et al: **Sarcopenia: european consensus on definition and diagnosis: report of the european working group on sarcopenia in older people.** *Age Ageing* 2010, **39**(4):412–423.
3. Parsons HA, Baracos VE, Dhillon N, Hong DS, Kurzrock R: **Body composition, symptoms, and survival in advanced cancer patients referred to a phase I service.** *PLoS One* 2012, **7**(1):e29330.
4. Prado CM, Baracos VE, McCargar LJ, Reiman T, Mourtzakis M, Tonkin K, Mackey JR, Koski S, Pituskin E, Sawyer MB: **Sarcopenia as a determinant of chemotherapy toxicity and time to tumor progression in metastatic breast cancer patients receiving capecitabine treatment.** *Clin Cancer Res* 2009, **15**(8):2920–2926.
5. Nebeker JR, Barach P, Samore MH: **Clarifying adverse drug events: a clinician's guide to terminology, documentation, and reporting.** *Ann Intern Med* 2004, **140**(10):795–801.
6. Prado CM, Baracos VE, McCargar LJ, Mourtzakis M, Mulder KE, Reiman T, Butts CA, Scarfe AG, Sawyer MB: **Body composition as an independent determinant of 5-fluorouracil-based chemotherapy toxicity.** *Clin Cancer Res* 2007, **13**(11):3264–3268.
7. Gusella M, Toso S, Ferrazzi E, Ferrari M, Padrini R: **Relationships between body composition parameters and fluorouracil pharmacokinetics.** *Br J Clin Pharmacol* 2002, **54**(2):131–139.
8. Aslani A, Smith RC, Allen BJ, Pavlakis N, Levi JA: **The predictive value of body protein for chemotherapy-induced toxicity.** *Cancer* 2000, **88**(4):796–803.

9. Coetzee JF: **Allometric or lean body mass scaling of propofol pharmacokinetics: towards simplifying parameter sets for target-controlled infusions.** *Clin Pharmacokinet* 2012, **51**(3):137–145.
10. Heymsfield SB, Nunez C, Testolin C, Gallagher D: **Anthropometry and methods of body composition measurement for research and field application in the elderly.** *Eur J Clin Nutr* 2000, **54**(3):S26–32.
11. Kyle UG, Bosaeus I, De Lorenzo AD, Deurenberg P, Elia M, Gomez JM, Heitmann BL, Kent-Smith L, Melchior JC, Pirlich M, et al: **Bioelectrical impedance analysis–part I: review of principles and methods.** *Clin Nutr* 2004, **23**(5):1226–1243.
12. Janmahasatian S, Duffull SB, Ash S, Ward LC, Byrne NM, Green B: **Quantification of lean bodyweight.** *Clin Pharmacokinet* 2005, **44**(10):1051–1065.
13. Mourtzakis M, Prado CM, Lieffers JR, Reiman T, McCargar LJ, Baracos VE: **A practical and precise approach to quantification of body composition in cancer patients using computed tomography images acquired during routine care.** *Appl Physiol Nutr Metab* 2008, **33**(5):997–1006.
14. Mitchell SJ, Kirkpatrick CM, Le Couteur DG, Naganathan V, Sambrook PN, Seibel MJ, Blyth FM, Waite LM, Handelsman DJ, Cumming RG, et al: **Estimation of lean body weight in older community-dwelling men.** *Br J Clin Pharmacol* 2010, **69**(2):118–127.
15. Heitmann BL: **Evaluation of body fat estimated from body mass index, skinfolds and impedance. A comparative study.** *Eur J Clin Nutr* 1990, **44**(11):831–837.
16. Deurenberg P, Weststrate JA, Seidell JC: **Body mass index as a measure of body fatness: age- and sex-specific prediction formulas.** *Br J Nutr* 1991, **65**(2):105–114.
17. Norton JP, Clarkson PM, Graves JE, Litchfield P, Kirwan J: **Serum creatine kinase activity and body composition in males and females.** *Hum Biol* 1985, **57**(4):591–598.
18. Swaminathan R, Ho CS, Donnan SP: **Body composition and plasma creatine kinase activity.** *Ann Clin Biochem* 1988, **25**(Pt 4):389–391.
19. Visser M, Kritchevsky SB, Newman AB, Goodpaster BH, Tylavsky FA, Nevitt MC, Harris TB: **Lower serum albumin concentration and change in muscle mass: the health, aging and body composition study.** *Am J Clin Nutr* 2005, **82**(3):531–537.
20. Dent E, YU S, Visvanathan R, Piantadosi C, Adams R, Lange K, Chapman I: **Inflammatory cytokines and appetite in healthy people.** *J Ageing Res Clin Pract* 2012, **1**(1):40–43.
21. Tai K, Visvanathan R, Hammond AJ, Wishart JM, Horowitz M, Chapman IM: **Fasting ghrelin is related to skeletal muscle mass in healthy adults.** *Eur J Nutr* 2009, **48**(3):176–183.
22. Grant JF, Taylor AW, Ruffin RE, Wilson DH, Phillips PJ, Adams RJ, Price K: **Cohort profile: the north west adelaide health study (NWAHS).** *Int J Epidemiol* 2009, **38**(6):1479–1486.
23. Martin S, Haren M, Taylor A, Middleton S, Wittert G: **Cohort profile: the florey adelaide male ageing study (FAMAS).** *Int J Epidemiol* 2007, **36** (2):302–306.
24. Grant JF, Chittleborough CR, Taylor AW, Dal Grande E, Wilson DH, Phillips PJ, Adams RJ, Cheek J, Price K, Gill T, et al: **The north west adelaide health study: detailed methods and baseline segmentation of a cohort for selected chronic diseases.** *Epidemiol Perspect Innov* 2006, **3**:4.
25. Visvanathan R: *Under-nutrition and Older People.* Position Statement No. 6, http://www.anzsgm.org/posstate.asp.
26. **Obesity: preventing and managing the global epidemic. Report of a WHO consultation.** *World Health Organ Tech Rep Ser* 2000, **894**(i-xii):1–253.
27. Maple-Brown LJ, Hughes J, Piers LS, Ward LC, Meerkin J, Eisman JA, Center JR, Pocock NA, Jerums G, O'Dea K: **Increased bone mineral density in aboriginal and torres strait islander australians: impact of body composition differences.** *Bone* 2012, **51**(1):123–130.
28. Mazess RB, Barden HS: **Evaluation of differences between fan-beam and pencil-beam densitometers.** *Calcif Tissue Int* 2000, **67**(4):291–296.
29. Lin LI: **A concordance correlation coefficient to evaluate reproducibility.** *Biometrics* 1989, **45**(1):255–268.
30. Chumlea WC, Baumgartner RN: **Status of anthropometry and body composition data in elderly subjects.** *Am J Clin Nutr* 1989, **50**(5 Suppl):1158–1166. discussion 1231–1155.
31. Bland JM, Altman DG: **Measuring agreement in method comparison studies.** *Stat Methods Med Res* 1999, **8**(2):135–160.
32. Sheiner LB, Beal SL: **Some suggestions for measuring predictive performance.** *J Pharmacokinet Biopharm* 1981, **9**(4):503–512.

33. Omran ML, Morley JE: Assessment of protein energy malnutrition in older persons. Part II: laboratory evaluation. *Nutrition* 2000, **16**(2):131–140.

34. Tothill P, Hannan WJ: Comparisons between hologic QDR 1000W, QDR 4500A, and lunar expert dual-energy X-ray absorptiometry scanners used for measuring total body bone and soft tissue. *Ann N Y Acad Sci* 2000, **904**:63–71.

23

Label-free integrative pharmacology on-target of opioid ligands at the opioid receptor family

Megan Morse[1], Haiyan Sun[2], Elizabeth Tran[2], Robert Levenson[1*] and Ye Fang[2*]

Abstract

Background: *In vitro* pharmacology of ligands is typically assessed using a variety of molecular assays based on predetermined molecular events in living cells. Many ligands including opioid ligands pose the ability to bind more than one receptor, and can also provide distinct operational bias to activate a specific receptor. Generating an integrative overview of the binding and functional selectivity of ligands for a receptor family is a critical but difficult step in drug discovery and development. Here we applied a newly developed label-free integrative pharmacology on-target (iPOT) approach to systematically survey the selectivity of a library of fifty-five opioid ligands against the opioid receptor family. All ligands were interrogated using dynamic mass redistribution (DMR) assays in both recombinant and native cell lines that express specific opioid receptor(s). The cells were modified with a set of probe molecules to manifest the binding and functional selectivity of ligands. DMR profiles were collected and translated to numerical coordinates that was subject to similarity analysis. A specific set of opioid ligands were then selected for quantitative pharmacology determination.

Results: Results showed that among fifty-five opioid ligands examined most ligands displayed agonist activity in at least one opioid receptor expressing cell line under different conditions. Further, many ligands exhibited pathway biased agonism.

Conclusion: We demonstrate that the iPOT effectively sorts the ligands into distinct clusters based on their binding and functional selectivity at the opioid receptor family.

Keywords: Opioid receptor, Functional selectivity, Label-free biosensor

Background

Historically, drug selectivity is described as the differential binding affinity of drug molecules to distinct receptors. The discovery of ligand-directed functional selectivity or biased agonism has led to new avenues for achieving desired drug selectivity. Functional selectivity describes the differential ability of drug molecules to activate one of the multiple downstream pathways to which the receptor is coupled [1-4]. Opioid receptors exemplify many aspects of functional selectivity, with the dependency of receptor-mediated events on ligands used and the cellular or *in vivo* environments examined [5]. Functional selectivity of opioid drugs has been postulated to be related to their clinical profiles, particularly the progression of analgesic tolerance after their extended use [6].

However, integrating functional selectivity into the drug development process remains a challenging problem. The wide spectrum of signaling events mediated by a receptor [7], coupled with the differences in signaling components in distinct types of cells [8], makes it extremely difficult to fully discover and quantify the functional selectivity of drug molecules using conventional molecular assays. Also, these molecular assays screen drug molecules based on a predetermined molecular hypothesis, but such a hypothesis may or may not be relevant to the pathogenesis of a disease [9]. A further complication is the existence of signaling readout- and cell background-dependent potency and efficacy, which is inherited from the operational bias of drug molecules on a receptor [3]. The possibility that a drug may have multidimensional efficacy makes it difficult to optimize and prioritize drug candidate molecules. In many instances, the efficacy profiles obtained for a candidate drug may not be good predictors of their *in vivo*

* Correspondence: rlevenson@hmc.psu.edu; fangy2@corning.com
[1]Department of Pharmacology, Pennsylvania State University College of Medicine, Hershey, PA, USA
Full list of author information is available at the end of the article

therapeutic impacts, and it may be difficult to sort out which molecular mode of action leads to a desired therapeutic impact. Thus, assays that are phenotypic in nature yet allow mechanistic descriptions of drug actions would be advantageous.

With the ability to interrogate wide pathway coverage utilizing a single assay and to mechanistically delineate drug pharmacology at the whole cell or cell system level, label-free receptor assays have emerged as promising platforms for drug discovery [10-14]. Here, we applied a recently developed label-free integrative pharmacology on-target (iPOT) approach [15,16] to systematically survey the binding and functional selectivity of a library of opioid ligands. This comparative pharmacological approach is centered on similarity analysis of DMR profiles of drugs obtained in model cell lines that have been pretreated with a wide variety of probe chemicals. The probe molecules are chosen to modify pathways downstream of activated receptors, so that the sensitivity of drugs to the pathway modulation can be surveyed at the whole cell level. After translating DMR profiles into multidimensional coordinates, similarity analysis is used to categorize drugs into distinct clusters. We found that the iPOT approach provides an integrative display of the binding and functional selectivity of a library of opioid ligands at the family of opioid receptors.

Methods

Materials and reagents

Pertussis toxin (PTX), cholera toxin (CTX), forskolin and dimethyl sulfoxide (DMSO) were purchased from Sigma-Aldrich (St. Louis, MO). DAMGO, DPDPE, BRL-52537, CTOP, naltrindole hydrochloride, norbinaltorphimine, U0126, SB202190, SP600125, and LY294002 were purchased from Tocris Biosciences (Ellisville, MO). The Opioid Compound Library consisting of 64 compounds of pan-specific and receptor subtype-specific agonists and antagonists, each at 10 mM in DMSO, was obtained from Enzo Life Sciences (Plymouth Meeting, PA). All tissue culture media and reagents were purchased from Invitrogen (Calrsbad, CA). Both fibronectin-coated and tissue culture treated (TCT) Epic® biosensor microplates, as well as polypropylene compound source plates were obtained from Corning Inc (Corning, NY).

Cell culture

We used five distinct cell lines including human neuroblastoma cell line SH-SY5Y, human embryonic kidney HEK293 cells, and three engineered HEK 293 cell lines for label-free pharmacology profiling. HEK293 cells and SH-SY5Y cells were obtained from American Type Tissue Culture (Manassas, VA) and cultured in Dulbecco's modified Eagle's medium (DMEM GlutaMAX-I) supplemented with 10% non-heated inactivated fetal bovine serum, 100

units/ml penicillin, and 100 g/ml streptomycin. Both HEK-MOR and HEK-DOR cell lines were a generous gift from Dr. Mark von Zastrow (University of California, San Francisco). The HEK-KOR cell line was donated from Dr. Lee-Yuen Lui-Chen (Temple University).

The HEK-MOR stably expresses FLAG-tagged wild type human mu opioid receptor (MOR1) with a Bmax of 2.5 pmoles/mg cell protein [16,17]. The HEK-DOR stably expresses FLAG-tagged wild type human delta opioid receptor with a Bmax of 0.8 pmoles/mg cell protein [18]. The HEK-KOR cell line stably expresses FLAG-tagged wild type human kappa opioid receptor with an unknown Bmax [19]. SH-SY5Y is a dopaminergic neuronal cell line which has been used as an *in vitro* model for assessment of functional responses of the MOR. SH-SY5Y is known to express both MOR and DOR with a protein ratio of approximately 4.5:1 [20], and the Bmax for the DOR was estimated to be 35 to 100 fmol/mg protein [21,22]. SH-SH5Y is also known to endogenously express several splice variants of opioid receptors including a single TM protein (MOR1S) resulting from an exon-skipping variant [23,24], an alternatively spliced isoform MOR1K that is a 6TM GPCR variant without the N-terminal extracellular and first transmembrane domains and is preferentially coupled to $G_{\alpha s}$ [25], and a splice variant of δ opioid receptor that lacks the third cytoplasmic loop of the native receptor [26]. This short δ receptor appeared to be associated with human malignoma, although its biological functions remain unknown.

These cells were grown in complete DMEM GlutaMAX-I containing 400 µg/ml geneticin. For cell culture in the fibronectin-coated Epic® biosensor microplates, cells were seeded at a density of 16,000 cells/40 µL/well for HEK293 cells, and 20,000 cells/40 µL/well for both HEK-DOR and HEK-KOR cells. For SH-SY5Y cells, cells were seeded at 15,000 cells/40 µL/well onto Epic® tissue culture compatible microplates. After seeding the biosensor microplates were incubated for 30 min at room temperature, and then transferred to a humidified incubator (37°C, 5% CO_2) for 20–24 hrs for HEK cells, or 48 hours for SH-SY5Y cells.

Dynamic mass redistribution (DMR) assays

DMR assays were performed using Epic® system as previously described [27]. Epic® system from Corning is a wavelength interrogation reader system tailored for resonant waveguide grating biosensors in microplates. This system consists of a temperature-control unit (26°C), an optical detection unit, and an on-board liquid handling unit with robotics. The detection unit is centered on integrated fiber optics, and enables kinetic measures of cellular responses with a time interval of ~15 sec.

For DMR assays, once reached high confluency (~95%) the cells were washed twice with assay buffer (1× Hank's balanced salt solution with 20 mM HEPES, pH7.1) and transferred to the Epic® reader for 1 hr at 26°C so a steady baseline was reached. DMR was monitored in real time with a temporal resolution of ~15 sec throughout the assays. A typical DMR proceeded with a 2-min baseline, followed by a real time kinetic response after the compound additions using the onboard liquid handler. The DMR was recorded as a shift in resonant wavelength (picometer, pm). Different DMR assay formats were used for profiling opioid ligands. DMR agonist assays were used to directly record the DMR signal arising from a ligand itself. DMR antagonist assays were used to record the DMR arising from an agonist at a fixed dose (usually its EC_{100}) after pretreatment with an inhibitor or a ligand. An EC_{100} value was used to ensure maximal activation of respective receptor for follow-up potency studies in order to have greater antagonism differentiation power than the dose at its EC_{50}.

For iPOT profiling, all ligands were examined at 10 µM. This was based on three obvious reasons. First, different ligands often display a wide range of affinities binding to a specific receptor, and a specific ligand often displays distinct affinities binding to different opioid receptors (Additional file 1). Furthermore, the binding affinity of a ligand often does not directly translate to its potency to activate the receptor at the whole cell level [27,28], so it is practically difficult to choose ligand-specific concentrations for our systematic profiling. Second, the main purpose of the present study is to determine both binding and functional selectivity of the same family of ligands against the opioid receptor family, and almost all ligands examined displayed agonist activity in at least one of the five cell lines profiled (see results below). Thus, it is necessary to use a high concentration to saturate the receptor sites and to maximize the functional activation of the receptors induced by most, if not all, of the ligands examined. Third, 10 µM is the most commonly used concentration for high throughput screening and profiling.

To manifest the specificity, relative potency and efficacy, and modes of action of the drugs, a variety of probe molecules were used to achieve a wide range of chemical environments for each cell line through alteration of cellular signaling protein(s) in the signaling pathways of opioid receptors. Here, the cells were pretreated offline with several probe molecules by incubating the cells with a probe molecule at the indicated dose for the indicated period of time (Table 1). After the pretreatment with the probe molecules the cells were then stimulated with an opioid ligand, whose responses were recorded in real time and used for similarity and correlation analysis. Specifically, cells were pretreated with either 0.1% DMSO (the positive control), 10 µM opioid ligand in the library, 100 ng/ml PTx, 400 ng/ml CTX, 10 µM forskolin, 10 µM U0126, 10 µM SB202190, 10 µM SP600125, or 10 µM LY294002 for the times indicated. Since the primary purpose of the iPOT profiling of opioid ligands was to identify interesting ligands for quantitative pharmacology assessment, all kinase inhibitors at 10 µM were used to manifest the sensitivity of the label-free profiles of opioid ligands to the pathway modulation. PTX binds to $G_{\alpha i}$, resulting in inhibition of $G_{\alpha i}$ by ADP ribosylation of a Cys residue and uncoupling of the G protein from the receptor [29]. CTX binds to $G_{\alpha s}$, resulting in activation of $G_{\alpha s}$ by ADP ribosylation of an Arg residue and cAMP production [30]. Forskolin is an activator of adenylyl cyclase and is widely used for cell-based screening due to its ability to increase $G_{\alpha i}$-mediated signaling but desensitize $G_{\alpha s}$-mediated signaling [31]. U0126, SB202190, SP600125, and LY294002 are known kinase pathway inhibitors for MEK1/2, p38

Table 1 Assay protocols and DMR signals used for similarity analysis

Cell	Probe, pretreatment duration	DMR readout	Labels used in clustering	Figures
HEK293	0.1% DMSO in buffer, 1 hr	Ligand, 10 µM	HEK-3, 9, 30	Additional file 1: Figure S1, S2
Opioid*	0.1% DMSO in buffer, 1hr	Ligand, 10 µM	Buffer-3, 9, 30	Figures 1 5 6 7
HEK-MOR	10 µM ligand, 1 hr	DAMGO, 10 µM	MOR-3, 9, 30	Additional file 1: Figures S2 & S3
HEK-DOR	10 µM ligand, 1 hr	DPDPE, 10 µM	DOR-3, 9, 30	Figure 5
HEK-KOR	10 µM ligand, 1 hr	BRL-57532, 10 µM	KOR-3, 9, 30	Figure 6
SH-SY5Y	10 µM ligand, 1 hr	DAMGO, 10 µM	5Y-3, 9, 30	Figure 7
Opioid*	100 ng/ml PTX, 20 hr	Ligand, 10 µM	PTX-3, 9, 30	Figures 5 6 and 7
Opioid*	400 ng/ml CTX, 20 hr	Ligand, 10 µM	CTX-3, 9, 30	Figures 5 6 and 7
Opioid*	10 µM forskolin, 1 hr	Ligand, 10 µM	FSK-3, 9, 30	Figures 5 6 and 7
Opioid*	10 µM U0126, 1 hr	Ligand, 10 µM	U0126-3, 9, 30	Figures 5 6 and 7
Opioid*	10 µM SB202190, 1 hr	Ligand, 10 µM	SB-3, 9, 30	Figures 5 6 and 7
Opioid*	10 µM SP600125, 1 hr	Ligand, 10 µM	SP-3, 9, 30	Figures 5 6 and 7
Opioid*	10 µM LY294002, 1 hr	Ligand, 10 µM	LY-3, 9, 30	Figures 5 6 and 7

* Opioid receptor expressing cell lines wherein the same assay protocol was applied.

MAPK, JNK, and PI3K, respectively [32,33]. It has been suggested that opioid ligands often exhibit functional selectivity on these pathways [5,6,34]. It is worthy of noting that the results obtained using this approach may not directly translate into a pathway-specific biased agonism, given that many, if not all kinase inhibitors, display polypharmacology (that is, the ability to bind to more than one targets).

We screened a library of 64 opioid ligands. Literature mining revealed that fifty-five of the opioid ligands in the library had previously been shown to possess binding affinity for at least one member of the classic opioid receptor family (Additional file 1: Tables S1–S3), and thus chosen for analysis in this study.

Quantitative real-time PCR

Total RNA was extracted from SH-SY5Y or HEK293 cells using an RNeasy mini kit (Qiagen, Cat#74104). To eliminate genomic DNA contamination, on-column DNase digestion was performed using RNase-free DNase set from Qiagen (Valencia, CA). The concentration and quality of total RNA were determined using a Nanodrop 8000 from Thermo Scientific. Customized PCR-array plates for 352 GPCR genes and reagents were ordered from SABiosciences (Frederick, MD). About 1 µg total RNA was used for each 96-well PCR-array. The PCR-array was performed on an ABI 7300 Real-Time PCR System following the manufacturer's instructions.

Data visualization and clustering

For each opioid ligand in a cell line, ten DMR assays were performed that measured receptor specificity, G-protein coupling, and downstream kinase pathway selectivity. DMR assay offers a texture rich readout for ligand-receptor interactions at the whole cell level [11-13]. Originating from distinct functional selectivity and polypharmacology, the DMR signals of different ligands could be diverse in a specific cell [35]. To classify ligands, we adopt similarity analysis, a technology to cluster molecules through determination of the similarity and distances among a large set of different biological data [36-38]. For effective similarity analysis the real responses at three distinct time points (3 min, 9 min, and 30 min post-stimulation) were extracted from each kinetic DMR signal and used to rewrite the DMR pharmacology of each ligand. Combining DMR parameters from multiple assays and/or cells formed a numerical descriptor containing multi-dimensional coordinates for each ligand, which was then subject to similarity analysis. At least duplicate data for each assay were collected to generate an averaged response. For visualization, the real-time responses were color coded to illustrate relative differences in DMR signal strength. The red color refers to a positive value, the black a value near zero,

and the green color represents a negative value. Differences in color intensity illustrate differences in signal strength. In the ligand matrix, each column represents one DMR response at a particular time under a specific assay condition, and each row represents one ligand. Every row and column carries equal weight. The Ward hierarchical clustering algorithm and Euclidean distance metrics [15,16] were used for generating heat maps and clustering the DMR profiles. To assist with direct visualization of DMR characteristics of each ligand in an assay, we did not carry out similarity analysis among distinct columns, except for the analysis based on real time responses (Figure 1). Each assay was arranged in three consecutive columns to form a column group for clear understanding of the key characteristics of a DMR.

Statistical analysis

For profiling, two independent measurements, each done in duplicate, were performed. All replicates passed the 2 sigma coefficient of variation test in order to be included in the analysis. Drugs whose DMR responses failed the statistical test were re-screened. At least two replicates were included for the final analysis. For dose responses, at least two independent measurements, each done at least in duplicate, were performed to calculate the mean responses and the standard deviations (s.d.).

Results

Expression of endogenous opioid receptors

We performed quantitative real time PCR to determine the expression of endogenous opioid receptors in the parental HEK293 cell line as well as SH-SY5Y cells. Results showed that HEK293 expresses low levels of mRNAs for ORL1 (cycle threshold, C_t, 29.3), but little or no mRNAs for MOR (C_t, undetected), DOR (C_t, 35.3), and KOR (C_t, 33.1). As controls, the C_t values for hypoxanthine phosphoribosyltransferase 1 (HPRT1) and glyceraldehyde-3-phosphate dehydrogenase (GADPH) in HEK293 were found to be 19.6 and 16.1, respectively. Our quantitative real time PCR results also showed that SH-SY5Y expresses mRNAs for MOR (C_t, 23.2) and ORL1 (C_t, 25.8), low levels of mRNAs for DOR (C_t, 30.9), and no detectable mRNAs for KOR (C_t, undetected). The C_t values for controls were 21.3 for HPRT1, and 15.8 for GADPH. This is consistent with previous studies showing that SH-SY5Y expresses both MOR and DOR proteins at a ratio of approximately 4.5:1 [20].

Label-free integrative pharmacology profiling and data visualization

We adopted the newly developed iPOT approach to determine the binding and functional selectivity of a family of ligands against the opioid receptor family. This study begun with the preparation of a library consisting of

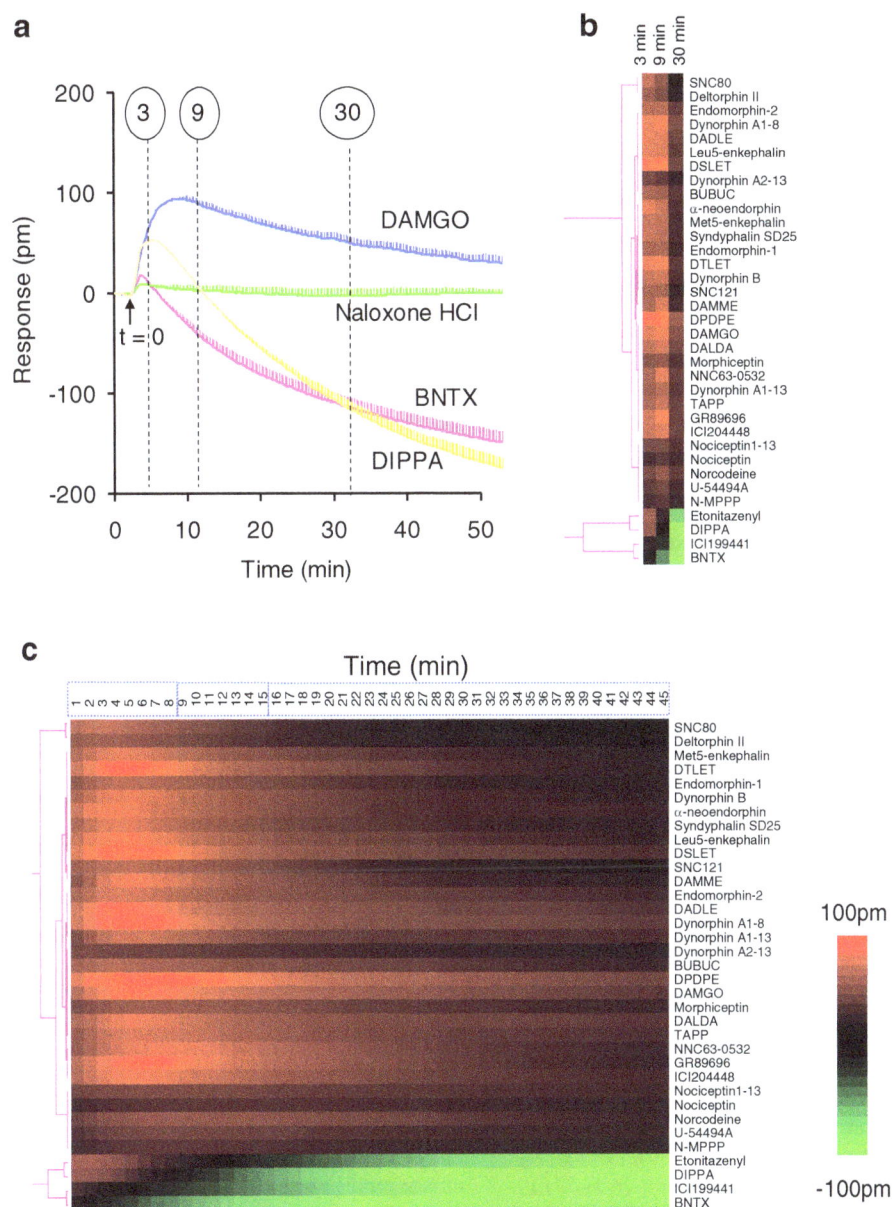

Figure 1 Extracting DMR parameters for effective similarity analysis. (a) Representative DMR signals of opioid ligands in native SH-SY5Y cells. The data represents the mean ± s.d. of 2 independent measurements, each in duplicate (n = 4). Responses at three time points (3 min, 9 min, and 30 min post-stimulation) were extracted to represent each DMR signal. The solid arrow indicates the time when ligands were added (t =0). **(b)** A colored heat map of opioid ligand-induced DMR in native SH-SY5Y cells based on the responses at the three time points. **(c)** A colored heat map based on the real time DMR signals of all opioid ligands that gave rise to a detectable DMR. The real time responses showed was reduced to every minute. Three time domains were evident.

fifty-five opioid ligands, followed by whole cell DMR profiling under different conditions and similarity analysis of respective DMR signals (Table 1). Ligands with interesting label-free profiles were then identified and selected for quantitative pharmacology assessment.

Interrogating SH-SY5Y cells with the library of opioid ligands identified three types of DMR signals (Figure 1a). Out of the fifty-five ligands tested, twenty ligands including naloxone-HCl were silent in this cell line, leading to

a net-zero DMR. Conversely, thirty-one ligands including DAMGO produced a positive DMR signal that consists of an initial positive DMR (P-DMR) event followed by a negative DMR (N-DMR) event. The N-DMR event eventually decayed back to a steady level that is still above the baseline at 1 hr poststimulation. The remaining four ligands, DIPPA, etonitazenyl isothiocyanate, BNTX, and ICI 199441, produced a biphasic DMR response whose late N-DMR event eventually decayed below the baseline.

We adopt similarity analysis to classify ligands based on DMR responses. Given that a DMR is a kinetic response and consists of over 200 dimensions due to its high temporal resolution, it is practically impossible to include all time points of a DMR signal for similarity analysis of all ligands under all conditions. Thus, we first reduced the DMR dimensions to three distinct time points (3, 9, and 30 min post-stimulation) for similarity analysis (Figure 1b). This dimensional reduction is based on the clustering of time domains of the DMR responses from all opioid ligands in each of the five cell lines examined. For SH-SY5Y cells, similarity analysis using the unsupervised Ward hierarchical clustering algorithm and Euclidean distance metrics [15,16] showed that all DMR signals with an amplitude greater than 30 pm generally propagate with three distinct time periods: immediate (1–8 min), early (9–15 min), and late responses (15–50 min post-stimulation) (Figure 1c). Clustering based on the entire kinetic response or the reduced three time-points led to similar clusters of ligands in SH-SY5Y cells (comparing Figure 1c with b), although clustering based on the entire kinetic response expectedly gave rise to better resolution than by using the reduced time-points. Therefore, we chose to limit our analysis to the three time point parameters (3, 9, and 30 min) for each DMR response.

Selectivity of opioid agonists at the opioid receptor family

We first determined the selective agonist activity of opioid ligands in five distinct cell lines using DMR agonist assays, based on their ability to trigger DMR signals in respective cell lines. For the four opioid receptor-expressing cell lines, we included both positive and negative controls to define the range of responses for classification of ligand agonism. For the negative controls (that is, the assay buffer containing equal amount of DMSO), the DMR responses at 9 min poststimulation were found to be 3 ± 12 pm, -4 ± 14 pm, 5 ± 11 pm and 3 ± 5 pm (n = 16) for HEK-MOR, HEK-DOR, HEK-KOR and SH-SH5Y cells, respectively. For the positive controls, the DMR responses at 9 min poststimulation were found to be 240 ± 17 pm, 321 ± 26 pm, 213 ± 21 pm, and 87 ± 9 pm (n = 32) for 10 μM DAMGO in HEK-MOR, 10 μM DPDPE in HEK-DOR, 10 μM BRL52537 in HEK-KOR, and 10 μM DAMGO in SH-SH5Y cells, respectively. For a given cell line, a ligand whose DMR amplitude was within the mean$\pm2\sigma$ of its positive control was considered to be a full agonist, while a ligand whose DMR amplitude was smaller the mean-2σ of its positive control and greater than 50 pm was considered to be a partial agonist, and a ligand whose DMR amplitude was smaller than 50 pm was considered to be inactive. A ligand that led to a detectable DMR in HEK293 was viewed to have off-target effect(s).

Table 2 summarizes the agonist activity of all opioid ligands in the five different cell lines. Out of the fifty-five ligands tested, six off-target ligands including BNTX, β-funaltrexamine, etonitazenyl isothiocyanate, ICI 199441, dynorphin A 2–13 and nocicepin 1–13 gave rise to a noticeable DMR in the parental HEK293 cells (Additional file 1: Figure S1). Among the six ligands only BNTX led to an N-DMR in all five cell lines, while the others produced a P-DMR signal in the four opioid receptor-expressing cell lines.

Out of the fifty-five ligands tested, four ligands including naloxone was inactive in all cell lines, while the other forty-nine ligands gave rise to agonist activity in at least one of the four opioid receptor-expressing cell lines. Several ligands that are believed to be opioid antagonists also produced noticeable DMR in at least one of the engineered cell lines, but not in SH-SH5Y cells. Specifically, nalbuphine and β-funaltrexamine acted as partial agonists at MOR, DOR, and KOR sites, while levallorphan, SKF10047 and N-benzylnaltrindole specific to both DOR and KOR sites, and naloxonazine and naltrexone specific to the KOR.

The pattern of agonist activity in SH-SY5Y cells (Additional file 1: Figure S2) cannot be explained by the solo activation of endogenous MOR, and/or by the differential expression levels of the MOR between SH-SY5Y and HEK-MOR cells. This is expected given that SH-SY5Y expresses both MOR and DOR. This conclusion was supported by correlation analysis between the two cell lines (Figure 2). This analysis excluded the six off-target ligands, and all other responses were normalized to the DAMGO response in respective cell line. Results showed that SNC 121, SNC80 and deltrophin II had no or little activity in the HEK-MOR, but active in SH-SY5Y cells. In contrast, tramadol was active in HEK-MOR, but inactive in SH-SY5Y cells. Similarly, a group of ligands including U-50488H, U62066, DIPPA and (−)U-50488H were active in the three transfected cell lines, but not in SH-SY5Y cells. Furthermore, DPDPE and GR89696 behaved as partial agonists in HEK-MOR cells, but full agonists in SH-SY5Y cells.

Selectivity of opioid ligands to block the DMR response produced by the activation of opioid receptors

We used a two-step DMR assay (i.e., an antagonist assay) to determine the ability of opioid ligands to block or desensitize the DMR responses resulting from the activation of opioid receptors. The antagonist or desensitization assay was performed in two sequential steps, each lasting about one hour. Cells were pretreated with a ligand from the opioid library, followed by treatment with a fixed dose of a known opioid agonist. A ligand that does not trigger a DMR but blocks the DMR of the known agonist is termed an antagonist. Conversely, a ligand that leads to noticeable

Table 2 Classification of opioid ligands based on their DMR agonist activity in the five distinct cell lines

Name	HEK	MOR	DOR	KOR	SH-SY5Y	Literature classification
β-Funaltrexamine	off-target	Partial agonist	Partial agonist	Partial agonist		Mu antagonist
BNTX	off-target	off-target	off-target	off-target	off-target	Delta antagonist
Dynorphin A (2–13)	off-target		Partial agonist	Partial agonist		Kappa agonist
Etonitazenyl	off-target	Partial agonist		Partial agonist		Mu agonist
ICI 199,441	off-target	Full agonist	Partial agonist	Full agonist		Kappa agonist
Nociceptin (1–13)	off-target	Partial agonist		Partial agonist		ORL1 agonist
α-Neoendorphin		Partial agonist	Full agonist	Full agonist	Full agonist	Kappa agonist
BRL-52537			Partial agonist	Full agonist		Kappa agonist
BUBUC		Partial agonist	Full agonist	Partial agonist	Partial agonist	Delta agonist
DADLE		Partial agonist	Full agonist	Partial agonist	Full agonist	Delta agonist
DALDA		Partial agonist			Full agonist	Mu agonist
DAMGO		Full agonist	Partial agonist	Partial agonist	Full agonist	Mu agonist
DAMME		Full agonist	Full agonist	Partial agonist	Full agonist	Mu/Delta agonist
Deltorphin II		Partial agonist	Full agonist			Delta agonist
DIPPA		Partial agonist	Partial agonist	Full agonist		Kappa antagonist
DPDPE		Partial agonist	Full agonist	Partial agonist	Full agonist	Delta agonist
DSLET		Full agonist	Full agonist	Partial agonist	Full agonist	Delta agonist
DTLET		Full agonist	Full agonist	Partial agonist	Full agonist	Delta agonist
Dynorphin A (1–13)		Full agonist	Full agonist	Full agonist	Partial agonist	Kappa agonist
Dynorphin A (1–8)		Full agonist	Full agonist	Full agonist	Full agonist	Kappa agonist
Dynorphin B		Partial agonist	Full agonist	Full agonist	Full agonist	Kappa agonist
Endomorphin-1		Partial agonist	Partial agonist		Partial agonist	Mu agonist
Endomorphin-2		Partial agonist	Partial agonist	Partial agonist	Full agonist	Mu agonist
(Leu5)-Enkephalin		Full agonist	Full agonist	Partial agonist	Full agonist	Mu/Delta agonist
(Met5)-Enkephalin		Full agonist	Full agonist	Partial agonist	Full agonist	Mu/Delta agonist
GR 89696		Partial agonist	Partial agonist	Full agonist	Full agonist	Kappa agonist
ICI 204,448		Partial agonist	Partial agonist	Full agonist	Full agonist	Kappa agonist
Levallorphan			Partial agonist	Partial agonist		Partial Mu/delta agonist
Morphiceptin		Partial agonist			Partial agonist	Mu agonist
Nalbuphine		Partial agonist	Partial agonist	Partial agonist		Partial Mu/kappa agonist
Naloxonazine				Partial agonist		Mu antagonist
Naloxone HCl						Opioid antagonist
Naloxone methiodide						Opioid antagonist
Naltrexone				Partial agonist		Opioid antagonist
Naltriben						Delta antagonist
Naltrindole						Delta antagonist
N-Benzylnaltrindole			Partial agonist	Partial agonist		Delta antagonist
N-MPPP		Partial agonist	Partial agonist	Full agonist		Kappa agonist
NNC 63-0532		Partial agonist	Partial agonist	Partial agonist	Full agonist	ORL1 agonist
Nociceptin				Partial agonist		ORL1 agonist
Nor-Binaltorphimine						Kappa antagonist
(−)-Norcodeine		Partial agonist		Partial agonist	Partial agonist	Opioid antagonist
Salvinorin A		Partial agonist		Full agonist		Kappa agonist
SKF10047			Partial agonist	Partial agonist		Opioid agonist/antagonist

Table 2 Classification of opioid ligands based on their DMR agonist activity in the five distinct cell lines *(Continued)*

SNC 121		Partial agonist	Partial agonist	Partial agonist	Delta agonist
SNC 80	Partial agonist	Partial agonist	Partial agonist	Partial agonist	Delta agonist
Syndyphalin SD-25	Full agonist	Partial agonist	Partial agonist	Partial agonist	Mu agonist
TAPP	Partial agonist	Partial agonist	Partial agonist	Full agonist	Mu agonist
Tramadol	Partial agonist				Weak Mu agonist
(−)-U-50488	Partial agonist	Partial agonist	Full agonist		Kappa partial agonist
(+)-U-50488			Full agonist		Kappa partial agonist
U-50,488H	Partial agonist	Partial agonist	Full agonist		Kappa agonist
U-54494A	Partial agonist	Partial agonist	Partial agonist		Kappa agonist
U-62066	Partial agonist		Full agonist		Kappa agonist
U-69593	Partial agonist	Partial agonist	Full agonist		Kappa agonist

The blank indicates that the ligand did not result in any noticeable DMR.

DMR response but desensitizes the cells responding to the succeeding agonist is termed an agonist.

We first determined the DMR potency of a known agonist for each cell line: DAMGO for HEK-MOR, DPDPE for HEK-DOR, BRL-52537 for HEK-KOR, and DAMGO for SH-SY5Y cells, based on their respective maximal amplitudes. We have previously shown that DAMGO produces a mono-phasic dose response in HEK-MOR cells with an EC_{50} of 0.93 ± 0.12 nM [16]. In HEK-DOR cells, DPDPE produced biphasic dose response with two distinct EC_{50}'s of 0.15 ± 0.03 nM, and 2.8 ± 0.09 nM (2 independent measurements, n =4) (Figure 3a and b). In HEK-KOR cells, BRL-52537 also produced a biphasic dose response with two distinct EC_{50}'s of 35.6 ± 3.1 pM, and 26.0 ± 1.9 nM (2 independent measurements, n =4) (Figure 3c and d). Conversely, in SH-SY5Y cells DAMGO produced a monophasic dose response with an

EC_{50} of 4.5 ± 0.3 nM (2 independent measurements, n =4) (Figure 3e and f).

We next performed cluster analysis of the known agonist DMR responses after pretreatment with the library ligands using unsupervised Ward hierarchical clustering algorithm and Euclidean distance metrics. To achieve high resolution to differentiate the relative potency of opioid ligands to block or desensitize the agonist DMR response at each receptor site we employed a high dose for each agonist tested (10 μM DAMGO for HEK-MOR cells, 10 μM DPDPE for HEK-DOR cells, 10 μM BRL-52537 for HEK-KOR cells, and 10 μM DAMGO for SH-SY5Y cells). The DMR of each known agonist in its respective cell line was shown to be specific to the activation of its respective receptor. Results showed that the cluster analysis separated these ligands into different clusters (Additional file 1: Figure S3), and most of the ligands in each subcluster exhibited DMR characteristics in general agreement with their previously described pharmacology and classifications (Table 2 and Additional file 1: Tables S1–S3).

We further examined the DMR responses of DAMGO in SH-SY5Y cells with and without pretreatment with the library ligands, based on reported affinities of opioid ligands (Additional file 1: Tables S1 to S3) [39]. Results show that the ligands blocking the DAMGO-elicited DMR in HEK-MOR also blocked the DAMGO DMR in SH-SY5Y cells, suggesting that the DAMGO response in SH-SY5Y is mostly originated from the activation of the MOR. However, the extent of the DAMGO-induced DMR observed after pretreatment with the library of opioid ligands in SH-SY5Y cells cannot be explained by the known affinities of these ligands binding to MOR or the DOR sites (Figure 4a and b). To best illustrate this, we first assumed that the DAMGO DMR in SH-SY5Y cells is originated from the activation of MOR or DOR alone, and then compared the actual DAMGO response with the calculated one for each ligand based on its

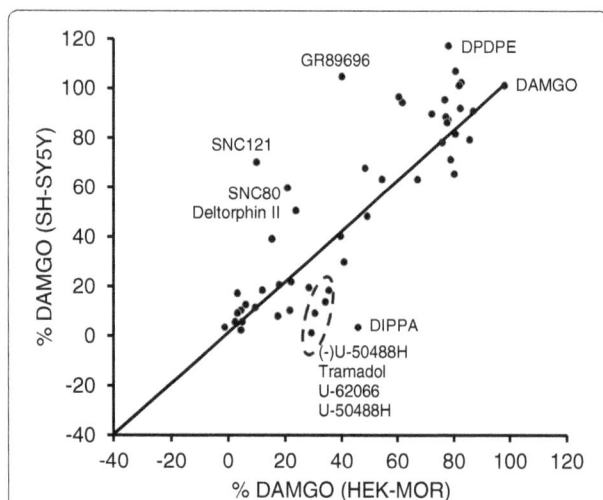

Figure 2 The correlation analysis of the DMR of forty-nine opiate ligands in HEK-MOR cells versus SH-SY5Y cells after normalized to the DAMGO DMR. All ligands were assayed at 10 μM.

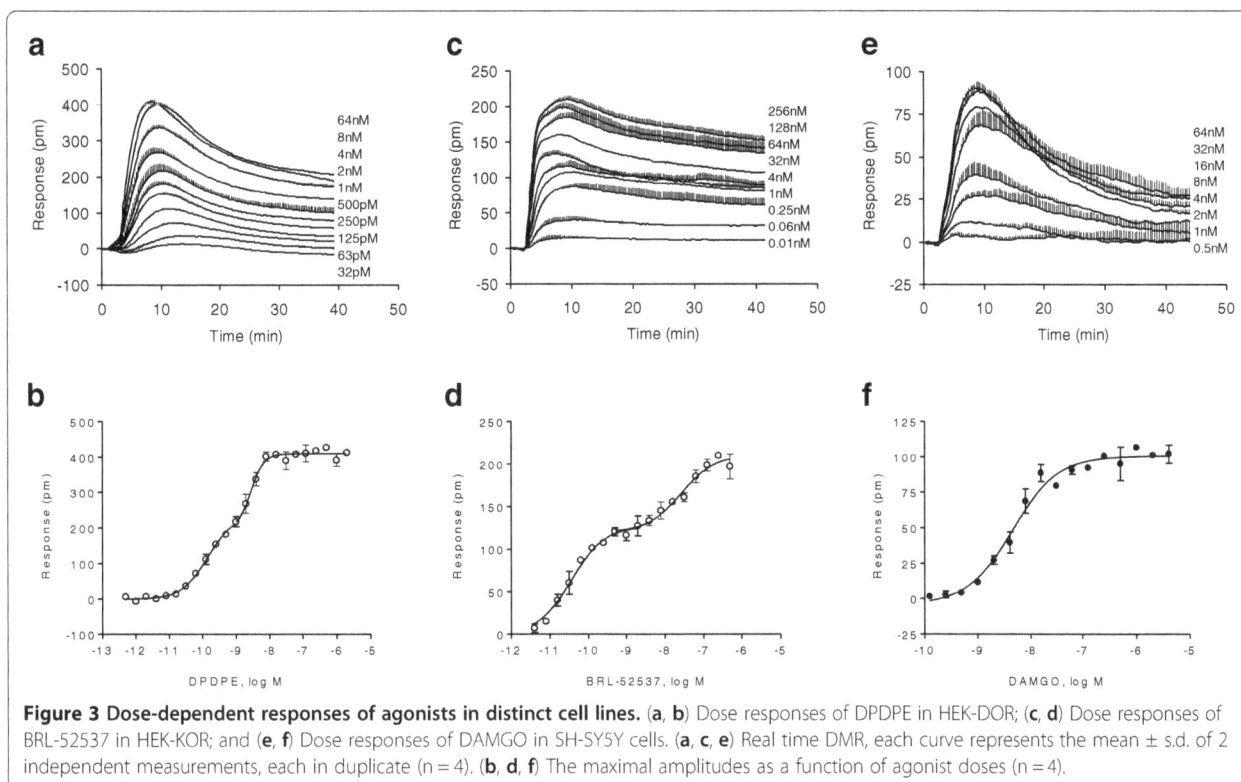

Figure 3 Dose-dependent responses of agonists in distinct cell lines. (**a**, **b**) Dose responses of DPDPE in HEK-DOR; (**c**, **d**) Dose responses of BRL-52537 in HEK-KOR; and (**e**, **f**) Dose responses of DAMGO in SH-SY5Y cells. (**a**, **c**, **e**) Real time DMR, each curve represents the mean ± s.d. of 2 independent measurements, each in duplicate (n = 4). (**b**, **d**, **f**) The maximal amplitudes as a function of agonist doses (n = 4).

reported affinity for the MOR (Figure 4a) or DOR (Figure 4b), respectively. This analysis showed that three potent MOR antagonists, β-funaltrexamine, levallorphan and nor-binaltorphimine, appeared to be less potent to block the DAMGO-induced DMR in SH-SY5Y cells than that would be expected at MOR binding sites; conversely, three agonists including SKF10047, ICI 199,441 and DIPPA desensitized SH-SY5Y cells with greater potency than their reported affinities at the MOR, and the remaining ligands gave rise to expected results (Figure 4a). This suggests that the DAMGO response has additional signaling component beside the MOR. Further, the DOR-selective agonists including deltorphin II, SNC121, BUBUC, SNC80 and DPDPE desensitized SH-SY5Y cells with lower potency than that would be expected at DOR binding sites, but the rest ligands behaved as expected at DOR binding sites (Figure 4b), suggesting that the DAMGO response in SH-SY5Y cells has additional signaling component beside the DOR. As comparison, the DAMGO induced DMR in HEK-MOR cells after pretreatment with library ligands was correlated well with their known binding affinities, with an exception of a group of antagonists including nor-binaltorphimine, N-benzylnatrindole, naloxone methiodide, naltrindole, and naltriben (Figure 4c). Similarly, the DPDPE-induced DMR in HEK-DOR cells after the ligand pretreatment was mostly correlated well with their known binding affinities, except for a group of opioid antagonists

including naloxone HCl (Figure 4d). The partial blockage of the DAMGO response in HEK-MOR, or of the DPDPE response in HEK-DOR by these antagonists is partially due to the use of high dose agonists used (10 μM for both agonists). Other factors such as receptor dimerization or differing cellular contexts may also contribute to these differences. Nonetheless, these results suggest that ligand pharmacology at the whole cell level is different from the *in vitro* binding profiles.

Functional selectivity of opioid ligands at the opioid receptors

We hypothesized that functional selectivity of a ligand at the whole cell level is reflected by the sensitivity of its DMR response to pretreatment of cells with various probe molecules [15,16]. We excluded BNTX, β-funaltrexamine, etonitazenyl isothiocyanate, ICI 199441, dynorphin A2-13 and nocicepin 1–13 from biased agonism analysis because of their off-target activity. To effectively visualize the effect of the probe pretreatments, we used the net change of the DMR response of a ligand (*i.e.*, Its DMR in a probe molecule pretreated cells minus its DMR in DMSO treated cells) for similarity analysis. This was done for all assay conditions except for PTX pretreatment wherein the raw DMR were used, since these DMR are generally small with amplitudes similar to the net change in other probe-treated cells – an important consideration for accurate clustering. The

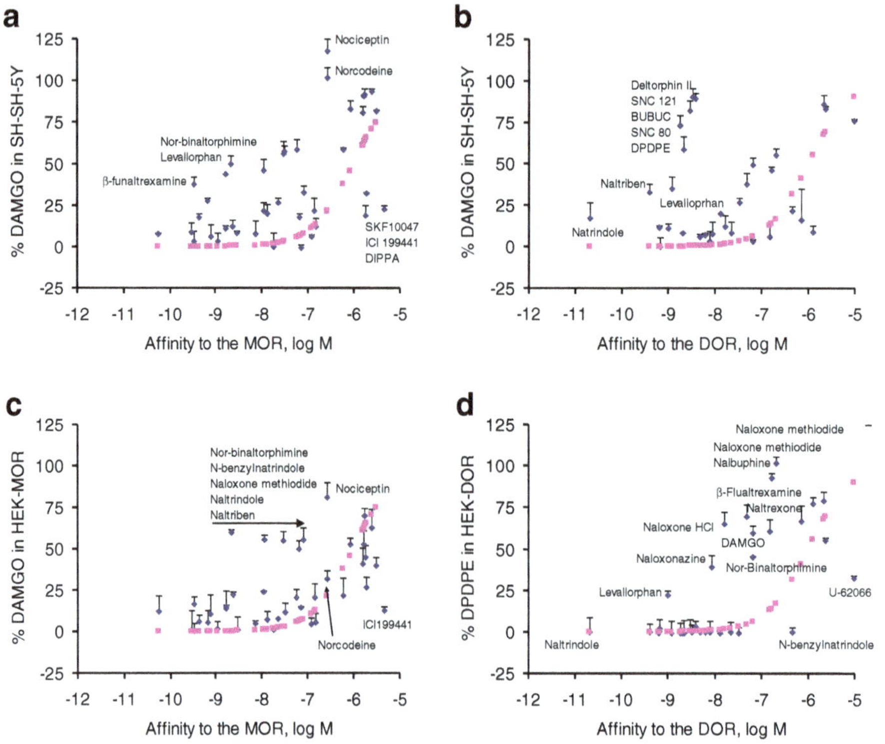

Figure 4 The inhibition pattern by opioid ligands. (a) The percentage of DAMGO responses in SH-SY5Y cells as a function of the binding affinity of opioid ligands to the MOR. **(b)** The percentage of DAMGO responses in SH-SY5Y cells as a function of the binding affinity of opioid ligands to the DOR. **(c)** The percentage of DAMGO responses in HEK-MOR cells as a function of the binding affinity of opioid ligands to the MOR. **(d)** The percentage of DPDPE responses in HEK-DOR cells as a function of the binding affinity of opioid ligands to the DOR. The percentage of agonist responses after pretreatment with ligands in the library were calculated based on the normalization of the agonist response in the presence of a ligand to the positive control (*i.e.*, the agonist response after pretreatment with the vehicle buffer only). The data points in pink were calculated based on the known binding affinity of each ligand against the specific receptor using% agonist response = 1/[1 + 10^log (X − K_i)], wherein X is the concentration of each ligand, and K_i the binding affinity obtained in literature. Included in this analysis are ligands whose binding affinities at specific receptor sites are known.

DMR in the DMSO treated cells were also included as references. A positive net change indicates that the probe pretreatment potentiates a ligand-induced DMR response, while a negative net change indicates a decrease in a ligand-induced DMR response by the probe pretreatment. The averaged responses of at least 2 experiments were used. Statistical analysis showed that for a total of 2× 3960 DMR data points obtained (3 cell lines × 8 assay conditions × 55 ligands × 3 time points), 97.1% gave rise to an absolute difference between replicates for a ligand under one condition that was smaller than 10 pm, and the remaining 2.9% (115 parameters, all of which occurred in either HEK-DOR or HEK-KOR cells) was between 10 and 20 pm. Thus, a net change induced by a probe pretreatment greater than 30 pm was considered to be significant for both HEK-DOR and HEK-KOR cells, while a net change greater than 20 pm was to be significant for SH-SY5Y cells.

Profiling HEK-DOR cells after pretreatment with seven probe molecules produced a heat map which grouped the ligands into two large superclusters (Figure 5). Notably, all ligands gave rise to a P-DMR response under at least one assay condition. The first supercluster consists of antagonists and ligands that were inactive in the untreated HEK-DOR cells, except for endomorphin-1 which acted as a partial agonist in the control HEK-DOR cells (*i.e.*, the cells pretreated with the vehicle only). All ligands in this supercluster exhibited a small P-DMR in the forskolin-pretreated cells, suggesting that these ligands gave rise to weak partial agonist activity when the basal cAMP level is high. The second supercluster can be further subdivided into three subclusters, one for ligands such as DPDPE who appear to act as full agonists, and two others comprised of ligands that appear to act as partial agonists. For the full agonist subcluster, these ligands still triggered a noticeable DMR response in PTX-pretreated cells; CTX pretreatment generally increased their DMR; forskolin only increased their early DMR response but suppressed their late DMR response (*i.e.*, 30 min post-stimulation); U0126, SP600125

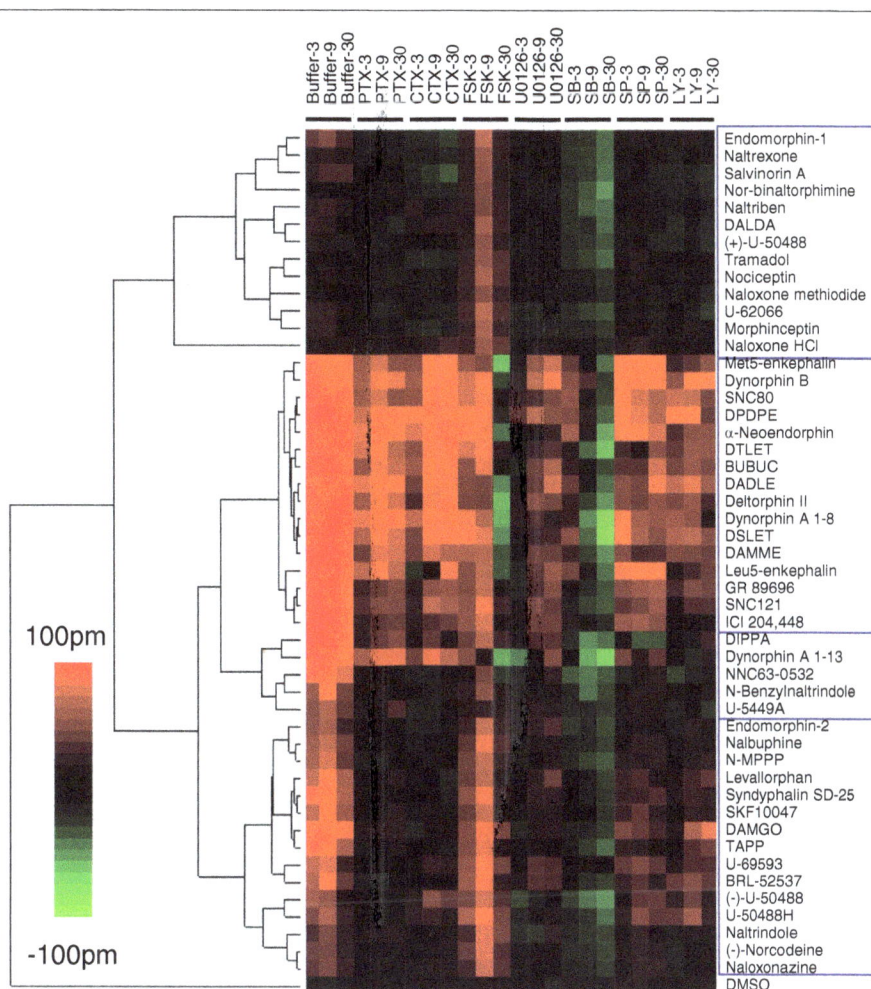

Figure 5 A colored heat map based on the functional selectivity of opioid ligands at the DOR. The DMR signals of ligands in HEK-DOR cells with and without (*i.e.,* buffer) pretreatment with probe molecules including PTX, CTX, U0126, SB202190, SP600125 and LY294002 were used to generate the heat map. All of the ligands in the library were assayed at 10 μM. The negative control (DMSO) was also included. To effectively visualize the impact of probe molecules, the net change for each ligand after pretreatment was obtained via subtraction, except for both the positive control (*i.e.,* DMR in cells pretreated with the buffer vehicle only) and the ligand DMR in PTX-pretreated cells for which the raw data were used.

and LY294002 generally increased their DMR; but SB202190 suppressed their DMR. The second subcluster was comprised of DIPPA, dynorphin A 1–13, NNC63-0532, N-benzylnaltrindole, and U-5449A, all of which were insensitive to U0126, SP600125 and LY294002 pretreatment. However, only DIPPA and dynorphin A 1–13 produced a noticeable DMR response in PTX treated cells and led to an increased DMR in the CTX or forskolin treated cells. Forskolin pretreatment selectively suppressed the late DMR of dynorphin A 1–13, and SB202190 only suppressed the DMR of DIPPA, dynorphin A 1–13, NNC63-0532, N-benzylnaltrindole. The third subcluster consists of fifteen ligands including endomorphin-2, none of which produced any DMR response in PTX- treated cells. All ligands in this subcluster were insensitive to the pretreatment with CTX, U0126 or SB202190, but were

increased by forskolin pretreatment. Together, these results suggest that the opioid ligands are divergent in their biased agonism at the DOR.

The DMR profiles obtained in HEK-KOR cells under the eight assay conditions produced a heat map that also separated the ligands into two superclusters (Figure 6). The first cluster consists of the DMSO negative control and nor-binaltorphimine. The absence of any DMR under all conditions suggests that nor-binaltorphimine behaved as a true neutral antagonist at the KOR. The second supercluster can be further subdivided into multiple subclusters, each of which produced a P-DMR signal under at least one assay condition. Agonists that produced a detectable P-DMR in the PTX pretreated cells include DIPPA, dynorphin B, α-neoendorphin, dynorphin A 1–8, dynorphin A 1–13, (–)-U-50488, U-50488H, salvinorin A,

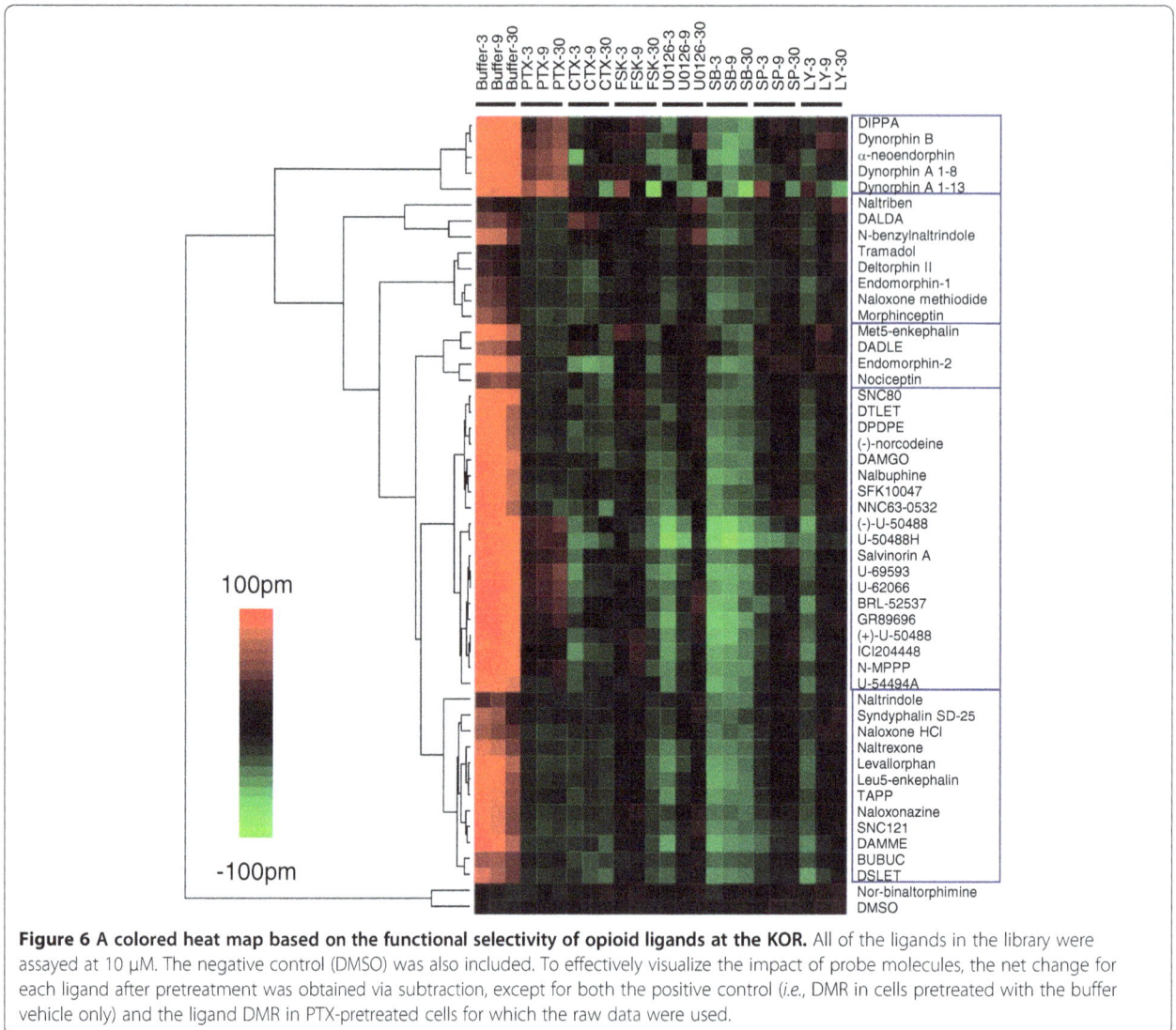

Figure 6 A colored heat map based on the functional selectivity of opioid ligands at the KOR. All of the ligands in the library were assayed at 10 µM. The negative control (DMSO) was also included. To effectively visualize the impact of probe molecules, the net change for each ligand after pretreatment was obtained via subtraction, except for both the positive control (*i.e.*, DMR in cells pretreated with the buffer vehicle only) and the ligand DMR in PTX-pretreated cells for which the raw data were used.

U-69595, U-62066, BRL-52537, and GR89696. Unlike the situation in HEK-MOR and HEK-DOR cells, the DMR responses of almost all agonists were found to be insensitive to both CTX- and forkolin-pretreatment in HEK-KOR cells. A similar pattern was observed for both SP600125- and LY294002-treatment. However, pretreatment of HEK-KOR cells with SB202190 suppressed the ligand-library DMR response induced by virtually all agonists, with U-50488H exhibiting the most significant suppression. Further, U0126 selectively suppressed the DMR of (−)-U-50488 and U-50488H. Together, these results suggest that p38 MAPK pathway may play a more significant role in the KOR signaling than any of the other kinase pathways.

We next profiled the opioid library ligands using SH-SY5Y cells under the eight different assay conditions. Results showed that SH-SY5Y cells led to different patterns for the library ligands (Figure 7). Ligands in the agonist supercluster typically behaved as would be expected.

However, some ligands, most notably DIPPA, produced unique DMR responses – DIPPA triggered a biphasic DMR response which eventually decayed below the baseline in the native SH-SY5Y cells, while PTX pretreatment suppressed both the early and late DMR response; both CTX and forskolin potentiated the DMR response; U0126 converted the DMR response to a single phase N-DMR; and SB202190 delayed the time to reach its peak. This unique pattern suggests that DIPPA activates both $G_{\alpha i}$-dependent and independent pathways. Except for DAMGO and TAPP, ligands in the agonist supercluster led to little or no DMR in the PTX-treated cells. Both CTX and forskolin suppressed the DMR of dynorphin A 1–8, DPDPE or DALDA. Forskolin also suppressed the DMR of Leu5-enkephalin, DSLET and DAMME. In general, the kinase inhibitors mostly suppressed the same group of agonists which included dynorphin A 1–8, DPDPE, DALDA, GR89696 and DAMME. These results suggest that ligand

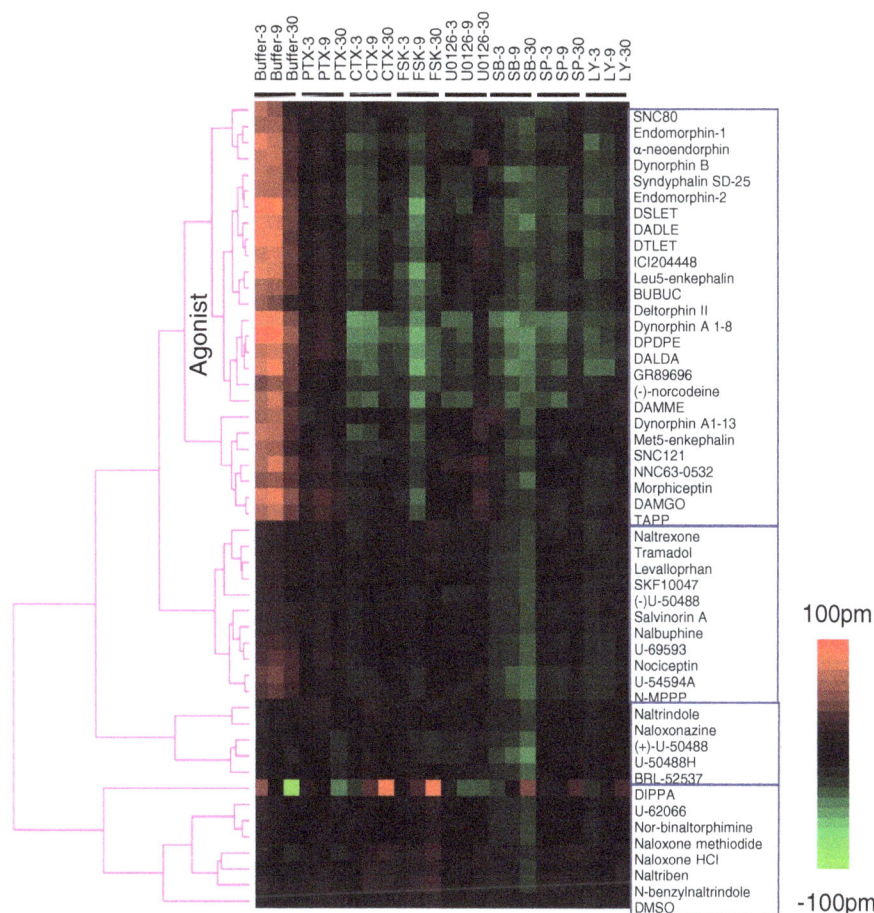

Figure 7 A colored heat map based on the functional selectivity of opioid ligands at the endogenous receptor in SH-SY5Y cells. All of the ligands in the library were assayed at 10 μM. The negative control (DMSO) was also included. To effectively visualize the impact of probe molecules, the net change for each ligand after pretreatment was obtained via subtraction, except for both the positive control (*i.e.*, DMR in cells pretreated with the buffer vehicle only) and the ligand DMR in PTX-pretreated cells for which the raw data were used.

pharmacology in SH-SY5Y cells is distinct from those in both HEK-MOR and HEK-DOR.

Potency and efficacy of opioid ligands at distinct opioid receptors

Based on the iPOT profiles, we further examined the dose responses of selected ligands at distinct opioid receptors. For HEK-DOR cells, besides DPDPE five additional ligands were profiled using both DMR 1-step agonist and 2-step antagonist assays. The agonist DMR assays showed that four of these ligands including DPDPE, DAMGO, ICI 199441 and naltrindole, gave rise to dose-dependent responses in HEK-DOR cells (Figure 8a) while naltriben and naloxone HCl were silent in HEK-DOR cells. DPDPE resulted in a biphasic dose response, resulting to two saturable amplitudes, 279±11 pm and 415±17 pm (n =16), respectively (Figure 3a and b). However, all other agonists led to a monophasic dose response, yielding an EC_{50} of 281.1±21.3 nM (n =4), 104.8±4.9 nM (n =4) and 6.1±0.9 nM (n =4) for ICI 199441, DAMGO

and naltrindole, respectively (Figure 8a). The corresponding maximal amplitudes were found to be 300±23 pm (n =16), 235±13 pm (n =16) and 82±9 pm (n =16).

The DMR antagonist assay showed that distinct ligands differentially blocked the succeeding DPDPE-induced DMR response in HEK-DOR cells (Figure 8b and c). The dose-dependent desensitization by DPDPE is best fitted with single phase sigmoidal non-linear regression, leading to an IC_{50} of 1.25±0.10 nM (n = 4). Similar monophasic inhibitory dose-responses were obtained for naltrindole (IC_{50}, 8.87±0.39 nM; n =4), ICI 199441 (IC_{50}, 753±67 nM; n = 4), and naltriben (IC_{50}, 5.30±0.36 nM; n = 4). However, a biphasic dose-dependent inhibition of the DPDPE-induced DMR was observed for the partial agonist DAMGO (IC_{50}: 368±51 nM and 7.58±1.32 μM; n =4), and the antagonist naloxone HCl (IC_{50}: 135.1±14.9 nM and 6.41±0.75 μM; n =4).

We next characterized the KOR using four opioid ligands, including BRL-52537. The DMR agonist assay showed that all four ligands triggered dose-dependent

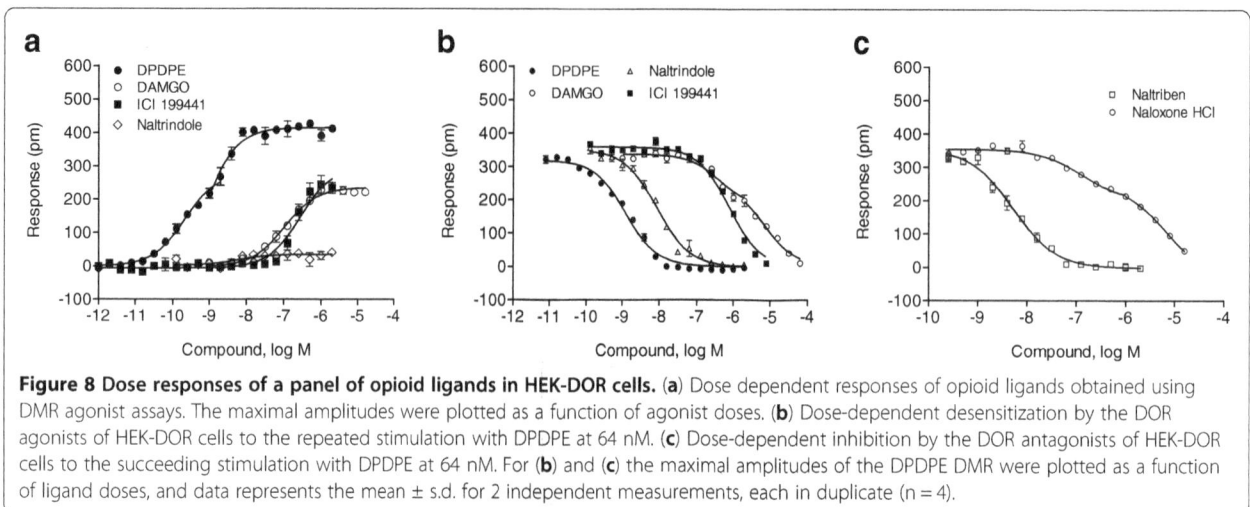

Figure 8 Dose responses of a panel of opioid ligands in HEK-DOR cells. (a) Dose dependent responses of opioid ligands obtained using DMR agonist assays. The maximal amplitudes were plotted as a function of agonist doses. **(b)** Dose-dependent desensitization by the DOR agonists of HEK-DOR cells to the repeated stimulation with DPDPE at 64 nM. **(c)** Dose-dependent inhibition by the DOR antagonists of HEK-DOR cells to the succeeding stimulation with DPDPE at 64 nM. For **(b)** and **(c)** the maximal amplitudes of the DPDPE DMR were plotted as a function of ligand doses, and data represents the mean ± s.d. for 2 independent measurements, each in duplicate (n = 4).

DMR signals (Figure 9a), similar to BRL-52537 (Figure 3b). Like BRL-52537, DIPPA and DAMGO all yielded biphasic dose responses. This analysis revealed EC_{50} values of 13.4 ±1.5 nM and 239.6±11.2 nM (n = 4) for DIPPA, and 93.8 ±7.4 nM and 4.5±1.1 µM (n =4) for DAMGO. The two saturable amplitudes were 120±6 pm and 207±13 pm (n = 4) for BRL-52537, 138±8 pm and 205±9 pm (n = 4) for DIPPA, and 139±6 pm and 200±8 pm (n = 4) for DAMGO. In contrast, the partial agonist naloxone HCl yielded a monophasic dose response with an EC_{50} of 1.4 ±0.2 nM, with a maximal response of 69±5 pm (n = 4). Further, the two-step DMR antagonist assay showed that distinct ligands differentially inhibited the HEK-KOR cells responding to repeated stimulation with 64 nM BRL-52537 (Figure 9b). DIPPA, DAMGO and BRL-52537 each inhibited the BRL-52537 response with single phase sigmoidal non-linear regression producing IC_{50} values of 454.9±32.3 nM (n = 4), 2.21±0.51 µM, and 4.1±0.23 nM, respectively. In contrast, the dose-dependent inhibition by the antagonist naloxone HCl was best fitted with a biphasic sigmoidal non-linear regression, which exhibited biphasic IC_{50}'s of 67.2±5.6 nM and 2.05±0.0.54 µM (n = 4).

Lastly, we characterized the DMR response elicited by opioid receptors in SH-SY5Y cells utilizing seven known agonists and antagonists. Results from the DMR agonist assay showed that all ligands yielded dose-dependent P-DMR signals, except for naloxone HCl, which did not produce any observable DMR response in SH-SY5Y cells (Figure 10a). Similar to DAMGO (Figure 3e), the dose-dependent activation responses were best fitted using a single phase sigmoidal non-linear regression, revealing EC_{50} values of 26.5±2.1 nM (n = 4), 1.4±0.2 nM (n = 4), 2.4±0.2 nM (n = 4), 1.2±0.1 nM (n = 4), and 2.8±0.3 nM (n = 4) for morphine, fentanyl, endomorphin-1, endomorphin-2 and CTOP, respectively (Figure 10a). The maximal DMR responses were found to be 102±8 pm, 94±5 pm, 105±7 pm,

102±6 pm, 102±7 pm, and 31±4 pm (n = 16 for all) for DAMGO, morphine, fentanyl, endomorphin-1, endomorphin-2 and CTOP, respectively. The two-step DMR antagonist assay showed that all ligands blocked the DMR produced by 64 nM DAMGO in a dose-dependent fashion. Single IC_{50} values of 1.0±0.1 nM, 115.8±14.7 nM, 4.2±0.3 nM, 10.0±0.9 nM, 5.8±0.4 nM, 475.5±39.7 nM, and 231.4±21.5 nM were obtained for DAMGO, morphine, fentanyl, endomorphin-1, endomorphin-2, CTOP, and naloxone HCl, respectively (Figure 10b). Together, these results suggest that the family of opioid receptors exhibit complex pharmacology.

Discussion

Functional selectivity represents the underlying basis for drug selectivity, one of the most important pharmacological properties of drug molecules which assist to determine their *in vivo* efficacy and therapeutic index. However, functional selectivity has not been fully integrated into the mainstream drug discovery and development processes. This is partly because of the simplistic molecular assays conventionally used to characterize the pharmacological properties of many drug molecules and partly because of unknown molecular mode(s) of action that is critical to *in vivo* efficacy or *in vivo* side effects of drugs. This issue is exemplified by opioid ligands. Molecular assays have revealed a wide array of biased agonism demonstrated by opioid ligands which appear to be cell-systems and assay technology dependent [5,6,34]. However, multidimensional biased agonism makes it difficult to rank candidate compounds for *in vivo* testing and to relate a specific biased agonism of drug molecules to their *in vivo* profiles.

Many opioid ligands often display relatively poor selectivity binding to different opioid receptor family members [39,40]. This problem is exacerbated by the fact that the binding affinity profiles of opioid ligands do

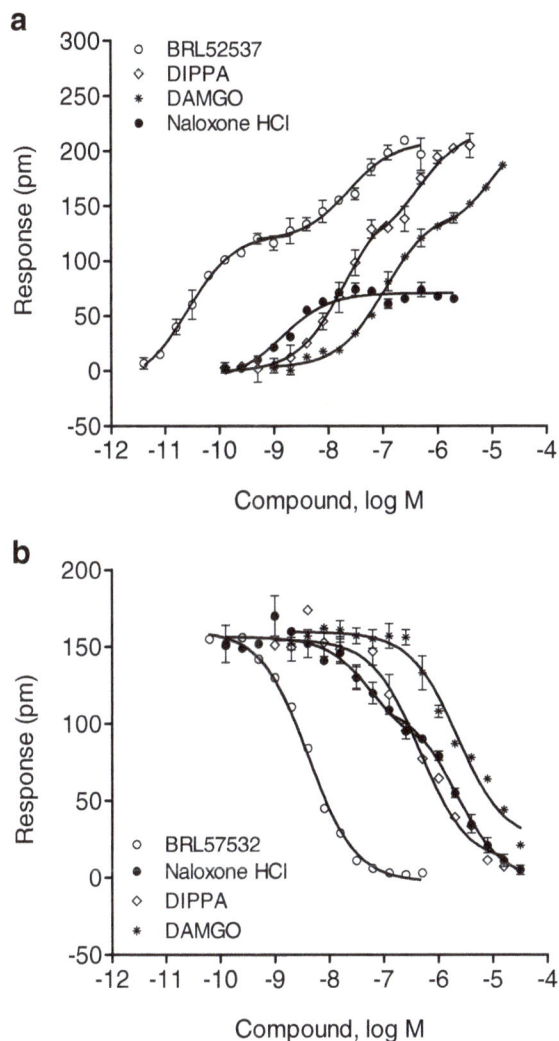

Figure 9 Dose responses of a panel of opioid ligands in HEK-KOR cells. (**a**) Dose dependent responses of opioid ligands obtained using DMR agonist assays. The maximal amplitudes were plotted as a function of agonist doses. Data represents the mean ± s.d. for 2 independent measurements, each in duplicate (n = 4). (**b**) Dose-dependent inhibition of the DMR of 64 nM BRL-57532 by opioid ligands. The maximal amplitudes of the BRL-57532 DMR were plotted as a function of ligand doses. Data represents the mean ± s. d. for 2 independent measurements, each in duplicate (n = 4).

Figure 10 Dose responses of a panel of opioid ligands in SH-SY5Y cells. (**a**) Dose dependent responses of opioid ligands obtained using DMR agonist assays. The maximal amplitudes were plotted as a function of agonist doses. (**b**) Dose-dependent inhibition of the DMR of 64 nM DAMGO by opioid ligands. The maximal amplitudes of the DAMGO DMR were plotted as a function of ligand doses. For (**a**) and (**b**) data represents the mean ± s.d. for 2 independent measurements, each in duplicate (n = 4).

not directly translate into their selectivity in cellular and *in vivo* environments due to the expression of more than one opioid receptor or its splice variants in native cells, as well as the possibility that opioid receptors may present in different oligomerizational states [41-45]. Thus, an effective means to differentiate drug candidate molecules based on both binding and functional selectivity in native cells would be beneficial to identify and prioritize lead compounds, and to relate *in vitro* results to *in vivo* profiles.

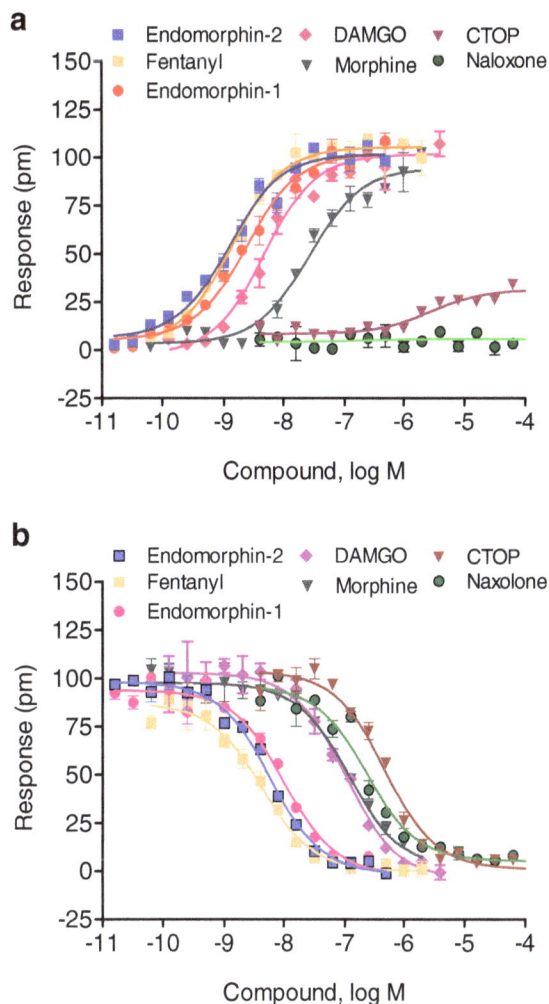

Recently, we have developed a label-free iPOT approach and applied it to differentiate individual ligands in libraries for both β_2-adrenergic receptor [15] and the MOR [16]. High resolution heat maps obtained allowed us to sort these ligands into distinct clusters based on their cellular binding profiles and pathway biased agonism. Here, we extended this approach to survey the entire classic opioid receptor family (mu-, kappa- and delta-receptors). Both recombinant and native cells expressing opioid receptors were used to generate DMR profiles of a library of opioid ligands using a battery of DMR assay formats. The DMR profiles for all the ligands were translated into numerical coordinates which were subject to similarity analysis to determine the similarity and distance between ligand pairs. The results obtained were visualized using a color-coded heat map with a distance-dendrogram. Here, a variety of probe molecules such as a kinase inhibitor (e.g., SB202190) were used to pretreat the cells in order to manifest the sensitivity of a ligand-induced DMR to the altered cellular background. Such sensitivity is primarily used as a differentiating factor for ligand classification, rather than for determining the exact cellular mechanism of functional selectivity at a specific pathway (e.g., p38 MAPK activation). This is because kinase inhibitors such as SB202190 are known to inhibit multiple targets, and DMR is a whole cell response. On the other hand, MOR, KOR and DOR all can result in p38 MAPK activation in a cell context dependent manner, and kinase cascades have been proposed to be a basis to differentiate ligand-directed signaling at opioid receptors [34]. Our data indicate that compared to those in HEK-MOR, HEK-DOR and native SH-SH5Y cells, the DMR of almost all agonists in the HEK-KOR cells exhibited much higher sensitivity to the SB202190 pretreatment, suggesting that p38 MAPK pathway may be more important in the KOR signaling. However, the biological implications still need further elucidation.

This methodology led to several interesting findings. First, the off-target activity of a subset of ligands including BNTX, β-funaltrexamine, etonitazenyl isothiocyanate, ICI 199,441, dynorphin A 2–13 and nociceptin 1–13 was visualized in both HEK293 and SH-SY5Y cells, indicating that DMR assays are indeed capable of characterizing molecules with much wider pathway coverage than conventional pharmacological or molecular assays.

Second, opiate ligands were found to display distinct pharmacology in MOR or DOR stably expressed cell lines versus the native SH-SY5Y cells. Such a cellular background-dependent pharmacology, termed phenotypic pharmacology, is common to many GPCR ligands [46], and is believed to be originated from many different factors [47-49]. The specific cellular mechanisms causing the differential pharmacology of these ligands in different opioid receptor expressing cells are unknown, and further studies are warranted.

Third, almost all ligands in the library behaved as agonists in at least one opioid receptor expressing cell line with or without pretreatment with probe molecules. Using the DMR agonist assay, we found that out fifty-five opioid ligands testes, forty-nine displayed agonist activity in at least one opioid receptor-expressing cell line (Table 2). This is significant since as many as thirteen ligands in the library were classified as opioid receptor antagonists (Table 2, Additional file 1: Tables S1–S3). Furthermore, all ligands displayed agonist activity in at least one opioid receptor expressing cell lines under one

condition. In HEK-KOR cells, nor-binaltorphimine was distinct as it did not trigger any DMR response under any conditions, leading us to conclude that nor-binaltorphimine was a true neutral antagonist for the KOR.

Fourth, pathway biased agonism was also visualized for many ligands. First, $G_{\alpha i}$-independent signaling was evident in the DMR produced by a subset of ligands in PTX-treated cells. Generally full agonists and strong partial agonists for each receptor led to a detectable DMR response in PTX-treated cells, indicative of activating $G_{\alpha i}$-independent signaling. An alternative mechanism is that PTX treatment unnaturally shifts receptor signaling to a different signal transduction pathway. As such the lack of a complete blockade of signal with PTX does not necessarily mean that under naïve conditions (when functional $G_{\alpha i}$ is present) a ligand signals through $G_{\alpha i}$-independent pathways. Second, CTX and forskolin pretreatment generally increased the DMR response induced by opioid agonists in both HEK-MOR [16] and HEK-DOR cells (Figure 5), but clearly suppressed the DMR of a subset of opioid ligands in HEK-KOR and SH-SY5Y cells (Figures 6 and 7, respectively). These patterns suggest that the KOR in HEK-KOR cells and the opioid receptors in SH-SY5Y may also signal via a pathway distinct from $G_{\alpha i}$.

Lastly, the iPOT analysis of opioid ligands further indicates the complexity of opioid ligand pharmacology. First, the difference in ligand specificity between HEK-MOR and SH-SY5Y cells, or between HEK-DOR and SH-SY5Y cells (Figure 4) cannot be explained solely by the known affinity of these ligands for the MOR or for the DOR, respectively [39]. Such a difference seems to be reflective of the presence of different populations of endogenous opioid receptors or the different level and complement of second messengers and signal transduction components in SH-SY5Y cells. Second, the dose-dependent efficacy and potency of panels of ligands to activate opioid receptors, together with the dose-dependent desensitization/inhibition of the activation of opioid receptors, clearly shows that different ligands produce very different types of dose responses. These responses may be monophasic or biphasic in a ligand- and cell-dependent manner. The biphasic dose responses in opioid receptor expressing cells observed for certain agonists may be related to dual modes of action of the ligands acting at a receptor; that is, the ligands at low doses are biased to a specific pathway, but at higher doses the ligands activate a broader range of pathways [50]. Alternatively, a biphasic dose response for agonists and antagonists may be associated with the existence of different receptor states such as functional monomers and oligomers [51]. A ligand may have different potency to activate or deactivate distinct receptor populations. Nonetheless, the present study represents the first study using label-free cellular assays to assess the binding and functional selectivity of opioid ligands across the entire classic opioid receptor family.

We are still at the early phase to understand how label-free mirrors the innate complexity of drug-target interactions in living cells or cell systems. To elucidate biased agonism, several different approaches have been proposed. Owing to wide pathway coverage, label free is quickly realized to be able to manifest the biased agonism through producing pathway-dependent variations in the whole cell phenotypic profile of different ligands [15]. Multi-parameter analysis based on kinetics can be used to sort ligands into different clusters [13]. Profiling of the same set of ligands in different cellular backgrounds has been attempted to determine biased agonism [52], while comparing label-free with molecular assay results also manifests biased agonism within the same cell background [53]. Controlling the duration of agonist exposure and receptor resensitization using microfluidics offers additional levers to determine ligand-directed functional selectivity [54]. The iPOT approach represents the next step toward deeper and broader elucidation of the biological complexity of drug-target interactions. This approach leverages the signaling capacity of a receptor and the sensitivity of label-free profiles to cell preconditioning via pathway modulation. Owing to the same measurement (that is, the label-free profiling), similarity analysis can be performed and used to sort ligands into different clusters based on their ontarget and off-target pharmacology. A rationale way for lead selection based on the iPOT is to select a few representative ligands from each cluster for *in vivo* testing. The future of label-free is dependent on the identification of an *in vitro* label-free profile that is linked to the *in vivo* action of drug molecules. Nonetheless, the high resolution heat maps and pharmacological characterization of the opioid receptor family using DMR response assays suggest that the iPOT is powerful new approach for elucidating of the complex and multifaceted efficacy of GPCR ligands, and label-free cellular assays are uniquely sensitive to the complexities of receptor mediated signal transduction at the whole-cell level, and as such inform the process of drug discovery in ways that other assay technologies cannot. The power of the iPOT to differentiate ligands can be further improved by using optimizing the algorithm for similarity analysis, in particular methods that take both time domain and signal amplitude into account [35]. The iPOT approach offers a unique platform for drug development when functional selectivity is important.

Conclusions

In conclusion, we have applied label-free DMR whole cell profile-centred iPOT approach to systematically survey a fifty-five ligand library against the opioid receptor family members in both native and engineered cell backgrounds. The off-target activity, binding and functional selectivity of these ligands have been clearly evident. Notable is that all ligands display certain agonist activity under specific conditions, and opioid ligands exhibit complex pharmacology in both receptor and cell background dependent manner. These label-free profiling results also suggest the necessity to reclassify the ligands. The profiling approach presented here may be useful for lead compound selection.

Additional file

Additional file 1: Figure S1. DMR characteristics of a subset of ligands in parental HEK293 cells, **Figure S2**: A colored heat map based on the DMR of opioid ligands in five different cell lines, **Figure S3**: A colored heat map based on the selectivity of opioid ligands to block the DMR of control agonists in respective cell lines, **Table S1**: Opioid ligands and their affinity binding to the MOR, **Table S2**: Opioid ligands and their affinity binding to the DOR, and **Table S3**: Opioid ligands and their affinity binding to the KOR.

Abbreviation

Ct: Cycle threshold; CTX: Cholera toxin; DMR: Dynamic mass redistribution; DOR: Delta opioid receptor; GADPH: Glyceraldehyde-3-phosphate dehydrogenase; GPCR: G protein-coupled receptor; HPRT1: Hypoxanthine phosphoribosyltransferase 1; iPOT: Integrative pharmacology on-target; KOR: Kappa opioid receptor; MOR: Mu opioid receptor; ORL1: Opioid-like receptor-1; PTX: Pertussis toxin.

Competing interests

ET, and YF are employees and shareholders of Corning Inc. HS was an employee of Corning Inc. MM and RL received sponsored research funding from Corning Inc. Epic system is a marketed product. DMR assays are patented. There are no other patents, products in development, or marketed products to declare. This does not alter the authors' adherence to all the BMC Pharmacology policies on sharing data and materials.

Authors' contributions

YF, MM, RL conceived and designed the experiments; MM, SH, ET performed the experiments; MM and YF analyzed the data; MM, HS, ET, YF, RL contributed reagents/materials/analysis tools; YF, MM, RL wrote the paper; YF designed the software used in analysis. All authors have read and approved the manuscript.

Acknowledgements

MM and RL received sponsored research funding from Corning Inc. for this study.

Author details

[1]Department of Pharmacology, Pennsylvania State University College of Medicine, Hershey, PA, USA. [2]Biochemical Technologies, Science and Technology Division, Corning Inc., Corning, NY, USA.

References

1. Kenakin T: **New concepts in drug discovery: collateral efficacy and permissive antagonism.** *Nat Rev Drug Discov* 2005, **4**:919–927.
2. Mailman RB: **GPCR functional selectivity has therapeutic impact.** *Trends Pharmacol Sci* 2007, **28**:390–396.
3. Galandrin S, Oligny-Longpre G, Bouvier M: **The evasive nature of drug efficacy: implications for drug discovery.** *Trends Pharmacol Sci* 2007, **8**:423–430.

4. Urban JD, Clarke WP, von Zastrow M, Nichols DE, Kobilka B, et al: Functional selectivity and classical concepts of quantitative pharmacology. J Pharmacol Exp Ther 2007, 320:1–13.

5. Neve KA: Functional selectivity of G protein-coupled receptor ligands. New York: Humana; 2009.

6. Raehal KM, Schmid CL, Groer CE, Bohn LM: Functional selectivity at the µ-opioid receptor: implications for understanding opioid analgesia and tolerance. Pharmacol Rev 2011, 63:1001–1019.

7. Law PY, Wong YH, Loh HH: Molecular mechanisms and regulation of opioid receptor signaling. Ann Rev Pharmacol Toxicol 2000, 40:389–430.

8. Kenakin T, Miller LJ: Seven transmembrane receptors as shapeshifting proteins: the impact of allosteric modulation and functional selectivity on new drug discovery. Pharmacol Rev 2010, 62:265–304.

9. Swinney DC, Anthony J: How were new medicines discovered? Nat Rev Drug Discov 2011, 10:507–519.

10. Fang Y, Ferrie AM, Fontaine NH, Mauro J, Balakrishnan J: Resonant waveguide grating biosensor for living cell sensing. Biophys J 2006, 91:1925–1940.

11. Fang Y, Li G, Ferrie AM: Non-invasive optical biosensor for assaying endogenous G protein-coupled receptors in adherent cells. J Pharamcol Toxicol Methods 2007, 55:314–322.

12. Kenakin T: Cellular assays as portals to seven-transmembrane receptor-based drug discovery. Nat Rev Drug Discov 2009, 8:617–626.

13. Fang Y: Label-free receptor assays. Drug Discov Today Technol 2010, 7:e5–e11.

14. Scott CW, Peters MF: Label-free whole-cell assays: expanding the scope of GPCR screening. Drug Discov Today 2010, 15:704–716.

15. Ferrie AM, Sun H, Fang Y: Label-free integrative pharmacology on-target of drugs at the β_2-adrenergic receptor. Sci Rep 2011, 1:33.

16. Morse M, Tran E, Sun H, Levenson R, Fang Y: Ligand-directed functional selectivity at the mu opioid receptor revealed by label-free integrative pharmacology on-target. PLoS One 2011, 6:e25643.

17. He L, Fong J, von Zastrow M, Whistler JL: Regulation of opioid receptor trafficking and morphine tolerance by receptor oligomerization. Cell 2002, 108:271–282.

18. Tsao PI, von Zastrow M: Type-specific sorting on G protein-coupled receptors after endocytosis. J Biol Chem 2000, 275:11130–11140.

19. Li JG, Zhang F, Jin XL, Liu-Chen LY: Differential regulation of the human κ opioid receptor by agonists: etorphin and levorphanol reduced dynorphin-A and U50,488H-induced internalization and phosphorylation. J Pharmacol Exp Ther 2003, 305:531–540.

20. Yu VC, Elger S, Duan DS, Lameh J, Sadée W: Regulation of cyclic AMP by the µ-opioid receptor in human neuroblastoma SH-SY5Y cells. J Neurochem 1990, 55:1390–1396.

21. Kazmi SMI, Mishra RK: Comparative pharmacological properties and functional coupling of mu and delta opioid receptor sites in human neuroblastoma SH-SY5Y cells. Mol Pharmacol 1987, 32:109–118.

22. Zadina JE, Harrison LM, Ge LJ, Kastin AJ, Chang SL: Differential regulation of mu and delta opiate receptors by morphine, selective agonists and antagonists and differentiating agents in SH-SY5Y human neuroblastoma cells. J Pharmacol Exp Therap 1994, 270:1086–1096.

23. Du YL, Elliot K, Pan YX, Pasternak GW, Inturrisi CE: A splice variant of the mu opioid receptor is present in human SHSY-5Y cells. Soc Neurosci Asbtr 1997, 23:1206.

24. Pan YX: Diversity and complexity of the mu opioid receptor gene: alternative pre-mRNA splicing and promoters. DNA Cell Biol 2005, 24:736–750.

25. Gris P, Gauthier J, Cheng P, Gibson DG, Gris D, et al: A novel alternatively spliced isoform of the mu-opioid receptor: functional antagonism. Mol Pain 2010, 6:33.

26. Mayer P, Tischmeyer H, Jayasinghe M, Bonnekoh B, Gollnick H, et al: A δ opioid receptor lacking the third cytoplasmic loop is generated by atypical mRNA processing in human malignomas. FEBS Lett 2000, 480:156–160.

27. Fang Y, Ferrie AM: Label-free optical biosensor for ligand-directed functional selectivity of acting on β_2 adrenoceptor in living cells. FEBS Lett 2008, 582:558–564.

28. Kenakin T: Being mindful of seven-transmembrane receptor 'guests' when assessing agonist selectivity. Br J Pharmacol 2010, 160:1045–1047.

29. Barbieri JT, Cortina G: ADP-ribosyltransferase mutations in the catalytic S-1 subunit of pertussis toxin. Infect Immun 1988, 56:1934–1941.

30. Gill DMM, Meren R: ADP-ribosylation of membrane proteins catalyzed by cholera toxin: basis of the activation of adenylate cyclase. Proc Natl Acad Sci USA 1978, 75:3050–3054.

31. Tran E, Fang Y: Label-free optical biosensor for probing integrative role of adenylyl cyclase in G protein-coupled receptor signaling. J Recept Signal Transduct Res 2009, 29:154–162.

32. Karaman MW, Herrgard S, Treiber DK, Gallant P, Atteridge CE, et al: A quantitative analysis of kinase inhibitor selectivity. Nat Biotechnol 2008, 26:127–132.

33. Davis MI, Hunt JP, Herrgard S, Ciceri P, Wodicka LM, et al: Comprehensive analysis of kinase inhibitor selectivity. Nat Biotechnol 2011, 29:1046–1051.

34. Bruchas MR, Chavkin C: Kinase cascades and ligand-directed signaling at the kappa opioid receptor. Psychopharmacology 2010, 210:137–147.

35. Fang Y: The development of label-free cellular assays for drug discovery. Exp Opin Drug Discov 2011, 6:1285–1298.

36. Eisen MB, Spellman PT, Brown PO, Botstein D: Cluster analysis and display of genome-wide expression patterns. Proc Natl Acad Sci USA 1998, 95:14863–14868.

37. Fang Y: Probing cancer signaling with resonant waveguide grating biosensors. Exp Opin Drug Discov 2010, 5:1237–1248.

38. Gehlenborg N, O'Donoghue SI, Baliga NS, Goesmann A, Hibbs MA, et al: Visualization of omics data for systems biology. Nat Methods 2010, 7:S56–S68.

39. PDSP Ki database. http://pdsp.med.unc.edu/pdsp.php.

40. Dietis N, Rowbotham DJ, Lambert DG: Opioid receptor subtypes: fact or artifact? Br J Anaesthesia 2011, 107:8–18. 37.

41. Dhawan BN, Cesselin F, Raghubir R, Reisine T, Bradley PB, et al: International Union of Pharmacology. XII. Classification of opioid receptors. Pharmacol Rev 1996, 48:567–592.

42. Jordan BA, Trapaidze N, Gomes I, Nivarthi R, Devi LA: Oligomerization of opioid receptors with β_2-adrenergic receptors: a role in trafficking and mitogen-activated protein kinase activation. Proc Natl Acad Sci USA 2001, 98:343–348.

43. Jordan BA, Devi LA: G-protein-coupled receptor heterodimerization modulates receptor function. Nature 1999, 399:697–700.

44. Gomes I, Gupta A, Filipovska J, Szeto HH, Pintar JE, et al: A role for heterodimerization of µ and δ opioid receptors in enhancing morphine analgesia. Proc Natl Acad Sci USA 2004, 101:5135–5139.

45. van Rijn RM, Whistler JL, Waldhoer M: Opioid-receptor-heteromer-specific trafficking and pharmacology. Curr Opin Pharmacol 2010, 10:73–79.

46. Nelson CP, Challiss RA: "Phenotypic" pharmacology: the influence of cellular environment on G protein-coupled receptor antagonist and inverse agonist pharmacology. Biochem Pharmacol 2007, 73:737–751.

47. Kinzer-Ursem TL, Linderman JJ: Both ligand- and cell-specific parameters control ligand agonism in a kinetic model of G protein-coupled receptor signaling. PLoS Comput Biol 2007, 3:e6.

48. Tran E, Sun H, Fang Y: Dynamic mass redistribution assays decodes surface influence on signaling of endogenous purinergic receptors. Assay Drug Dev Technol 2012, 10:37–45.

49. Kenakin T: The potential for selective pharmacological therapies through biased receptor signaling. BMC Pharmacol Toxicol 2012, 13:3.

50. Sun Y, Huang J, Xiang Y, Bastepe M, Juppner H, et al: Dosage-dependent switch from G protein-coupled to G protein-independent signaling by a GPCR. EMBO J 2007, 26:53–64.

51. Giraldo J: On the fitting of binding data when receptor dimerization is suspected. Br J Pharmacol 2008, 155:17–23.

52. Peters MF, Scott CW: Evaluating cellular impedance assays for detection of GPCR pleiotropic signaling and functional selectivity. J Biomol Screen 2009, 14:246–255.

53. McLaughlin JN, Shen L, Holinstat M, Brooks JD, DiBenedetto E, Hamm HE: Functional selectivity of G protein signaling by agonist peptides and thrombin for the protease-activated receptor-1. J Biol Chem 2005, 280:25048–25059.

54. Goral V, Jin Y, Sun H, Ferrie AM, Wu Q, Fang Y: Agonist-directed desensitization of the β_2-adrenergic receptor. PLoS One 2011, 6:e19282.

24

The current status and trend of clinical pharmacology in developing countries

Andrew Walubo

Abstract

Background: Several international forums for promoting clinical pharmacology in developing countries have been held since 1980, and several clinical pharmacology programmes targeting developing countries were instituted such that the status of clinical pharmacology in developing countries is not where it was 50 years ago. Therefore, a survey and an appraisal of the literature on the current status of clinical pharmacology in developing countries were undertaken with a hope that it would enable development of appropriate strategies for further promotion of clinical pharmacology in these countries.

Methods: First, nine determinants (or enabling factors) for running a successful clinical pharmacology programme were identified, i.e., disease burden, drug situation, economic growth, clinical pharmacology activities, recognition, human capital, government support, international collaboration, and support for traditional/alternative medicines. These factors were then evaluated with regard to their current status in the developing countries that responded to an electronic questionnaire, and their historical perspective, using the literature appraisal. From these, a projected trend was constructed with recommendations on the way forward.

Results: Clinical pharmacology services, research and teaching in developing countries have improved over the past 50 years with over 90% of countries having the appropriate policies for regulation and rational use of medicines in place. Unfortunately, policy implementation remains a challenge, owing to a worsening disease burden and drug situation, versus fewer clinical pharmacologists and other competing priorities for the national budgets. This has led to a preference for training 'a physician clinical pharmacologist' in programmes emphasizing local relevancy and for a shorter time, and the training of other professionals in therapeutics for endemic diseases (task shifting), as the most promising strategies of ensuring rational use of medicines.

Conclusion: Clinical pharmacology in developing countries is advancing in a different way to that in the developed world and continuing support for these efforts will go a long way in promoting improved health for all.

Keywords: Clinical pharmacology, Developing countries, Trend, Clinical pharmacologist, Research, IUPHAR and World Health Organisation

Background

The need for special focus on clinical pharmacology in developing countries was expressed in several workshops at the first World Congress of Clinical Pharmacology in 1980, and later by Fraser in 1981 [1,2]. Soon after, another international forum aimed at promoting clinical pharmacology in developing countries was held in 1984 under the auspices of the IUPHAR and the Clinical Section of the British Pharmacological Society [3]. This

was followed by several communications as well as physical meetings by different stakeholders including IUPHAR and the World Health Organisation (WHO). Wide ranging proposals were made with regard to training, research and service in clinical pharmacology in developing countries by the developed world, including private industry. Since then, several clinical pharmacology programmes targeting developing countries have been instituted [4-8]. These clinical pharmacology programmes were augmented by developments in other sectors particularly economic growth that enabled the construction of essential facilities such as medical schools. These

Correspondence: waluboa@ufs.ac.za
Department of Pharmacology, University of the Free State, P. O. Box 339 (G6),
Bloemfontein 9300, South Africa

institutions have been the major focus of collaborative programmes on clinical pharmacology by the international community, and many graduates from these institutions have used them as spring boards to further training in clinical pharmacology in the developed countries. Unfortunately, despite such investment, reports on clinical pharmacology in developing countries over the past 50 years have been characterized by the same tone, gloomy: i.e., the discipline still remains in infancy, and that the need for clinical pharmacology here is bigger than anywhere else [1-3,9-11].

In response to such reports, the IUPHAR's division of clinical pharmacology, through its subcommittee on 'clinical pharmacology in the developing countries', embarked on a mission to make visible progress in the development of clinical pharmacology in these countries. Accordingly, the status of clinical pharmacology in developing countries was a subject of a focus conference at the World Congress of Pharmacology 2010 in Copenhagen, in which various speakers expressed their opinions. Again, it was clear that the status of clinical pharmacology in developing countries was not where it was 50 years ago, and that its development had not followed the same path as in the developed world. Later, in its subsequent meeting, the same IUPHAR subcommittee expressed the need for an accurate report on the current status of clinical pharmacology in developing countries, as a pre-requisite to development of appropriate strategies for promotion of clinical pharmacology in these countries.

Unfortunately, most of the information on clinical pharmacology in developing countries is not available in the main stream literature. It is contained in different communications, mainly experts' reports, for organisations such as the WHO, where it has not been associated with clinical pharmacology. Secondly, these reports are often so detailed and address a variety of multidisciplinary issues such that they are often not suitable for publication in a scientific journal. Here is presented a pragmatic report on the current status of clinical pharmacology in developing countries based on information obtained by a survey on clinical pharmacology activities in some of the developing countries, supplemented by a comprehensive appraisal of the literature. It is hoped that this information will enable formulation of appropriate interventions to foster rational use of medicines in the developing countries.

Methods

Nine factors were identified as the major determinants (or enabling factors) for running a successful clinical pharmacology programme. They were: the disease burden, the drug situation, economic growth, clinical pharmacology activities (training, research and service), recognition of clinical pharmacology, human capital (clinical

pharmacologists and affiliated personnel), local or government support, international support/collaboration and support for traditional/alternative medicines. A survey was undertaken to assess the status and/or existence of some of these enabling factors with a hope that their status would form a useful index for measuring the state of clinical pharmacology at any point in time. The study was approved by the Ethics Committee of University of the Free State (ECUFS ref: 148/2013).

This was a one page questionnaire. After a successful piloting in three institutions, the questionnaire was distributed electronically (by e-mail) worldwide to heads of departments of pharmacology with a help of regional volunteers in Asia, L. America and, Eastern Europe and Africa. It took approximately 15–20 min to complete the questionnaire. Developing countries were determined according to the United Nations Development Programme (UNDP) and World Bank classification of countries [12,13].

Respondents were asked whether clinical pharmacology is a recognised specialty in their country, and if yes, to name the certifying body. It also sought to know whether the respective institution had a dedicated clinical pharmacology department or unit, and if so, the number of professionals serving as clinical pharmacologists and their respective qualifications, i.e., the number of pharmacologists with M.B.Ch.B. and B. Pharm. or equivalent, as well as those with a Ph.D. or equivalent. The questionnaire also probed for presence of scientific forums for pharmacologists, such as a pharmacology society or other, and how often it holds conferences. For information on clinical pharmacology services, respondents were asked to indicate the main clinical pharmacology services undertaken at their departments/units by selecting from a given list, i.e., research, undergraduate teaching, research (clinical trials), postgraduate training, pharmacovigilance, drug utilization, therapeutic patient care/consultation, drug policy or drug regulation, poison information service and other. Respondents were asked to indicate the affiliated personnel with whom the clinical pharmacologists worked (staff members of the units/departments), i.e., medical doctors, pharmacists, nurses, laboratory personnel, poison information officers and others. Regarding training, the questionnaire sought for whether the respective clinical pharmacology departments or units undertake undergraduate and postgraduate training in clinical pharmacology, and for the latter, what qualification was awarded to these graduates, i.e., M.Sc., Ph.D., D.M., M. Med, F.C.P., D.Sc., Dip. The questionnaires also asked whether the institution had adequate number of patients and the disease profile to enable adequate training of clinical pharmacologists, and whether the institution had the appropriate drugs to meet its patient requirements. For those countries that had a drug regulatory authority, it sought the opinion as to whether the respondent was satisfied with the effectiveness of the respective drug regulatory authority, and what fraction (percentage) of drugs on market were made locally versus those imported.

Data was captured on an Excel® data sheet, where the responses were coded and summarised as a percentage of respondents that answered a specific question in a similar way. The result was reported for each status of enabling factors for running a successful clinical pharmacology programme that was evaluated, i.e., clinical pharmacology training, recognition of clinical pharmacology, human capital: clinical pharmacologists and affiliated personnel, local support (government) and international support.

Literature review

Because some aspects of the enabling factors could not reasonably be determined by the survey, particularly the historical perspectives, information from the literature and relevant experts' reports from agencies such as WHO and UNAIDS (United Nations Programme on HIV/AIDS), were used to supplement the survey. This was also important for determination of 'trends in clinical pharmacology'.

Results

Of the 52 institutions approached, there were 21 respondents (40.4%) despite repeated reminders, i.e., Africa (11), Asia (8), Latin America (3) and Easter Europe (0). They comprised of medical schools (12), pharmacy schools (6), contract research organizations (2) and hospitals (1). Fortunately all the responses could be utilised.

Regarding the professional background of staff members serving as clinical pharmacologists, 34.5% of respondents indicated they had medical graduates (i.e., with M.B. Ch.B. or equivalent), 32.7% had pharmacy graduates, and altogether 38% of the medical and pharmacy graduates had Ph.D. or equivalent. These clinical pharmacologists worked with other personnel in their teams whereby 66.7% of the respondents indicated they had medical officers, 60% had pharmacists, 60% had laboratory personnel, 40% had nurses, and only 13.3% had poison information officers (Figure 1A).

Figure 1B illustrates the on-going clinical pharmacology activities in the study sample. There was wide variation in the clinical pharmacology activities and qualifications offered by different institutions, even from within the same country. Regarding clinical pharmacology services, 40% of respondents undertook bedside patient consultation, 53.3% had a pharmacovigilance programme, 20% offered medical & poison information services, and 40% participated in drug policy formulation or drug regulation. Regarding clinical pharmacology research, the majority

(93.3%) of respondents undertook research, but only 66.7% were doing clinical trials (or drug development clinical research), while 53.3% participated in drug utilization studies, and only 13.3% had international collaborative research projects. On clinical pharmacology training, 87% offered undergraduate training, while 60% offered post-graduate training in both basic and/or clinical pharmacology, with only 25% indicating they undertook postgraduate training in clinical pharmacology. Interestingly, there was wide variation in the names or codes used for the postgraduate qualifications in pharmacology and/or clinical pharmacology (M. Sc., Ph.D., D.M., M. Med, F. clinical pharmacology, D.Sc., Dip.), such that it was difficult to determine a basic and clinical pharmacology qualification by the code. In effect, there was no standard qualification for a Clinical Pharmacologist in developing countries.

Figure 1C reflects on the drug situation, whereby only 40% of respondents indicated they had the appropriate number and variety of drugs to meet their patients' requirements, and that 66% of these drugs were imported. Furthermore, of the 96.3% who indicated that they had a national Drug Regulatory Authority, 46.7% indicated that it was ineffective. These results reflect a situation of chronic drug shortage in the developing countries.

On clinical pharmacology recognition and local support (Figure 1D), 53.3% of respondents indicated that clinical pharmacology is recognised as a specialty by their governments, but, within the institutions, only 40% indicated that they had a dedicated clinical pharmacology division or department. Furthermore, lack of visibility of clinical pharmacology was indicated by the few forums for clinical pharmacology knowledge exchange, whereby only 7% had Colleges of Clinical Pharmacologists and only 27% indicated that clinical pharmacology is part of their national pharmacology society that meets annually.

Discussion

In general, the survey has articulated the status of the drug situation, clinical pharmacology activities, and extent of recognition and local support for clinical pharmacology in the developing countries. The response rate of 40.4% to the electronic questionnaire was within the expected range of 33.4 ± 9.4% for online surveys, in general [14], and was better than in a previous report on clinical pharmacology in developing countries [15]. Although most of the respondents were from Africa, confining the report to Africa would lead to loss of the contribution by the other half of the respondents, which countries have a lot in common with African countries of similar socioeconomic categorization. Furthermore, the categorization of the responding institutions into medical and pharmacy schools, etc., was to emphasize that clinical pharmacologists are not only found in medical schools. Nevertheless,

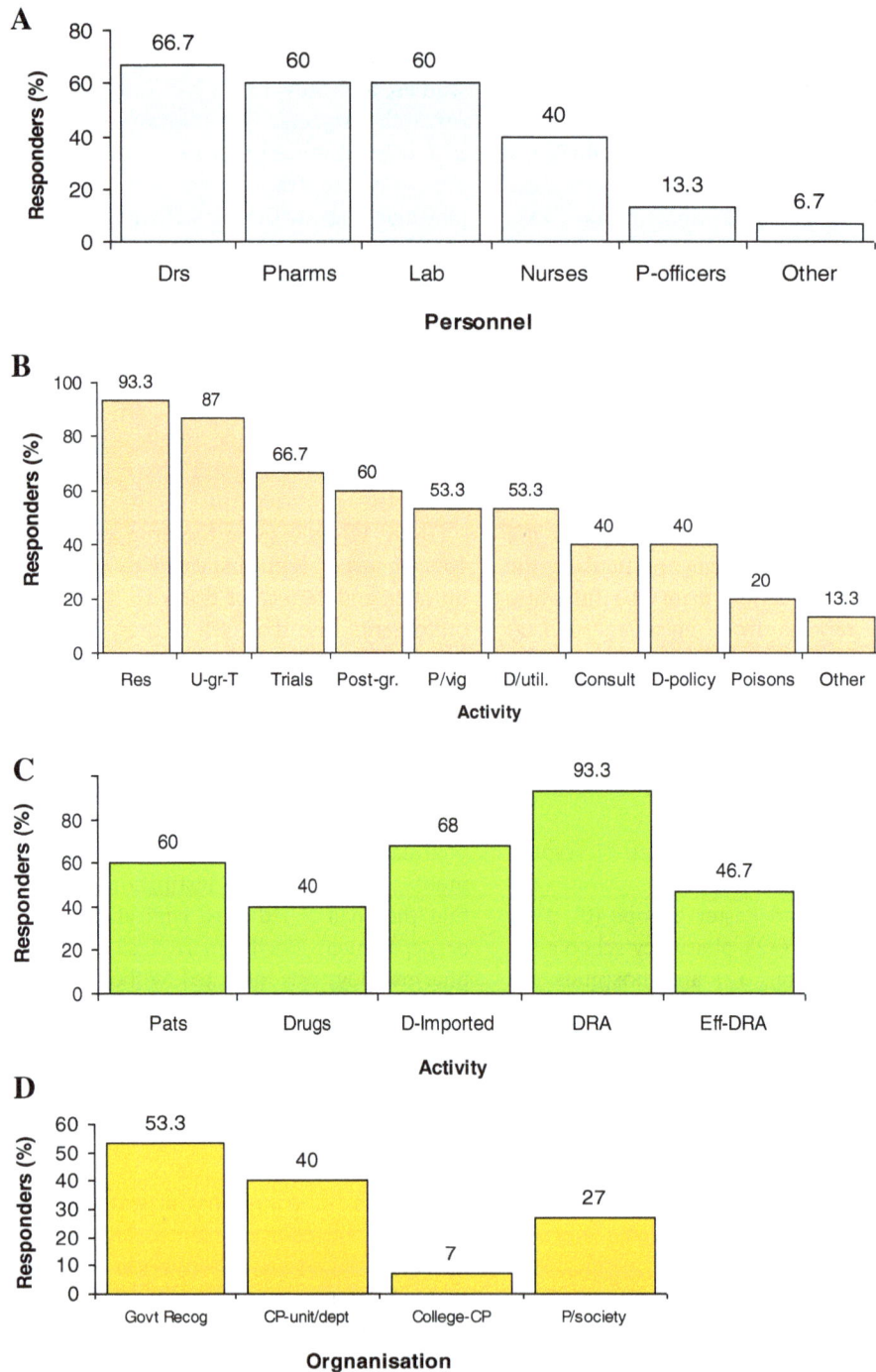

Figure 1 Enabling factors for clinical pharmacology. An Illustration of the proportion (%) of respondents regarding: composition of the personnel (**A**), clinical pharmacology activities (**B**), drug situation (**C**) and clinical pharmacology recognition (**D**). Key: A: Drs = medical officers; Lab = laboratory personnel; Other = other health workers. Pharms = pharmacists; P-officers = poison information officers; **B**: Consult = consultations; D/util. = drug utilization; D-policy = drug policy; Other = other services; P/vig = pharmacovigilance; Poisons = poison information services; Post-gr. = post graduate training; Res = research; Trials = clinical trials; U-gra-T = undergraduate training; **C**: D-imported = most drug are imported; DRA = have a drug regulatory authority; Drugs = drugs meet patient requirements; Eff-DRA = ineffective DRA; Pats = had appropriate mix of patients for training purposes; **D**: College-CP = had a College of Clinical pharmacologists; CP-unit/dept = had a clinical pharmacology unit/department; Govt-recog = Clinical pharmacology recognised by government; P/society = had a pharmacology society.

the response rate was still low, as such, the survey data should be regarded as preliminary hoping for confirmation in a larger study. Also, during the preparation of this manuscript, it emerged that the European Association of Clinical Pharmacology and Therapeutics (EACPT) has undertaken a study on clinical pharmacology in Europe but most of this has been communicated only at its congresses.

Clinical pharmacology activities

Clinical pharmacology activities include clinical pharmacology services, training and research. The scope of these activities is well explained in the recent WHO handbook and the IUPHAR position statement on clinical pharmacology in health care, research and teaching [16,17]. Nevertheless, whereas the two resources are appropriate for understanding the role of clinical pharmacology in health care, research and teaching, they don't illustrate the scale to which these activities are running, and how much more is needed.

From the survey, it is clear that training and research were the major functions of the clinical pharmacologists in the respondent's institutions. However, the survey could not determine whether the training was in clinical or basic pharmacology. The challenges of clinical pharmacologists in the developing countries include being trained from overseas in programmes with limited local content or relevancy, lack of appropriate clinical pharmacology training resources that appeal to the conditions in developing countries, limited incentives to clinical pharmacology training, and lack of close partnerships and collaboration among clinical pharmacologists in the developing countries. There is more collaboration with overseas institutions than amongst themselves.

Human capital

Lack of expertise is one of the biggest contributing factors to the poor clinical pharmacology services in the developing world. Worse still, human capital in any organisation is so dynamic that the results of this 2010-survey may not reflect the reality. Nevertheless, one can confidently say that, even though there was no recognition or accreditation for clinical pharmacologists in most of the developing countries, there is a small pool of clinical pharmacologists working in these countries. There is a need to organise these individuals into a regional or continental professional body that can be used to promote their plight.

Recognition of clinical pharmacology and local support

Recognition and local support for clinical pharmacology by government refers to the creation of posts and a career path for clinical pharmacologists, while recognition by the host institution gives the discipline a distinction indicated by presence of a clinical pharmacology department or unit in the respective institution. On the other hand, creation of a college of clinical pharmacologists ensures appropriate professional conduct, while forums such as clinical pharmacology society are important not only for sharing scientific information but also for advocacy.

Recognition by governments and professional visibility: Our search showed that by 2007, 84.8% (22/26) of the Eastern Europe countries had successfully recognised clinical pharmacology as a specialty. Furthermore, of the 26 countries in Easter Europe, 14 (50%) had a clinical pharmacology forum or society (Table 1). This was in sharp contrast to Africa where, of the 52 countries, only 5 (9.6%) had a pharmacology society. Even then, South Africa was the only country where clinical pharmacology was recognized as a specialty [18]. Of note, West African countries have opted for a regional society, the West Africa Pharmacology Society, which is dominated by Nigeria and Ghana. In Asia, of the 26 countries, 8 (31%) had a pharmacology society, and only three (Philippines, India and Thailand) had recognized clinical pharmacology as a specialty. In Latin America, of the 18 countries, 7 (39%) had a pharmacology society, and none recognized clinical pharmacology as a specialty. This poor rate of recognition as a specialty was also reflected in the survey.

It must be pointed out that government's recognition and local support for any speciality precedes the development of 'human capital' in that speciality. As such, it is only when a government recognises clinical pharmacology as a speciality that it creates an obligation to meet the training and employment needs of clinical pharmacologists. Unfortunately, although some governments have

Table 1 Developing countries that had a 'clinical pharmacology forum' separate or part of the broad national pharmacology society by 2007

AFRICA	L - AMERICA	ASIA	E - EUROPE
Egypt	Argentina	China	Bosnia & Herzegovina
Kenya	Brazil	Indian	Bulgaria
South Africa	Chile	Indonesian	Croatia
	Colombia	Korean	Czech Republic
	Cuba	Pakistan	Estonia
	Venezuela	Philippine	Georgia
	Mexico	Thailand	Hungary
		Malaysian	Latvia
			Lithuania
			Poland
			Romania
			Russia
			Serbia & Montenegro
			Slovakia

Key: L-America = Latin America; E-Europe = Eastern Europe.

recognized clinical pharmacology as a specialty, most governments are unwilling to do so owing to the contending priorities that supersede requirements for upcoming specialities such as clinical pharmacology. Nevertheless, appropriate local support should go beyond recognition by way of proclamation. Clinical pharmacology ought to be included in the competing priorities for national and institutional budgets aimed at establishing any facilities for health service, research and training.

International support

Developing countries have received considerable support from the international community for different purposes, and clinical pharmacology has been one of the main beneficiaries. The support ranges from sponsoring individuals to further their education and training overseas, and funding research capacity strengthening programmes, to direct intervention in running clinical pharmacology services by organisation such as the WHO, USP (United States Pharmacopeia), UNAIDS, to mention but a few. However, the IUPHAR and WHO, through their specialist divisions, remain the major advocates for clinical pharmacology development in the world.

Also, clinical pharmacology training opportunities have been offered in several countries: United Kingdom, United States of America, the Nordic Countries, Belgium, France, Germany, Australia, etc., and most of these have extensive collaborative Research Programmes with the many developing countries; i.e., the North–south collaboration through bilateral agreements, non-governmental organisations and specific institutions, and/or professional societies. The developing countries also benefited from many international private initiatives, specifically philanthropists and other private sponsors, as well as intergovernmental programmes.

As a result, there has been a significant increase in clinical pharmacology activities in many developing countries due to this international collaboration. For instance, in Serbia, there was an increased demand for clinical pharmacology services whereby the number of therapeutic consultations rose from less than 150 per year in 1995, to over 450 in 2003 [19]. From 1995 to 2006, the percentage growths in number of clinical trials was 200% for Africa, 400% for Asia, 800% and 1000% for Latin America [20]. In Russia alone, the number of clinical trials increased from 62 clinical trials run in 315 sites in 2003, to 158 clinical trials run in 863 sites in 2006 [21]. Nevertheless, there is still a need for improvement in clinical pharmacology programmes through increased local and international support.

The disease burden

The disease burden is a major determinant of the amount and type of medicines required by a given community,

and this, in turn, determines the scale of clinical pharmacology services required to ensure rational use of these medicines. From the survey, 60% of respondents indicated that they had adequate number of patients' disease profile to enable training of clinical pharmacologists (Figure 1D). Although this was a subjective question, the pilot study had shown that respondents understood they were to consider the number of patients and variety of disease conditions in their responses. Nevertheless, 60% is low, and this was most probably because the 'disease burden' in these countries is characterised by disease endemics rather than 'disease-variety' which the medical school seeks to meet its training requirements.

According to the UNAIDS (2008) report on the global AIDS epidemic, the HIV/AIDS, tuberculosis, malaria, and cardiovascular diseases were the leading causes of morbidity and mortality in the developing world [22]. They were characterized by an increased number of patients without treatment, an urgent need to increase number of patients on treatment, a need to provide lifelong therapy, a need to treat resistant cases and the inadequacy of funding.

Specifically, by end of 2010, there were 2.7 million new cases of HIV world-wide, of which 70% (1.9 million) were from sub-Sahara Africa [23]. Furthermore, the HIV/AIDS-related deaths between 2001 and 2010 increased more than 10-fold in the Eastern Europe and Central Asia, by 60% in the Middle East and North Africa, and more than doubled in East Asia. Regarding the need to treat more patients, only 20% of 34 million people with HIV/AIDS were on treatment. On the other hand, the tuberculosis epidemic posed a serious challenge to the developing world. In 2009, all the 22 high-tuberculosis-burdened countries were from the developing world, and they accounted for over 80% of the new cases of tuberculosis [24]. Worst still, the 27 countries with multi-drug resistant-tuberculosis were from the developing world, and they accounted for 84% of the new cases of multi-drug resistant-tuberculosis. Regarding malaria, in 2010, approximately 81% of the new malaria cases were in Africa and 13% were in the South-East Asia, and 91% of malaria deaths were in Africa [25]. It was estimated that the financial requirement for tuberculosis control is short by $1 billion dollars, while that for malaria is short by $3 billion dollars.

In general, this information shows that the developing world is still characterised by a high disease burden as indicated by several disease epidemics, and this is associated with increased use of medicines with the compounding requirements of rational prescribing and appropriate therapeutic monitoring, all of which require the expertise of a clinical pharmacologist.

Economic growth

Economic growth was a major determinant of progress in clinical pharmacology development because it enabled establishment of national infrastructures, essential health care facilities, attract and retain expertise, and increased availability of medicines. The best examples are the emerging markets of Eastern Europe where 86% of the countries had recognised clinical pharmacology as a specialty [26].

Since medical schools are in close association with teaching hospitals where most clinical pharmacology programmes are run, a comparison of the number of medical schools in developing and developed countries every 20 years since 1900 was made. This was then related to the level of development of clinical pharmacology programmes in the respective countries or regions. Of note, the WHO defines a medical school as 'any training institution for health professionals' and this includes schools of medicine, pharmacy, nursing and allied health sciences.

It was observed that, although presence of a medical school in a country or region was a pre-requisite to the existence of clinical pharmacology, the number of medical schools in a country did not correlate with the level of advancement in clinical pharmacology practice. Clinical pharmacology is well advanced in the United Kingdom, the United States of America and Germany, countries where the number of medical schools has remained consistently low for the past 100 years, and yet, the discipline remained stagnant in developing countries where

many new medical schools have been built in the past 50 years (Figure 2).

Specifically, most of the medical schools in the developed countries were built before 1900. By the year 1900, Germany had 19 medical schools, the United Kingdom had 20, the United State of America 53 and Japan 8, and there were virtually no new medical schools after 2000 in each of these countries (Figure 2A). On the contrary, both, the fast developing countries (Brazil, Russia, India and China; BRIC) and the less developed countries, had virtually no medical school before 1900 (Figure 2B and 2C). Medical schools in these countries were built after 1900: viz; in the BRIC countries, 234 new medicals schools were built between 1940 to 1960, and 164 between 1960 to 1980, while in the less developed countries, 174 new medical schools were built between 1960 to 1980 and 176 between 1980 to 2000.

Whereas by 2007 the number of medical schools in Germany, the United Kingdom, the United States of America and Japan increased only to double digits (19, 7, 82 and 75, respectively), the BRIC countries had a total of 629 medical schools (276 in China, 154 in India, 78 in Brazil, 67 in Russia and 54 in Mexico), while the less developed countries had a total of 528 medical schools (257 in Asia [excluding China and India], 101 in Eastern Europe, 90 in Latin America [excluding Brazil

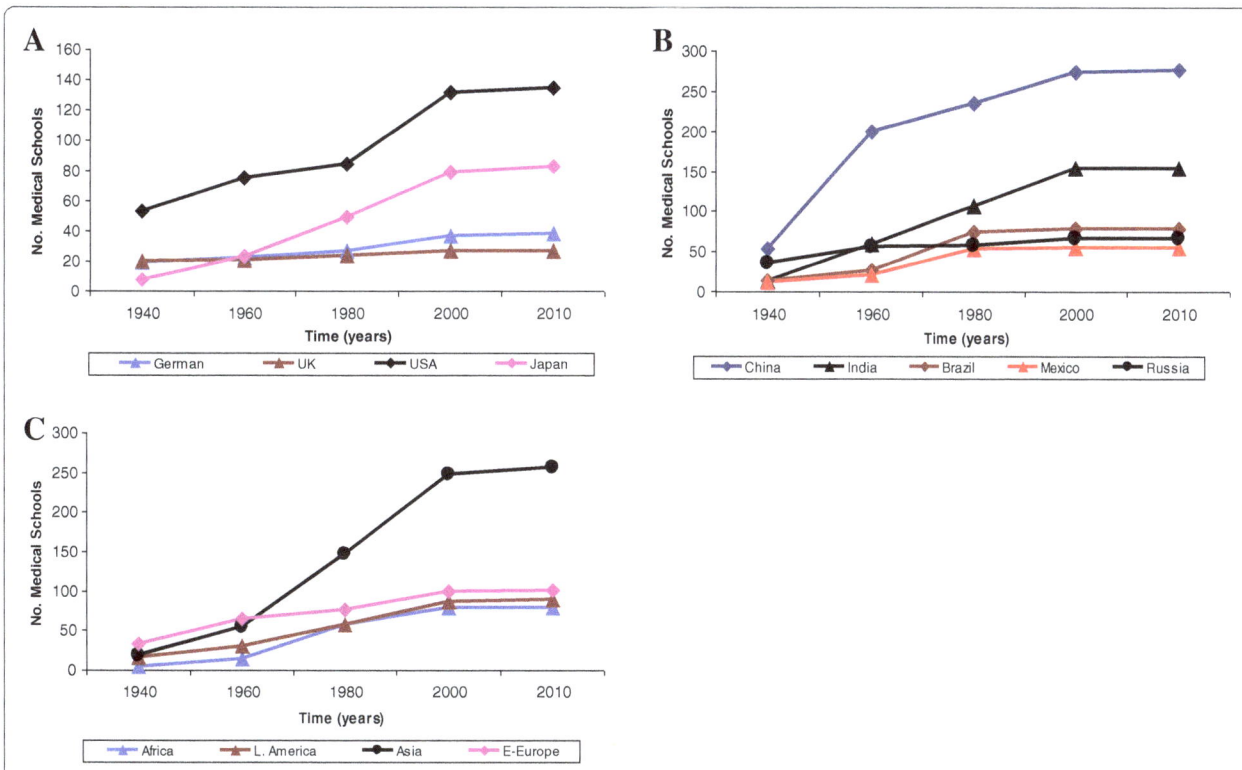

Figure 2 Medical schools and clinical pharmacology development. The total number of medical schools every 20 years over the past 100 years in the developed (**A**), fast developing (Brazil, Russia, India, China and Mexico; **B**) and least developed (**C**) countries [25].

and Mexico], and 80 in Africa). Again, it is not the number of medical schools that determine the development of clinical pharmacology, but most probably, the activities within these facilities. This is because these facilities were built to meet other priorities where clinical pharmacology was not included from the onset.

Nevertheless, the developing world exhibited a remarkable increase in the number of medical training facilities in the past 50 years, along with increased clinical pharmacology activities, particularly pharmacology training. This implies that despite the lack of clinical pharmacologists, there are professionals performing such work within these countries. This poses a question as to whether the current definition of a 'clinical pharmacologist' which emphasizes the training background of a specialist physician is universally applicable. As such, the claim that clinical pharmacology in the developing countries is still in infancy may be wrong because it ignores the reality that the professionals/practitioners in these countries are the clinical pharmacologists.

The drug situation

The 'drug situation' refers to the extent of utilisation of medicines to combat the disease burden through implementation of appropriate health care and medicines policies. In the developing world, the drug situation is characterised by severe drug shortages due to, among other things, wide spread drug misuse, limited access to drugs due to unaffordable cost and/or unavailability, too many unnecessary drugs, a complex medicine supply system and inadequate information to patients, etc., [27]. This situation was well expressed in the findings of the current survey. Nevertheless, all these problems can be addressed by developing appropriate medicines policies, which includes the policy on the 'rational use of medicines'.

Formulation and implementation of the fundamental policies of health-care

The major function of clinical pharmacologists is promotion of the rational use of medicines [28,29]. However, because implementation of the policy on rational use of medicines is guided by the national health care policies, clinical pharmacologists need to be part of the teams formulating these policies to ensure that they articulate with the policy on rational use of medicines (Figure 3). Such polices in include: A national health plan, a national medicine policy, a drug regulatory authority, a medicine supply policy, an access to medicine policy, a policy on rational use of medicines, a drug financing or pricing policy, a policy on production and sale of medicines, and a policy on intellectual property rights.

Regarding implementation, Table 2 illustrates the proportion of countries by income group that had established

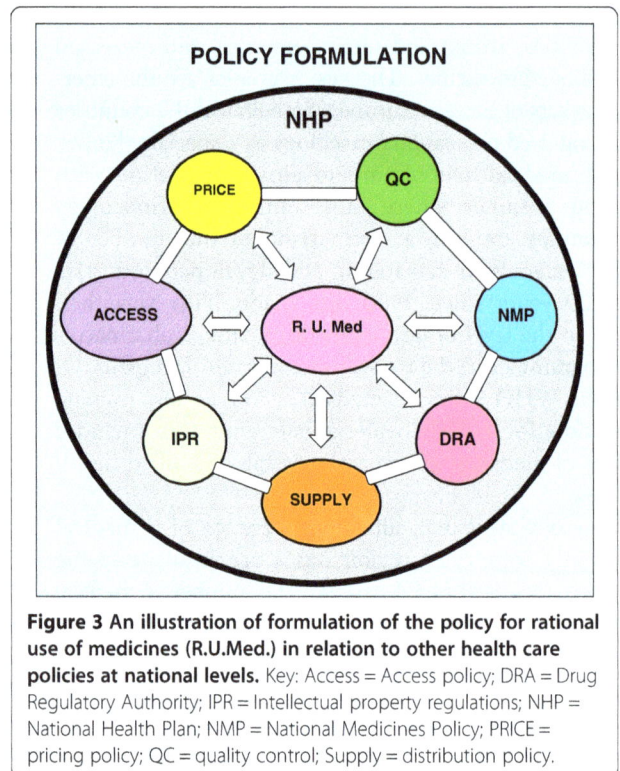

Figure 3 An illustration of formulation of the policy for rational use of medicines (R.U.Med.) in relation to other health care policies at national levels. Key: Access = Access policy; DRA = Drug Regulatory Authority; IPR = Intellectual property regulations; NHP = National Health Plan; NMP = National Medicines Policy; PRICE = pricing policy; QC = quality control; Supply = distribution policy.

seven of the above mentioned fundamental policies of health-care by 2007. Along side each policy are the respective performance indicators. Overall, 70% to 94% of low income countries had established (written) the health care policies that are fundamental to the development of clinical pharmacology (i.e., a national health plan, a drug regulatory authority, and policies on medicines' financing, supply, production and sales), and these percentages were not far from the corresponding values of the high income countries. However, the respective performance (or implementation) indicators for these policies in the low income countries lagged behind those of the high income countries. For instance, regarding the national health plan, less than 50% of the low income countries undertook a drug-situation analysis, prescribing audit' and 'evaluation of access to health care'. Also, the indicators for implementation of the sub-policies under the drug regulatory authority such as pharmacovigilance (50%) and quality control (68%) were still inadequate. Access to medicines was less than 20% in low income countries versus 75% in high income countries, while the medicines financing policy was only successful for anti-tuberculosis drugs, with research & development scoring an abysmal 16%.

Formulation and implementation of the policy for 'rational use of medicines'

From the afore-mentioned policies, more focused or subject specific policies are drawn to guide policy implemen-

Table 2 Comparison of the proportion (%) of countries that attained a particular policy or indicator in low, mid and high income countries by 2007 [30]

Parameter/Indicator	WHO-countries income category		
	Low income	Mid-income	High income
1. National Medicine Policy (NMP)	**94%**	**84%**	**74%**
Monitoring: Undertook assessment/audit of:			
• National assessment of NMP	80%	65%	81%
• Pharmaceutical/Drug situation	37%	48%	69%
• Prescriptions audit	39%	46%	71%
• Access	50%	52%	72%
2. Drug Regulatory Authority (DRA)	**89%**	**85%**	**97%**
• Marketing authorization of Medicines	88%	84%	94%
• Licensing of manuf., imp./expt. (av.)	91%	91%	99%
• Licensing of prescribers & pharmacies	94%	99%	100%
• Pharmacovigilance (ADR)	50%	64%	67%
• Quality control system in place	68%	69%	96%
3. Access to essential medicines: patients within 1-hr walking distance to a clinic, 2003			
• Very low Access (< 50%)	31%	6%	0%
• Low-Medium access (50 – 80%)	56%	38%	25%
• Medium-High access (81-95%)	10%	31%	0%
• Very high Access (< 95%)	2%	25%	75%
4. Medicine financing and/or pricing policy	**93%**	**100%**	**100%**
i) With health insurance policy? Medicines received for free:			
• All medicines	35%	59%	55%
• Malaria medicines	59%	72%	47%
• Tuberculosis medicines	100%	92%	94%
ii) Monitoring medicine retail prices:			
• Public sector	40%	58%	77%
• Private sector	36%	49%	78%
• NGO sector	17%	33%	71%
5. Medicines supply policy			
• Procurement policy for Ess. Meds	74%	90%	92%
6. Production and sale of medicines			
• R&D of new active substances	16%	27%	57%
• Repackaging of finished dos-forms	83%	78%	81%
• National legislation + TRIPS	55%	76%	86%
7. Rational use of medicines			

Key: *ADR*, adverse drug reactions; *AMR*, antimicrobial resistance; *CME*, continuing medical education; *DTC*, drug therapeutics committees; *Ess. Meds*, essential medicines; *HIC*, high income countries; *LIC*, low income countries; *MIC*, middle income countries; *NGO*, non-government organisation; *NMP*, National medicine policy; *R&D*, research and development; *TRIPS*, trade-related aspects of intellectual property rights.

tation (Figure 4). In this case, clinical pharmacologists are the leading professionals in the implementation of the policy on 'rational use of medicines'. This is also emphasized in the WHO recommendations that countries must encourage or ensure more appropriate (rational) use of medicines [29,31] by; establishing a national drug regulatory authority, formulating standard treatment guidelines, selecting an essential medicines' list, setting up

drug or pharmaceutical therapeutics committees, promoting training in good prescribing practices, enforcing continuing medical education, promoting prescribing audit or accredited standard of health care, providing unbiased medical information through medicines information centres and national drug formularies, promoting community education campaigns about medicines and patient package inserts, eliminating perverse financial incentives that lead

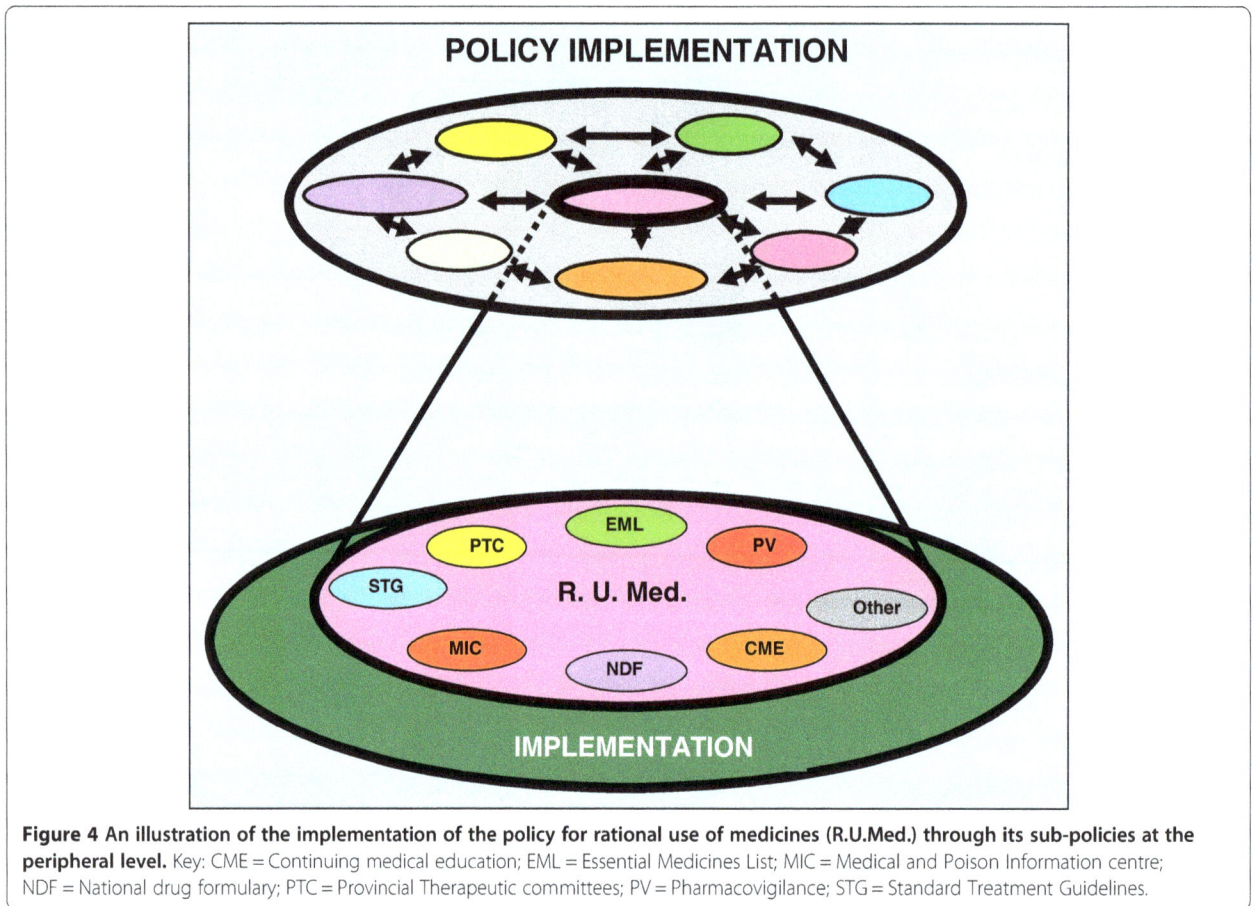

Figure 4 An illustration of the implementation of the policy for rational use of medicines (R.U.Med.) through its sub-policies at the **peripheral level.** Key: CME = Continuing medical education; EML = Essential Medicines List; MIC = Medical and Poison Information centre; NDF = National drug formulary; PTC = Provincial Therapeutic committees; PV = Pharmacovigilance; STG = Standard Treatment Guidelines.

to irrational prescribing, enforcing ethical medicinal drug promotion or advertising as adopted in resolution WHA 41.17, and advocate for adequate funding for health care.

Regarding implementation, Table 3 shows the proportion of countries by 'country income group' that had established nine of the sub-policies for promoting rational use of medicines by 2007. They are also accompanied by the respective indicators for implementation. Whereas the policy documents for promotion of rational use of medicines were available in more than 80% of the low income countries, their respective indicators for implementation were not impressive. Specifically, the proportion of low income countries with programmes for each of the nine indicators illustrated in Table 3 was far lower than that of high income countries. However, some of the respective performance indicators though low, were promising. For instance, the proportion of low income countries with appropriate prescribers at primary health care level, promoting generic substitution, and regulating medicines advertisement were almost similar to that of high income countries (> 85%).

Nevertheless, the poor implementation of the policy on rational prescribing should be expected in view of the fact that implementation of the fundamental health-care

policies was also low. The current drug situation in low income countries can be better appreciated when one considers the trend of events over the past 20 or more years. In fact, Figure 5 shows that policy formulation in the low income countries has been a fast process. The proportion of low income countries with a national medicines policy increased from less than 10% in 1985 to 94% in 2007, while the proportion with drug regulatory authorities increased from less than 40% in 1999 to 89% in 2007, and those with an essential medicines list increased from less than 10% in 1985 to 100% in 2007 [32-34]. Likewise, some indicators for policy implementation improved dramatically whereby the proportion of low income countries revising their essential medicines list every five years increased from less than 10% in 1985, to over 80% in 2007 (Figure 5).

Unfortunately, by 2007, the indicators for implementation of sub-policies that ensure rational use of medicines were not different from those of 2003 (Table 4) [31,35]. Whereas the increase in adverse drug reaction reporting (15%) and availability of standard treatment guidelines at national level (22%) were appreciated, these two indicators reflect availability rather than performance. In general, the required policy documents for health-care and rational

Table 3 Comparison of the proportion (%) of countries that attained a particular policy or indicator for rational use of medicines in low, mid and high income countries in 2007 [45]

Parameter/Indicator	WHO-countries income category		
	Low income	Mid-income	High income
1. Standard Treatment Guidelines (STG)	89%	75%	80%
2. Essential Medicines list (EML):	100%	86%	68%
• EML-Updated in <5 years	81%	74%	41%
3. Drug Therapeutics Committees (DTC):	38%	58%	74%
4. Prescribing policy or supervision/monitor prescribing			
i) Prescribers at primary care level in public sector			
• Doctors	98%	99%	100%
• Nurses	89%	60%	66%
• Pharmacists	37%	16%	3%
• Other	23%	9%	0%
ii) Policy on generic medicines in public sector			
• Obligatory use of generics	63%	62%	18%
• Generic substitution allowed	85%	87%	77%
• Incentives for prescribing generics	48%	26%	67%
iii) Prescriptions audit	39%	46%	71%
iv) Strategy for AMR containment	24%	46%	73%
5. Education and Training in CP: undergraduate and post graduate education (Includes training on EML, STG, pharmacotherapy & Rational prescribing)			
• Doctors	$62 \pm 3.7\%$	$73 \pm 7.1\%$	$88 \pm 17.4\%$
• Nurses	58 ± 10.8	$57 \pm 3.0\%$	$73 \pm 6.0\%$
• Pharmacists	$62 \pm 11.5\%$	$60 \pm 6.7\%$	$80 \pm 13.3\%$
• Other	$33 \pm 5.3\%$	$32 \pm 6.2\%$	$36 \pm 5.3\%$
6. Continuing Medical Education (CME): Obligatory CME for:			
• Doctors	51%	54%	70%
• Nurses + paramedics	53%	44%	65%
• Pharmacists	56%	51%	57%
7. Provision of information on Medicines:			
• Med. Information Centres	36%	52%	75%
• Medicines formulary	57%	69%	70%
8. Public/Consumer education and information on medicines			
• Education campaigns (A/biotic use)	44%	52%	62%
• Other rational medicine use topics	60%	56%	73%
9. Medicine promotion & advertising:			
• Regulate Drug prom/advertisement	85%	86%	100%

Key: *AMR*, antimicrobial resistance; *CME*, continuing medical education; *CP*, clinical pharmacology; *DTC*, drug therapeutics committees; *EML*, essential medicines; *HIC*, high income countries; *LIC*, low income countries; *MIC*, middle income countries; *STG*, standard treatment guidelines.

use of drugs were available in the majority of the developing countries, but their implementation remained poor.

Traditional medicines

With the majority of people in developing countries using traditional medicines for their health-care needs and concerns [36-38], there has been a growing recognition of traditional medicines as indicated by a worldwide increase in the number of countries with policies for regulation of traditional medicines, from 15 countries in 1986 to 110 in 2007 [39]. However, several challenges in the regulation of traditional medicines have been encountered. Specifically, the non-standardized classification of traditional medicines has made it more difficult to impose strict rules on their use. Traditional medicines are marketed as herbal medicines, herbal supplements,

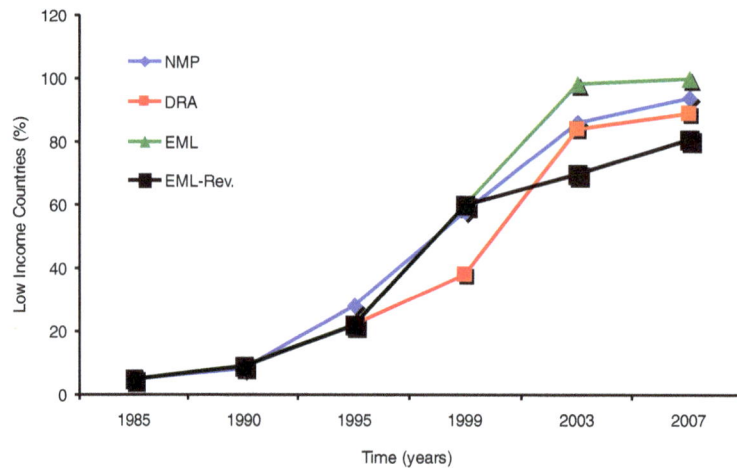

Figure 5 The proportion (%) of low income countries (LIC) that have formulated the relevant policies from 1985 to 2007 [30]. Key: DRA: Drug Regulatory Authority; EML = Essential Medicines List; EML-Rev. = Essential Medicines List-Revision; NMP National Medicines Policy.

herbal pharmaceuticals, phytoprotectants or phytotherapeutic agents, or even simply as medicines or as a foodstuff [40]. Also, since one product may be used for several diseases, it is may be sold as a prescription or over-the-counter medicine for self-medication, home remedies, dietary supplements, health foods, functional foods or by some other title [41]. Therefore, depending on the level of sophistication of the regulatory framework, a

Table 4 Indicators for policy implementation: comparison of the proportion (%) of low income countries that implemented the respective sub-policies for promoting rational use of medicines in 2003 and 2007 [30]

Year	2003	2007
Availability of STGs		
• STGs at National level	67.3%	89%
• STGs at Primary Health level	75%	72%
• NMF for EML	56.4%	57%
Education and information		
• EML in Med-Curriculum	67.3%	65.9%
• STG in Med-Curriculum	62.2%	59.5%
• CME for doctors	37.7%	51.1%
• Provided Med. Inform. to prescribers	32.1%	36.2%
• Public Education on Antibiotics	37.0%	44.4%
Key policies and regulations to promote rational drug use		
• ADR monitoring	32.7%	50.0%
• DTC in General Hospitals	38.8%	41.5%
• DTC in Regional Hospitals	36.2%	31.4%
• AMR-policy	23.6%	20.0%

Key: *ADR*, adverse drug reactions; *AMR*, antimicrobial resistance; *CME*, continuing medical education; *DTC*, drug therapeutics committees; *EML*, essential medicines list; *LIC*, low income countries; *NMF*, national medical formulary; *STG*, standard treatment guidelines.

single medicinal plant may be simultaneously defined and regulated under several different regulatory instruments. The WHO advises that countries must formulate national standards, policies and regulations governing the production and use of traditional medicines to promote and maintain good practice among appropriately-educated producers and practitioners for the benefit of the population [37,42].

Already, several clinical pharmacologists in the developing countries are involved in the establishment of appropriate specifications and standards for traditional medicines that will serve as the basis for consistency, quality control and the verification of safety [43-45], as well as establishment of a post-marketing surveillance system for the evaluation of potential toxicity and herb-herb/herb-drug interactions [32]. For instance, in China, 25% of the medical schools are for Chinese traditional medicines [26], and traditional herbal medicinal preparations constituted between 30% and 50% of the total consumption of medicines in 2005 [39].

The trend
A persistent need for clinical pharmacology
In a nut shell, there are several on-going clinical pharmacology activities in the developing world, but these activities are at different stages in the different countries depending on the level of economic advancement. The persistent epidemics of new and old diseases have led to increased demand for more medicines, which in turn, has increased the requirement for clinical pharmacology services. In the same perspective, the wide scope of clinical pharmacology activities enumerated here may be counter-productive by overstretching and thereby contributing to the scarcity of clinical pharmacologists. This is an appropriate concern, but this report was not on 'how to utilize

clinical pharmacologists'. However, clinical pharmacologists need not be full time employees in some of the roles indicated. In fact, some of the clinical pharmacology activities enumerated here, e.g., drug regulatory authority and national policy formulation, are run by other health care professionals whereby clinical pharmacologists only serve as temporary advisers. Therefore, the use of clinical pharmacologists in some of the clinical pharmacology activities will be determined by the availability of other experts for the respective tasks.

Task shifting

Although the number of medical schools do not predict advancement in clinical pharmacology activities, there has been considerable progress in developing clinical pharmacology through training, and running of clinical pharmacology services, particularly by non-governmental organisations such as the WHO and UNAIDS. In the WHO's programmes and other non-governmental organisations, clinical pharmacologists at their headquarters (located in the developed world) participate in the formulation of the clinical pharmacology policies and programmes, after which these programmes are run by professionals other than clinical pharmacologists, i.e., 'task shifting'. Specifically, 'task shifting' is where some of the allied health professionals (non-medical doctors) are trained in disease-specific therapeutics, e.g., HIV, tuberculosis, etc., to enable them prescribe some medicines under particular circumstances (Figure 6). 'Task shifting' is a challenging concept that requires careful planning in the selection, training and monitoring of the workers, patients and the condition in question, but

this is beyond the scope for this report. However, success in 'task shifting' has been made possible by the fact that, currently, many developing countries have developed and implemented several drug policies and guidelines for promoting rational drug use, which forms the basis for training other professionals.

Relevant training

For developing countries, the current training of an internationally recognised clinical pharmacologists with a Ph.D. takes too long. Such training often veers off the local requirements, and ventures into irrelevancy by emphasising highly specialised research over service delivery. Clinical pharmacology training for the developing countries needs to be modified to address local relevancy and within the optimum time. Therefore, it is no wonder that, currently, several developing countries have turned away from doctoral studies as the primary qualification for a clinical pharmacologist, to producing a physician in clinical pharmacology, whereby, after the primary medical degree (M.B.Ch.B.) and at least two years of practice, the candidate undertakes a four year training programme in clinical pharmacology, and graduates with a Masters' degree (M. Med.) or fellowship in clinical pharmacology (Figure 6). These professionals are employed in tertiary and peripheral hospitals where the government has created posts along side those of other clinical specialities. Even then, this does mean that doctoral studies are irrelevant. Therefore, as for other clinical specialties, these specialist clinical pharmacologists form a pool from which Ph.D. aspirants can be selected.

Advocacy

There is a need to promote recognition of clinical pharmacology by high advocacy both locally and internationally, particularly by intensifying IUPHAR's programmes in this regard. Intervention strategies need to take the stakeholders' interests into account so as to ensure cooperation. For instance, more government support is likely if the focus is on service based clinical pharmacologists, while international support is more likely with advanced training usually doctoral or research fellowship studies. Clinical pharmacology services should be extended to peripheral hospitals, and play a leading role in the formulation and implementation of drug policies. Besides clinical pharmacology consultation, the afore mentioned clinical pharmacology physicians should also provide special courses in clinical pharmacology (or rational prescribing) for medical students and other health workers as part of the continuing medical education.

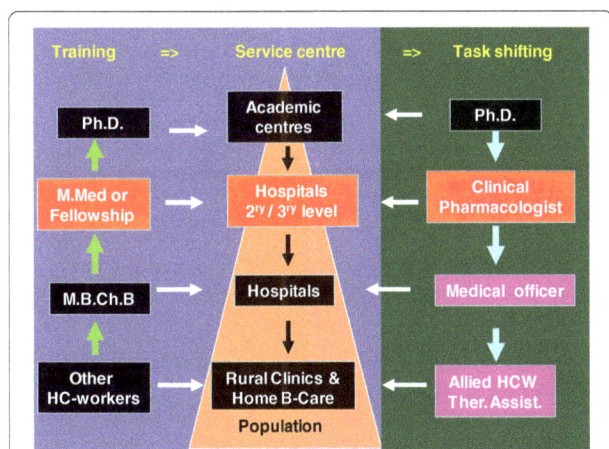

Figure 6 An illustration of the level of the preferred clinical pharmacologist physician (red box) with regard to level of training (masters), service delivery and task shifting (purple). Key: 2^{ry}/3^{ry} level = Secondary or tertiary level; HCW = Health care workers; HC-workers = Health care workers; Home B-care = Home based care; M.B.Ch.B. = Bachelor of Medicine & Bachelor of surgery; M.Med. = Master of Medicine; Ph.D. = Doctor of philosophy.

Conclusion

Circumstances in the developing countries foster promotion of 'a specialist clinical pharmacologist' and 'task shifting' for some endemic diseases as the most appropriate strategies to meet the current and future challenges to rational use of medicines in these countries. This implies that clinical pharmacology in developing countries is advancing in a different way to that in the developed world and that this does not, in any way, mean poor quality or no progress. Continuing support for these efforts will go a long way in promoting improved health for all.

Competing interests
The author declares that he had no competing interests.

Authors' information
Prof. Andrew Walubo M.B.Ch.B., M. Phil., M.D., MBA, FCP. Prof. Walubo is a chief clinical pharmacologist at Universitas academic hospital, and head of department of pharmacology of the University of the Free State. He completed his medical degree at Makerere University in Uganda, master's studies in Hong Kong, doctoral studies at the University of Cape Town and a postdoctoral fellowship in the Division of Clinical Pharmacology at Vanderbilt University USA.

Prof. Walubo has been instrumental in promotion of clinical pharmacology for a long time. He is a fellow of the American College of Clinical Pharmacology, and founder and 'Associate Member' of the 'The college of Clinical Pharmacologists of South Africa (CCP SA) which governs the training and examination of clinical pharmacology specialists in South Africa. He is a member of the Senate of the Colleges of Medicine of South Africa (CMSA), the Medicines Control Council (MCC; South Africa's drug regulatory authority) and the Executive committee of the South African Society for Basic and Clinical Pharmacology (SASBCP), to mention but a few. He is a co-author to the 2012 World Health Organization's (WHO) publication on 'Clinical Pharmacology in Health Care, Teaching and Research (http://www.who.int/medicines/areas/quality_safety/safety_efficacy/OMS-CIOMS-Report-20120913v4.pdf); to the IUPHAR 'position statement on Clinical Pharmacology' in 2010 (Basic Clin Pharmacol Toxicol 2010, 107: 531–559); and a leading author to the recent article (S. Afr.Med.J. 2013;103 (3):150–151) entitled 'Clinical pharmacology becomes a specialty in South Africa'. Among other things, Andrew is involved in assisting/organising clinical pharmacologists in some countries in Africa.

Acknowledgements
The author is grateful to all colleagues that helped to reach out in their respective institutions.

References

1. Turner P (Ed): *Proceedings of plenary lectures, symposia and therapeutic sessions of the First World Conference on Clinical Pharmacology and Therapeutics, 3–9 August 1980.* London, UK: Clinical Pharmacology & therapeutics: MacMillen Publishers; 1980.
2. Fraser HS: **Clinical pharmacology in developing countries.** *Br J clin Pharmacol* 1981, **11**:457–459.
3. Richens A, Routledge A: **Essentials of clinical pharmacology for education and research in developing countries.** *Br J clin Pharmacol* 1984, **18**:123–126.
4. Gyapong JO, Ofori-Adjei D: *Capacity building for relevant health research in developing countries;* 2009. http://www.inclentrust.org/uploadedbyfck/file/compile%20resourse/new-resourse-dr_-vishal/Capacity%20Building%20for%20Relevant%20Health%20Research%20in%20Developing%20Counties.pdf.
5. *International scholarship: for non-degree, undergraduate, postgraduate, PhD and post-doctoral students (website).* http://scholarization.blogspot.com/2011/01/phd-scholarship-in-medical-science.html.
6. Manabe YC, Katabira E, Brough RL, Coutinho AG, Sewankambo N, Merry C: **Developing independent investigators for clinical research relevant for**

7. **Africa.** *Health Res Policy Syst.* 2011, **9**:44–45. http://www.health-policy-systems.com/content/pdf/1478-4505-9-44.pdf.
8. Matee MI, Manyando C, Ndumbe PM, Corrah T, Jaoko WG, Kitua AY, *et al*: **European and developing countries clinical trials partnership (EDCTP): the path towards a true partnership.** *BMC Public Health* 2009, **9**:249.
9. Tomatis C, Taramona C, Rizo-Patrón E, Hernández F, Rodríguez P, Piscoya A, *et al*: **Evidence-based medicine training in a resource-poor country, the importance of leveraging personal and institutional relationships.** *J Eval Clin Pract* 2011, **17**:644–650.
10. Sadavongvivad C: **Challenge of clinical pharmacology in developing countries.** *J Clin Pharmacol* 1980, **20**:621–624.
11. Laing RO, Hogerzeil HV, Ross-Degnan D: **Ten recommendations to improve use of medicines in developing countries.** *Health Policy Planning* 2001, **16**:13–20.
12. Blaschke TF: **Global Challenges for clinical pharmacology in the developing world.** *Clin Pharmaco Ther* 2009, **85**:579–581.
13. Nielsen L: *Classifications of countries based on their level of development: How it is done and how it could be done. IMF working paper;* 2011. http://www.imf.org/external/pubs/ft/wp/2011/wp1131.pdf.
14. World Bank list of economies: *World Bank list of economies;* 2012. http://librarians.acm.org/sites/default/files/world%20bank%20List%20of%20Economies%20(as%20of%20July%202012)).pdf.
15. Nulty DD: **The adequacy of response rates to online and paper surveys: what can be done?** *Assess Eval Higher Educ* 2008, **33**:301–314. http://www.uaf.edu/files/uafgov/fsadmin-nulty5-19-10.pdf.
16. Suryawati S: **Contribution of clinical pharmacology to improve the use of medicines in developing countries.** *Int J Risk Safety Med* 2005, **17**:57–64.
17. Abernethy D, Birkett D, Brøsen K, Cascorbi I, Gustafsson LL, Hoppu K, *et al*: **Clinical Pharmacology in health care, teaching and research.** In Edited by Orme M, Sjöqvist F, Birkett D; 2012. http://www.who.int/medicines/areas/quality_safety/safety_efficacy/OMS-CIOMS-Report-20120913v4.pdf.
18. Birkett D, Brøsen K, Cascorbi I, Gustafsson LL, Maxwell S, Rago L, *et al*: **Clinical pharmacology in research, teaching and health care: Considerations by IUPHAR, the International Union of Basic and Clinical Pharmacology.** *Basic Clin Pharmacol Toxicol* 2010, **107**:531–559.
19. Walubo A, Barnes KI, Kwizera E, Greeff O, Rosenkranz B, Maartens G: **Clinical pharmacology becomes a speciality in South Africa.** *SAMJ* 2013, **301**:150–151.
20. Jankovic SM, Dragojevic'-Simic' V, Milovanovic' DR: **Impact of clinical pharmacology on health care: Serbian experience.** *Eur J Clin Pharmacol* 2005, **61**:787–788.
21. Kline D: *Clinical Trials in Latin America - White paper;* 2001. http://www.fast-track.com/pdfs/ClinicalTrialsLatinAmerica.pdf.
22. Synergy Research Group: *Clinical trials in Russia. Orange paper. No. 1/2007. Overview and Year;* 2006. http://www.appliedclinicaltrialsonline.com/applied clinicaltrials/data/articlestandard//appliedclinicaltrials/222007/430480/article.pdf.
23. UNAIDS: *Report on the global AIDS epidemic, 2008.* Geneva: UNAIDS; 2008. http://www.unaids.org/en/dataanalysis/knowyourepidemic/epidemiologypublications/2008reportontheglobalaidsepidemic/. ISBN 978 92 9 173711 6.
24. World Health Organization: *Global HIV/AIDS response - epidemic update and health sector progress towards universal access,* Progress Report 2011. Geneva: WHO/UNICEF/UNAIDS; 2011. http://www.unaids.org/en/media/unaids/contentassets/documents/unaidspublication/2011/20111130_ua_report_en.pdf.
25. World Health Organization report: *Global tuberculosis control.* Geneva: WHO; 2010. http://www.doh.state.fl.us/disease_ctrl/tb/trends-stats/Fact-Sheets/US-Global/WHO_Report2010_Global_TB_Control.pdf. ISBN 978 92 4 156406 9.
26. World Health Organization: *Global malaria programme. World malaria report: 2011.* Geneva: WHO; 2011. http://apps.who.int/iris/bitstream/10665/44792/2/9789241564403_eng_full.pdf. ISBN 978 92 4 156440 3.
27. World Health Organization: *World directory of medical schools.* University of Copenhagen. The AVICENNA directory of medicine; 2010. http://www.who.int/hrh/wdms/en/.
28. Smith AJ: **Unfinished business: clinical pharmacology and world health.** *Int J Risk Safety Med* 2005, **17**:65–71.
29. World Health Organization: *The rational use of drugs.* Geneva: Report of the conference of experts, Nairobi, 25–29 November 1985; 1987. http://apps.who.int/medicinedocs/documents/s17054e/s17054e.pdf.
30. World Health Organization: *Promoting rational use of medicines: Core components.* Geneva: WHO Policy Perspectives on Medicines, No.5; 2002. http://apps.who.int/medicinedocs/pdf/h3011e/h3011e.pdf.

30. Noller BN, Myers S, Abegaz B, Singh MM, Kronenberg F, Bodeker G: **Global forum on safety of herbal and traditional medicine: July 7, 2001, gold coast, Australia.** *J Altern Complement Med* 2001, **7**:583–601.

31. World Health Organization. **The World Medicines Situation 2011: Rational Use of Medicines.** In *The World Medicines Situation 2011: Rational Use of Medicines.* 3rd edition. Edited by Holloway K, van Dijk L. Geneva: WHO; 2011. http://apps.who.int/medicinedocs/documents/s16874e/s16874e.pdf.

32. World Health Organization: *Country pharmaceutical situations: Fact Book on WHO Level 1 indicators 2007.* Geneva: WHO Press; 2010. http://apps.who.int/medicinedocs/documents/s16874e/s16874e.pdf.

33. World Health Organization: *Using indicators to measure country pharmaceutical situations; Fact Book on WHO Level I and Level II monitoring indicators, 2003.* Geneva: WHO Press; 2006. http://www.who.int/medicines/publications/WHOTCM2006.2A.pdf.

34. World Health Organization: *The World Medicines Situation.* Geneva: WHO; 2004. http://apps.who.int/medicinedocs/pdf/s6160e/s6160e.pdf..

35. World Health Organization: **The world medicines situation 2011: Access to care and medicines, burden of health care expenditures, and risk protection: results from the world health survey.** In *Eds. A.K. Wagner, A.J. Graves, S.K. Reiss, R. LeCates, F. Zhang and D.s Ross-Degnan.* 3rd edition. Edited by Holloway K, van Dijk L. Geneva: WHO; 2011. http://apps.who.int/medicinedocs/documents/s16874e/s16874e.pdf.

36. World Health Organization: *WHO Traditional medicine strategy 2002–2005.* Geneva: WHO/EDM/TRM/2002.1; 2002. http://apps.who.int/medicinedocs/pdf/s2297e/s2297e.pdf.

37. World Health Organization: *Guidelines on registration of traditional medicines in the WHO African Region.* Brazzaville: World Health Organization Regional Office for Africa; 2004. (AFR/TRM/04.1). http://whqlibdoc.who.int/afro/2004/AFR_TRM_04.1.pdf.

38. UNAIDS: *AIDS Epidemic Update: December 2003.* Geneva: WHO; 2003. http://data.unaids.org/publications/irc-pub06/jc943-epiupdate2003_en.pdf.

39. World Health Organization: In *The World Medicines Situation 2011: Traditional Medicines: Global Situation, Issues and Challenges.* 3rd edition. Edited by Robinson MM, Zhang X. Geneva: WHO; 2011. http://digicollection.org/hss/documents/s18063en/s18063en.pdf.

40. World Health Organization: *Report of the Regional Meeting on Traditional Medicine and Herbal Medicines. Guatemala City, 18–20 February 2003.* Geneva; 2003.

41. World Health Organization: *National policy on traditional medicine and regulation of herbal medicines: Report of a WHO global survey.* Geneva: WHO; 2005. http://apps.who.int/medicinedocs/pdf/s7916e/s7916e.pdf.

42. World Health Organization: *Resolution WHA62.13.* Geneva: Traditional medicine; 2009. http://apps.who.int/gb/ebwha/pdf_files/WHA62-REC1/WHA62_REC1-en-P2.pdf.

43. Li S, Han Q, Qiao C, Song J, Cheng CL, Xu H: **Chemical markers for the quality control of herbal medicines: An overview.** *Chinese Med* 2008, **28**:7.

44. World Health Organization: *Guidelines on minimum requirements for the registration of herbal medicinal products in the Eastern Mediterranean Region.* Cairo: World Health Organization Regional Office for the Eastern Mediterranean; 2006. WHO-EM/EDB/048/E.

45. World Health Organization: *Guidelines for the regulation of herbal medicines in the South-East Asia Region.* New Delhi: World Health Organization Regional Office for South-East Asia; 2004. SEA-Trad. Med.-82.

25

Ecotoxicology inside the gut: impact of heavy metals on the mouse microbiome

Jérôme Breton[1], Sébastien Massart[2], Peter Vandamme[3], Evie De Brandt[3], Bruno Pot[1] and Benoît Foligné[1*]

Abstract

Background: The gut microbiota is critical for intestinal homeostasis. Recent studies have revealed the links between different types of dysbiosis and diseases inside and outside the intestine. Environmental exposure to pollutants (such as heavy metals) can also impair various physiological functions for good health. Here, we studied the impact of up to 8 weeks of oral lead and cadmium ingestion on the composition of the murine intestinal microbiome.

Results: Pyrosequencing of 16S RNA sequences revealed minor but specific changes in bacterial commensal communities (at both family and genus levels) following oral exposure to the heavy metals, with notably low numbers of *Lachnospiraceae* and high numbers levels of *Lactobacillaceae* and *Erysipelotrichaceacae* (mainly due to changes in *Turicibacter spp)*, relative to control animals.

Conclusions: Non-absorbed heavy metals have a direct impact on the gut microbiota. In turn, this may impact the alimentary tract and overall gut homeostasis. Our results may enable more accurate assessment of the risk of intestinal disease associated with heavy metal ingestion.

Keywords: Heavy metal exposure, Gut microbiota, Mice, 16S pyrosequencing, *Turicibacter*, Denaturing gradient gel electrophoresis (DGGE)

Background

Chronic ingestion of environmental heavy metals (HMs, such as lead (Pb) and cadmium (Cd)) is associated with the occurrence of various diseases. The underlying mechanism is thought to be related to excessive local and systemic oxidative stress or deregulation of immune responses. Intestinal absorption of HMs leads to accumulation in specific target organs, with severe detrimental effects on human health. However, high concentrations of non-absorbed HMs remain in the gut microenvironment, where they may have a direct impact on the gut ecosystem and its overall physiology [1,2]. The gut microbiota has been described as a complex "hidden" organ, which plays a key role in the maintenance of health; hence, the presence or absence of specific species can be essential for maintaining homeostasis both inside and outside the intestinal tract [3,4].

The gastrointestinal epithelium has several essential functions: constituting a physical barrier, ensuring mucosal immune responses and excluding or detoxifying harmful intestinal content. These processes are highly influenced by the microbiota via a complex interplay with the host [5-7]. Disturbance of the microbiota (dysbiosis) is associated with an increased risk of developing inflammatory diseases, allergic diseases and metabolic disorders; hence, it is of the utmost importance to understand microbiotal variability if we are to better understand disease states [8,9]. The most studied factors affecting microbiota composition are age, genetic background, diet and antibiotic consumption [10]. It has also been postulated that exposure to xenobiotic agents from the environment is an important factor shaping the gut microbiota. However, little attention has been given to the potential impact of bioavailable HMs on the commensal microbiota and intestinal homeostasis. We thus sought to characterize possible impact of environmental Pb and Cd on the microbial ecosystem in mice, in order to better understand

* Correspondence: benoit.foligne@ibl.fr

[1]Bactéries Lactiques & Immunité des Muqueuses, Centre d'Infection et d'Immunité de Lille, Institut Pasteur de Lille, U1019, UMR 8204, Université Lille Nord de France, 1 rue du Pr Calmette, Lille cedex BP 245, F-59019, France

Full list of author information is available at the end of the article

the potential role of environmental factors in the etiology and pathogenesis of gastrointestinal disorders in humans.

Methods

Animals and ethics statement

Twenty-five Balb/C female mice (aged 6 weeks on arrival) were obtained from Charles River (Saint-Germain-sur-l'Arbresle, France). The animals were randomly divided into groups of five and housed in a controlled environment (a temperature of 22°C, a 12 h/12 h light/dark cycle and with *ad libitum* access to food and water). All animal experiments were performed according to the guidelines of the Institut Pasteur de Lille Animal Care and Use Committee and in compliance with the Amsterdam Protocol on Animal Protection and Welfare and the Directive 86/609/EEC on the Protection of Animals Used for Experimental and Other Scientific Purposes (updated in the Council of Europe's Appendix A). The animal work was also compliant with French legislation (the French Act 87–848, dated 19-10-1987) and the European Communities Amendment of Cruelty to Animals Act 1976. The study's objectives and procedures were approved by the Ethic and Welfare Committee for Experiments on Animals in France's Nord-Pas-de-Calais region (approval number: 04/2011).

Animal exposure procedures and experimental set-up

Mice were exposed to doses of either Cd (20 or 100 ppm) or Pb (100 or 500 ppm), where ppm correspond to mg L^{-1}. The metals were administered continuously for 8 weeks by spiking the animals' drinking water with CdCl$_2$ or PbCl$_2$ solution, as previously described [11]. In order to cover both "environmentally relevant (low)" and "critical" doses of Cd exposure and to mimic Pb poisoning, the HM doses were selected according to the respective "lowest observed adverse effect" level (LOAEL) for chronic exposure in rodents. Control animals received water with no added CdCl$_2$ or PbCl$_2$. Fecal pellets and cecal content were collected in tubes and weighed. Samples were snap-frozen and then stored at –80°C until nucleic acid extraction was performed, as described previously [12].

DNA extraction and PCR amplification

16S rRNA genes were amplified using the PCR primers [13], which target the V5 and V6 hypervariable regions. The forward primer contained the sequence of the Titanium A adaptor (5′-CCATCTCATCCCTGCGTG TCTCCGACTCAG-3′) and a barcode sequence. The reverse primer contained the sequence of Titanium B adaptor primer B: (5′-CCTATCCCCTGTGTGCCTT G-3′). For each sample, a PCR mix of 100 µL contained 1 × PCR buffer, 2 U of KAPA HiFi Hotstart polymerase blend and dNTPs (Kapabiosystems, Cliniscience, Naterre,

France), 300 nM primers (Eurogentec, Liège, Belgium), and 60 ng per g DNA. Thermal cycling consisted of initial denaturation at 95°C for 5 min, followed by 25 cycles of denaturation at 98°C for 20 s, annealing at 56°C for 40 s and extension at 72°C for 20 s, plus final extension at 72°C for 5 min. Amplicons were visualized on 1% agarose. Gels were stained with GelGreen Nucleic Acid gel stain in 1x Tris-acetate-EDTA (TAE) buffer and then cleaned with Wizard SV Gel and PCR Clean-up System (Promega, Charbonnieres les Bains, France), according to the manufacturer's instructions.

Amplicon quantitation, pooling, and pyrosequencing

Amplicon DNA concentrations were determined using the Quant-iT PicoGreen dsDNA reagent and kit (Life Tech, Carlsbad, CA) following the manufacturer's instructions. Assays were carried out using 2 µL of cleaned PCR product in a total reaction volume of 200 µL in black, 96-well microtiter plates. Following quantitation, cleaned amplicons were combined in equimolar ratios in a single tube .The final pool of DNA was eluted in 100 µL of nuclease-free water and purified using an Agencourt Ampure XP Purification Systems, according to the manufacturer's instructions (Agencourt Biosciences Corporation-Beckman Coulter, Beverly, MA) and then resuspended in 100 µL of TAE 1x. The concentration of the purified pooled DNA was determined using the Quant-iT PicoGreen dsDNA reagent and kit (Life Tech, Carlsbad, CA), according to the manufacturer's instructions. Pyrosequencing was carried out using primer A on a 454 Life Sciences Genome Sequencer FLX instrument (Roche, Branford, CT) following titanium chemistry.

16S rRNA data analysis

The sequences were assigned to samples as a function of their sample-specific barcodes. The sequences were then checked for the following criteria [14]: (i) an almost perfect match with the barcode and primers; (ii) at least 240 nucleotides in length (not including barcodes and primers); and (iii) no more than two undetermined bases (denoted by N). By "an almost perfect match", we mean that one mismatch/deletion/insertion per barcode or per primer was allowed. Each pyrosequenced dataset that passed quality control was assigned to a family with the RDP classifier (version 2.1, http://rdp.cme.msu.edu) with a confidence threshold > 80%. The Chao richness estimate was calculated with the Mothur software package (for more details, see http://www.mothur.org/wiki/Chao).

Denaturing gradient gel electrophoresis (DGGE)

The variable V3 region of the 16S rRNA gene was amplified using the universal bacterial primers F357-GC and R518 [15,16]. The PCR and temperature program have been described elsewhere [17]. The resulting 16S rRNA amplicons were analyzed by DGGE fingerprinting analysis (the D-Code System from Bio-Rad, Nazareth, Belgium) using 35% to 70% denaturing gels, as previously described [16]. Each lane received 30 µl of PCR product and electrophoresis was performed at 70 V for 990 min. Next, the DGGE gels were stained for 30 min with 1 X SYBR Gold nucleic acid gel stain (S-11494; Invitrogen, Merelbeke, Belgium) in 1 X TAE buffer (Bio-Rad), and the band profiles were digitized and visualized with a charge-coupled device (CCD) camera and Quantity One software (Bio-Rad). Every fifth or sixth lane contains a reference sample (containing the V3-16S rRNA amplicons of a taxonomically well-characterized strain for each of 12 bacterial species) and fingerprint profiles were normalized using BioNumerics software (version 5.10, Applied Maths, Sint-Martens-Latem, Belgium).

Statistics and data analysis

All statistical analyses were performed by comparing experimental groups with the control group. A non-parametric one–way analysis of variance, Mann–Whitney U-tests or Student's t tests were used as appropriate. Bacterial count data are presented as the mean ± standard error of the mean (SEM). The threshold for statistical significance was set to $p < 0.05$.

Results and discussion

In the present study, groups of wild-type mice underwent up to of 8 weeks continuous exposure to $CdCl_2$ (20 or 100 ppm) or $PbCl_2$ (100 or 500 ppm) administered in their drinking water. In an earlier study, these HM levels were sub-toxic and not associated with hepatotoxicity or changes in behavior, organ weights (liver, spleen and kidneys), body weight or overall growth (when compared with regular water-treated mice, [11]. Furthermore, none of the HM treatments had a detectable impact on our animals' food intake, stool consistency or gut motility. Indeed, this was demonstrated by providing oral exogenous food-grade microorganisms (such as yeasts and lactic bacteria) as feces markers. All the animals exhibited similar transit times and persistence parameters (data not shown).

We measured the microbial communities' profiles in feces and cecal content. On the basis of the DGGE results, an 8-week treatment with either Cd or Pb did not significantly modify the murine microbiota at either sampling site (Figure 1). A discriminant analysis of band classes (performed with Bionumerics software) enabled us to distinguish between fecal and colonic samples (Figure 2) and between control samples and HM-treated samples but did not pinpoint systematic differences between Pb and Cd treatments or between low and high concentrations of the HMs (results not shown). This finding contrasts with a recent report in which oral Cd had harmful effects on the viability of some components of the mouse microbiota [18]. This disparity might be explained by the fact that Fazeli and coworkers used restrictive

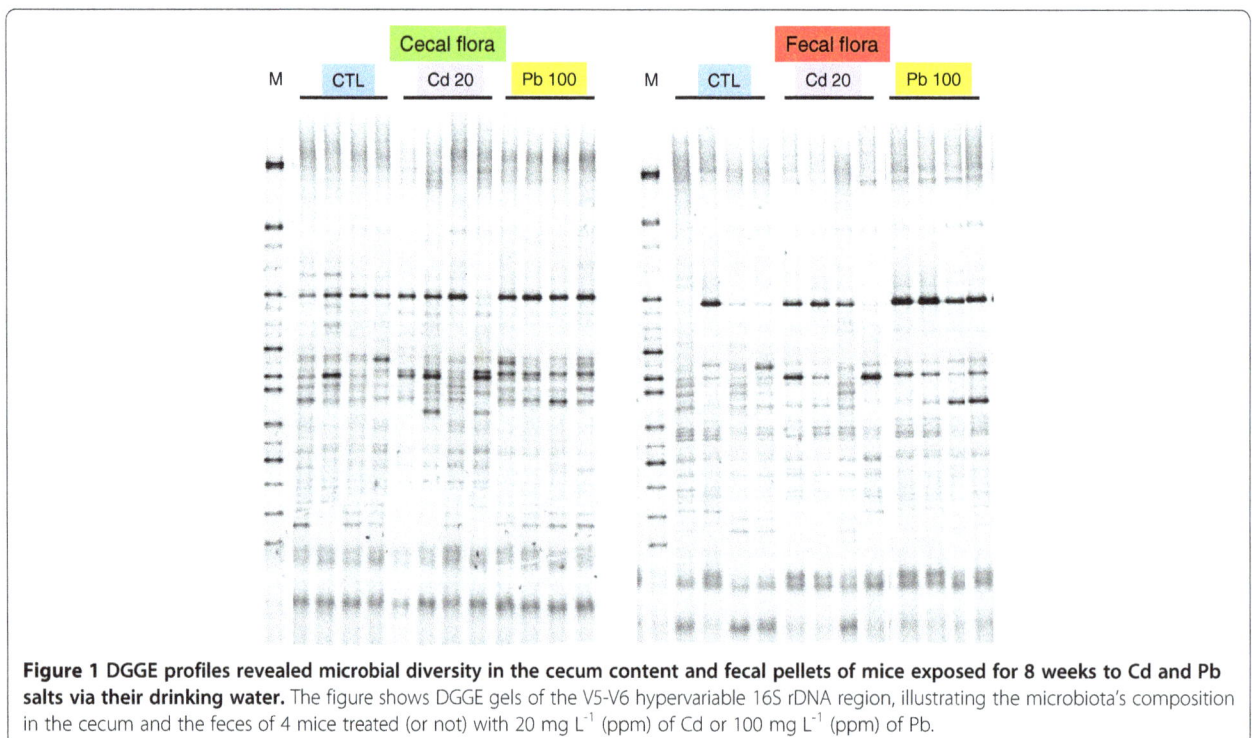

Figure 1 DGGE profiles revealed microbial diversity in the cecum content and fecal pellets of mice exposed for 8 weeks to Cd and Pb salts via their drinking water. The figure shows DGGE gels of the V5-V6 hypervariable 16S rDNA region, illustrating the microbiota's composition in the cecum and the feces of 4 mice treated (or not) with 20 mg L^{-1} (ppm) of Cd or 100 mg L^{-1} (ppm) of Pb.

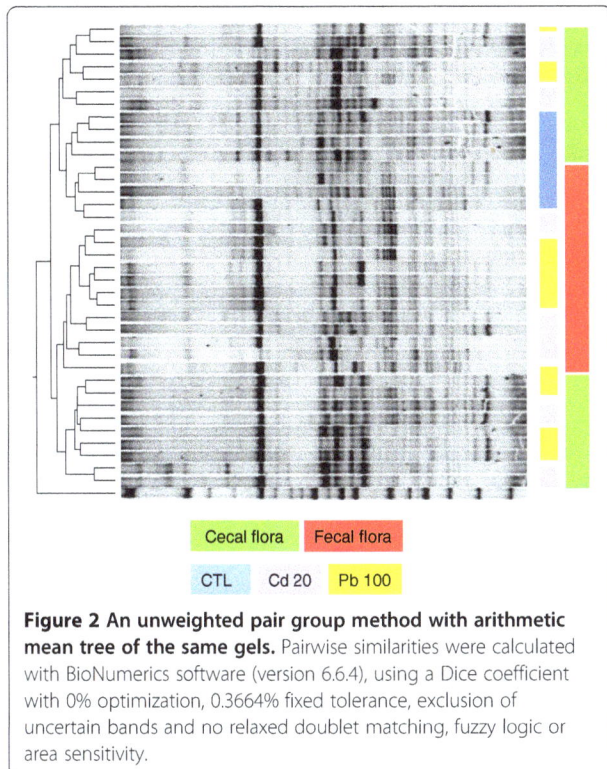

Figure 2 An unweighted pair group method with arithmetic mean tree of the same gels. Pairwise similarities were calculated with BioNumerics software (version 6.6.4), using a Dice coefficient with 0% optimization, 0.3664% fixed tolerance, exclusion of uncertain bands and no relaxed doublet matching, fuzzy logic or area sensitivity.

Cecal flora | Fecal flora

CTL | Cd 20 | Pb 100

conventional culture methods, whereas we used a molecular approach.

A more in-depth analysis of the cecal and fecal microbiome was carried out via 454 pyrosequencing of the V5-V6 region of the 16S rRNA (Table 1, Figures 3 and 4). We generated a dataset consisting of 197,143 filtered, high-quality 16S rRNA gene sequences (mean ± SD number of sequences per sample: 11,596 ± 6060). With operational taxonomic unit (OTU) cut-offs of 0.03, 0.05 or 0.10, the samples from the Cd, Pb and control groups did not differ significantly in terms of microbial richness (as estimated by the Chao richness index) or biodiversity (assessed by a nonparametric Shannon index). With an OTU cut-off of 0.03, the mean number of clusters was 1244 ± 381. The abundance of the two major phyla (the Firmicutes and Bacteroidetes) was similar in all three groups, whereas there were few Actinobacteria (Figure 3). In contrast, treatment with the two HMs was associated with a change in the composition of the colonic microbiota at both the family and genus levels. In fact, eight weeks of oral Cd or Pb treatment caused small but statistically significant differences in numbers of Prevotellaceae and Clostridiaceae (especially in the feces). Significant differences (p < 0.05) in the relative abundance of several other families in both cecal and fecal samples were observed, with low numbers of Lachnospiraceae and high numbers of Lactobacillaceae and Erysipelotrichaceae in the HM-treated groups

(Figure 4A). Within the Erysipelotrichaceae family, numbers of Turicibacter (Figure 4B), coprococci, streptococci, *Blautia, Barneselia* and *Allistipes* were higher in HM-treated groups than in controls. In general, we observed lower genus diversity in the HM-treated groups. Low bacterial diversity and low number of Lachnospiraceae have been linked to intestinal inflammation and considered as a predisposition to colitis [19,20]. Whether changes in Lachnospiraceae, Lactobacillaceae and Erysipelotrichaceae are consistently linked with inflammation remains to be established. However, the frequent literature reports on changes in the abundance of these groups in the mouse microbiome indicate that these groups are more sensitive to external factors than other, less abundant groups are. However, cautious interpretation is necessary because of the low family-level resolution of metagenomics, which prevents reliable microbial community analyses under in inflammatory conditions, for example [21].

The genus *Turicibacter* was previously detected in the ileal pouch of an ulcerative colitis patient [22], in human appendicitis [23] and in infectious states in piglets. Interestingly, high levels of *Turicibacter* were observed in mice fed an iron-free diet (in which these bacteria might favor anti-inflammatory effects) [24] and in colitis-resistant CD8-knock-out mice (where it is potentially involved in the anti-inflammatory phenotype) [25]. The ongoing sequencing of several *Turicibacter* spp genomes will hopefully clarify their function as part of the microbiota and elucidate their role(s) in the interaction between HM exposure and inflammation [26]. Lastly, the lactobacilli's apparent ability to tolerate HMs might be helpful for bioremediation purposes, since some microorganisms can bind labile metal ions and remove them from the environment [27]. In theory, HM-resistant, innocuous strains with anti-oxidant and anti-inflammatory properties could be used as probiotics by combining their chelating properties with targeted treatment of the xenobiotics' harmful effects on the host's microbiota [28,29].

Laboratory mice have a less complex gut microbiota than humans and there are only slight mouse-to-mouse variations when groups of individuals are housed together. Nevertheless, HM-associated differences in the microbiota were observed in all individual, exposed mice (data not shown). Our DGGE and metagenomics results confirmed a clear link between ingestion of HMs and the composition of the gut microbiota. The marked, environmentally-induced alteration in the gut microbiota also suggests a link between HM exposure and inflammation. However, the functional classification of groups of bacteria as "predisposing", "colitogenic" or even "protective" is hotly debated and difficult to investigate [23]. Besides producing quantitative and qualitative changes

Table 1 Relative distributions of bacterial phylotypes, families and genera in (i) the cecum content of mice orally exposed for 8 weeks to Cd (20 or 100 ppm) or Pb (100 or 500 ppm) salts and (ii) the fecal pellets for mice orally exposed for 8 weeks to Cd (20 ppm) or Pb (100 ppm)

Phylum	Cd0Pb0	Cd20	Cd100	Pb100	Pb500
Cecal content					
Actinobacteria	0.25%	0.59%	1.19%	2.27%	0.25%
(range)	(0.11-0.40)	(0.16-1.30)	(0.36-1.84)	(0.11-5.39)	(0.10-0.40)
SEM	0.049	0.210	0.272	1.113	0.161
P value	-	0.0775	0.0045	0.0537	0.478
Bacteroidetes	1.9%	2.58%	1.60%	1.47%	1.36%
(range)	s(1.29-2.28)	(0.35-7.66)	(0.31-4.97)	(0.30-3.36)	(0.8-2.40)
SEM	0.183	1.328	0.854	0.612	0.3
P value	-	0.3131	0.3697	0.2578	0.0869
Firmicutes	97.8%	96.77%	97.2%	96.24%	98.36%
(range)	(97.4-98.4)	(92.0-99.3)	(93.1-98.8)	(91.1-99.6)	(97.9-99.0)
SEM	0.187	1.297	1.037	1.739	0.272
P value	-	0.2269	0.2916	0.1986	0.1755
Fecal pellet					
Actinobacteria	0.30%	0.39%		0.24%	
(range)	(0.18-0.50)	(0.13-0.65)		(0.08-0.42)	
SEM	0.053	0.089		0.058	
P value	-	0.2304		0.2188	
Bacteroidetes	34.4%	38.8%		35.65%	
(range)	(12.5-50.8)	(30.1-7.5)		(22.4-51.5)	
SEM	6.56	10.84		8.65	
P value	-	0.3670		0.4553	
Firmicutes	64.7%	60.44%		63.85%	
(range)	(48.2-71.3)	(47.5-90.9)		(38.2-77.5)	
SEM	6.73	10.86		8.72	
P value	-	0.3736		0.4701	
Family	**Cd0Pb0**	**Cd20**	**Cd100**	**Pb100**	**Pb500**
Cecal content					
Lachnospiraceae	72.6%	53.17%	25.9%	43.7%	67.5%
(range)	(33.2-88.3)	(26.8-76.6)	(10.3-28.5)	(27.1-61.4)	(59.1-75.0)
SEM	10.01	9.24	4.15	6.09	2.62
P value	-	0.037	0.0081	0.0378	0.05859
Lactobacillaceae	22.34%	38.20%	54.68%	38.24%	26.1%
(range)	(5.6-64.9)	(19.01-60.6)	(41.6-81.6)	(28.7-67.1)	(19.2-32.1)
SEM	10.88	8.54	7.06	7.26	2.09
P value	-	0.05859	0.0379	0.0379	0.05859
Ruminococcaceae	1.82%	2.15%	2.64%	2.15%	1.14%
(range)	(0.72-3.01)	(0.76-5.91)	(0.81-7.21)	(0.63-3.22)	(0.58-1.67)
SEM	0.442	0.836	0.876	0.934	0.939
P value	-	0.3804	0.2627	0.3106	0.0997

Table 1 Relative distributions of bacterial phylotypes, families and genera in (i) the cecum content of mice orally exposed for 8 weeks to Cd (20 or 100 ppm) or Pb (100 or 500 ppm) salts and (ii) the fecal pellets for mice orally exposed for 8 weeks to Cd (20 ppm) or Pb (100 ppm) *(Continued)*

Porphyromonadaceae	0.42%	0.63%	0.42%	0.49%	0.41%
(range)	(0.0-1.25)	(0.0-2.24)	(0.0-1.41)	(0.0-1.65)	(0.05-1.24)
SEM	0.228	0.438	0.433	0.415	0.411
P value	-	*0.3152*	*0.4774*	*0.4139*	*0.0641*
Rikenellaceae	0.51%	0.42%	0.27%	0.21%	0.26%
(range)	(0.0-1.32)	(0.0-1.32)	(0.0-0.92)	(0.0-0.6)	
(0.0-0.47)					
SEM	0.250	0.245	0.259	0.174	0.174
P value	-	*0.3883*	*0.2216*	*0.1564*	*0.1800*
Coriobacteriaceae	0.49%	1.19%	2.38%	4.57%	0.36%
(range)	(0.2-0.76)	(0.23-2.6)	(0.69-4.35)	(0.2-11.75)	(0.1-0.51)
SEM	0.111	0.0939	0.107	0.433	0.138
P value	-	*0.1736*	*0.01414*	*0.0250*	*0.3*
Streptococcaceae	0.3%	0.14%	0.15%	0.24%	0.04%
(range)	(0.0-0.50)	(0.05-0.3)	(0.0-0.66)	(0–0.75)	(0–0.1)
SEM	0.102	0.0239	0.0983	0.0894	0.0581
P value	-	*0.0901*	*0.1905*	*0.3711*	*0.0164*
Erysipelotrichaceae	0.1%	2.32%	12.98%	6.89%	3.6%
(range)	(0.0-0.24)	(0.42-8.02)	(3.82-28.12)	(2.13-14)	(1.73-6.05)
SEM	0.044	0.232	0.219	0.268	0.02236
P value	-	*0.0182*	*0.0096*	*0.0096*	*0.00051*

Family	Cd0Pb0	Cd20		Pb100	
Fecal pellet					
Lachnospiraceae	37.36%	23.67%		12.55%	
(range)	(18.8-86.9)	1.77-82.9)		(3.52-26.6)	
SEM	12.81	14.14		17.28	
P value	-	*0.0453*		*0.023*	
Lactobacillaceae	32.99%	42.77%		50.88%	
(range)	(10.3-51.2)	(4.49-67.1)		(25.1-65.6)	
SEM	8.58	8.87		10.02	
P value	-	*0.2782*		*0.1121*	
Ruminococcaceae	1.70%	1.4%		0.83%	
(range)	(0.24-3.46)	(0.08-4.58)		(0.11-1.61)	
SEM	0.65	0.65		0.86	
P value	-	*0.3916*		*0.1275*	
Porphyromonadaceae	11.14%	13.01%		12%	
(range)	(3.46-16.25)	(1.60-22.04)		(4.88-19.6)	
SEM	2.22	3.11		3.84	
P value	-	*0.3447*		*0.4075*	
Rikenellaceae	8.36%	4.99%		5.82%	
(range)	(5.71-14.18)	(1.93-16.07)		(0.45-18.5)	
SEM	1.92	2.47		2.87	
P value	-	*0.1736*		*0.2626*	

Table 1 Relative distributions of bacterial phylotypes, families and genera in (i) the cecum content of mice orally exposed for 8 weeks to Cd (20 or 100 ppm) or Pb (100 or 500 ppm) salts and (ii) the fecal pellets for mice orally exposed for 8 weeks to Cd (20 ppm) or Pb (100 ppm) *(Continued)*

Coriobacteriaceae	0.68%	0.67%		0.41%	
(range)	(0.03-0.99)	(0.32-1.32)		(0.16-0.67)	
SEM	0.137	0.114		0.159	
P value	-	*0.4841*		*0.0677*	
Streptococcaceae	0.27%	0.26%		0.20%	
(range)	(0.0-0.68)	(0.02-0.69)		(0–0.36)	
SEM	0.127	0.129		0.09	
P value	-	*0.4969*		*0.3060*	
Erysipelotrichaceae	0.33%	4.05%		6.56%	
(range)	(0.0-0.89)	(0.48-15.53)		(0.44-20.7)	
SEM	0.158	0.399		0.4033	
P value	-	*0.0585*		*0.0107*	
Prevotellaceae	0.14%	1.06%		0.75%	
(range)	(0.0-0.25)	(0.08-4.14)		(0.11-1.22)	
SEM	0.058	0.806		0.812	
P value	-	*0.1345*		*0.049*	
Clostridiaceae	0.00%	0.675%		1.55%	
(range)	(0.0-0.00)	(0.0-2.17)		(0.0-3.06)	
SEM	0.0	0.094		0.0940	
P value	-	*0.0628*		*0.0086*	

Genus	CdOPb0	Cd20	Cd100	Pb100	Pb500
Cecal content					
Lactobacillus	75.28	84.57%	77.4%	74.8%	83.82%
(range)	(60–98.9)	(68–91.11)	(57.6-93.6)	(54.1-90.6)	(80.4-89.3)
SEM	7.554	4.419	5.97	7.741	1.589
P value	-	*0.2229*	*0.1248*	*0.1234*	*0.1503*
Blautia	5.39%	2.82%	0.36%	4.90%	0.78%
(range)	(0–12.6)	(0.45-8.8)	(0–0.97)	(0–9.2)	(0.3-1.22)
SEM	2.58	1.526	0.176	1.990	0.165
P value	-	*0.2456*	*0.1085*	*0.1136*	*0.2036*
Coprococcus	3.49%	3.06%	0.46%	1.65%	0.64%
(range)	(0–7.95)	(0.22-6.49)	(0.14-0.73)	(0.7-3.62)	(0.32-1.2)
SEM	1.651	1.172	0.110	0.521	0.151
P value	-	*0.1874*	*0.2086*	*0.2677*	*0.2757*
Alistipes	3.42%	1.40%	0.41%	0.40%	0.74%
(range)	(0.0-12.5)(0.0-4.0)	(0.0-1.49)	(0.0-1.16)	(0.0-1.34)	
SEM	2.40	0.725	0.273	0.232	0.221
P value	-	*0.2084*	*0.0439*	*0.4421*	*0.0461*
Steptococcus	2.84%	0.35%	0.24%	0.47%	0.11%
(range)	(0.0-6.67)	(0.11-0.80)	(0.0-1.05)	(0.0-1.45)	(0.0-0.24)
SEM	1.235	0.132	0.204	0.274	0.0514
P value	-	*0.4189*	*0.0522*	*0.1590*	*0.0616*

Table 1 Relative distributions of bacterial phylotypes, families and genera in (i) the cecum content of mice orally exposed for 8 weeks to Cd (20 or 100 ppm) or Pb (100 or 500 ppm) salts and (ii) the fecal pellets for mice orally exposed for 8 weeks to Cd (20 ppm) or Pb (100 ppm) *(Continued)*

Barnesiella	1.56%	0.34%	0.44%	0.66%	0.72%
(range)	(0.0-6.67)	(0.0-0.8)	(0.0-1.35)	(0.0-2.6)	(0.0-2.27)
SEM	1.295	0.152	0.244	0.503	0.404
P value	-	*0.1598*	*0.4157*	*0.4842*	*0.1505*
Bacteroides	0.95%	0.44%	0.09%	0.11%	0.36%
(range)	(0.0-3.33)	(0.0-1.6)	(0.0-0.37)	(0–0.54)	(0–1.29)
SEM	0.631	0.292	0.071	0.108	0.236
P value	-	*0.0401*	*0.0356*	*0.0489*	*0.0229*
Turicibacter	0.28%	4.02%	19.63%	14.34%	11.32%
(range)	(0.0-1.15)	(0.76-11.8)	(4.48-41.3)	(3.09-22.15)	(6.37-15.4)
SEM	0.222	1.987	6.566	4.599	1.749
P value	-	*0.0492*	*0.0092*	*0.0078*	*0.0001*

Genus	Cd0Pb0	Cd20		Pb100	
Fecal pellet					
Lactobacillus	49.31%	58.0%		63.07%	
(range)	(8.96-73.18)	(22.4-88.4)		(34.4-82.9)	
SEM	10.71	12.14		11.67	
P value	-	*0.3032*		*0.2053*	
Blautia	0.73%	0.75%		0.28%	
(range)	(0.0-2.99)	(0.0-3.28)		(0.0-0.64)	
SEM	0.570	0.634		0.143	
P value	-	*0.4873*		*0.2331*	
Coprococcus	1.61%	0.83%		0.14%	
(range)	(0.0-5.97)	(0.0-3.48)		(0.0-0.32)	
SEM	1.101	0.664		0.065	
P value	-	*0.2795*		*0.1091*	
Alistipes	17.5%	8.47%		7.20%	
(range)	(7.2-29.8)	(2.0-19.3)		(0.43-24.5)	
SEM	3.871	3.822		4.454	
P value	-	*0.0678*		*0.0495*	
Steptococcus	0.50%	0.38%		0.28%	
(range)	(0.0-1.44)	(0.1-0.87)		(0.0-0.5)	
SEM	0.263	0.152		0.094	
P value	-	*0.3494*		*0.2254*	
Barnesiella	14.18%	9.13%		7.38%	
(range)	(6.8-25.3)	(5.12-16.7)		(2.4-11.8)	
SEM	3.049	2.216		1.711	
P value	-	*0.1086*		*0.0438*	
Bacteroides	11.17%	12.32%		10.46%	
(range)	(4.7-19.6)	(2.08-39.9)		(3.76-24.8)	
SEM	3.175	7.419		4.364	
P value	-	*0.4448*		*0.4492*	

Table 1 Relative distributions of bacterial phylotypes, families and genera in (i) the cecum content of mice orally exposed for 8 weeks to Cd (20 or 100 ppm) or Pb (100 or 500 ppm) salts and (ii) the fecal pellets for mice orally exposed for 8 weeks to Cd (20 ppm) or Pb (100 ppm) *(Continued)*

Turicibacter	0.75%	4.81%	8.71%
(range)	(0.0-1.49)	(0.82-17.6)	(2.84-28.24)
SEM	0.307	3.236	4.996
P value	-	*0.0483*	*0.0281*

Data are expressed as the mean, range and SEM percentage abundance of the total assignment (n = 5 animals per group) and the corresponding p value is given in italics. The threshold for statistical significance was set to p < 0.05.

in the gut microbiota, HMs also impact (directly or indirectly) intestinal homeostasis through their many local effects (on the epithelia mucosa) and systemic effects. Indeed, we previously reported that chronic ingestion of Cd and Pb induced (i) anemia and tissue iron loss from tissues, (ii) slight but consistent changes in the expression of transport-related genes, (iii) the small intestine and colon's oxidative and inflammatory status and (iv) genotoxicity [11]. It is difficult to predict the net inflammatory balance in this context, since both harmful and adaptive events occur together. We also recently emphasized the key role of the microbiota in the process of HM absorption and dissemination throughout the body - illustrating the complex metal-microbe-host interplay that operates [30]. Our present ecotoxicological results complement that first attempt to identify the impact of HMs on the gut's microbial ecology. This is in line with the need to develop a more comprehensive view of environmental exposure, i.e. one that is not restricted

to the mere entry of xenobiotics into the body but also takes account of inflammation, oxidative stress, other gut flora, metabolic processes and a continually fluctuating chemical environment. Defining this type of integrated "exposome" may provide a way of causally linking long-term exposure to the occurrence of chronic disease [31].

Conclusions

Non-absorbed heavy metals have a direct impact on the gut microbiota. In turn, this may impact the alimentary tract and overall gut homeostasis. Our results may enable more accurate assessment of the risk of intestinal disease associated with heavy metal ingestion. Further studies are needed to understand the complex crosstalk between the gut microbiota and the host, interpret the clinical consequences of exposure to xenobiotics and assess the relationship between the environment and disease susceptibility.

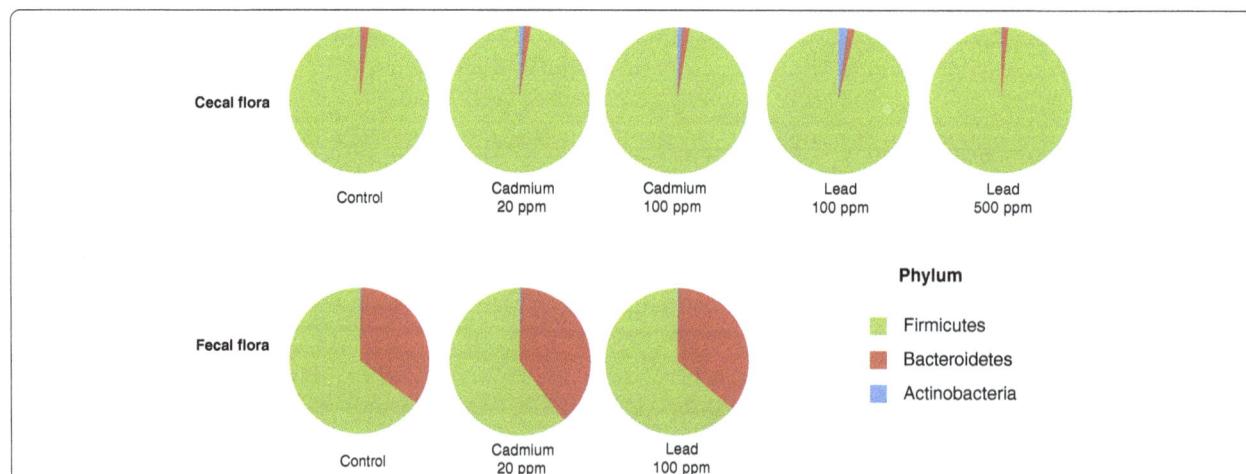

Figure 3 Distribution of bacterial phylotypes in the cecum content and fecal pellets of mice exposed for 8 weeks to Cd (20 or 100 ppm) or Pb (100 or 500 ppm) salts via their drinking water. 16S rRNA-base analyses were derived from 454/Roche multitag pyrosequencing. Data are expressed as the mean percentage abundance of the total assignment (n = 5 animals per group). In line with the literature data, most of the bacteria in untreated (control) mice belonged to Firmicutes or the Bacteroidetes, whereas Actinobacteria were very rare.

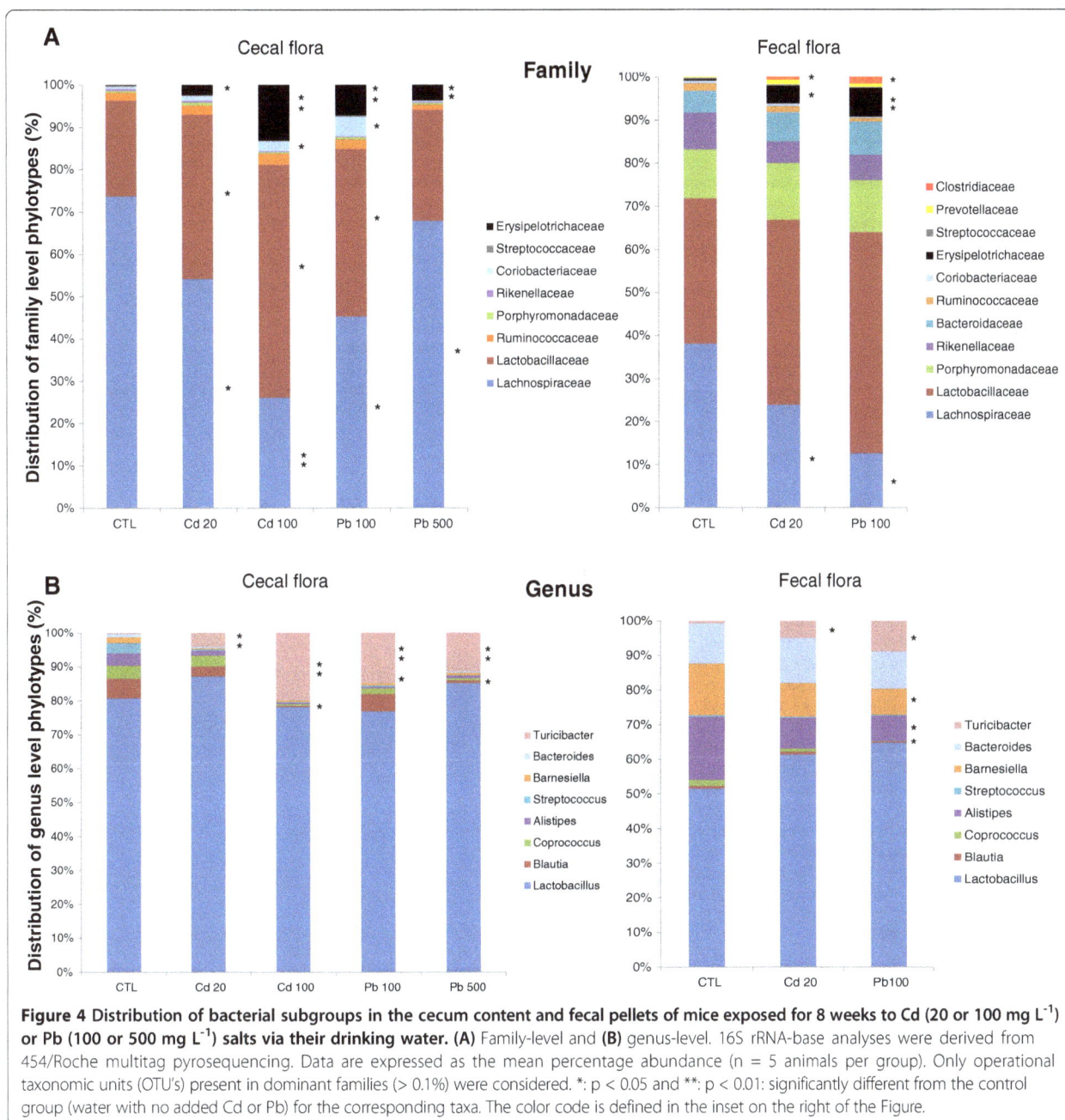

Figure 4 Distribution of bacterial subgroups in the cecum content and fecal pellets of mice exposed for 8 weeks to Cd (20 or 100 mg L^{-1}) or Pb (100 or 500 mg L^{-1}) salts via their drinking water. **(A)** Family-level and **(B)** genus-level. 16S rRNA-base analyses were derived from 454/Roche multitag pyrosequencing. Data are expressed as the mean percentage abundance (n = 5 animals per group). Only operational taxonomic units (OTU's) present in dominant families (> 0.1%) were considered. *: p < 0.05 and **: p < 0.01: significantly different from the control group (water with no added Cd or Pb) for the corresponding taxa. The color code is defined in the inset on the right of the Figure.

Competing interests

None of all authors have conflicts of interest to declare.

Authors' contributions

BF and BP: study conception and design and drafting of the manuscript; BF, JB, SM, EDB and PVD: data acquisition; BF, SM, PVD and BP: data analysis and interpretation. All authors read and approved the final manuscript.

Acknowledgments

This study was funded by a grant from the French National Research Agency (ANR-09-CES-016: Mélodie-Reve). The authors thank Dr Fabienne Jean for her assistance with project management and Humphrey Bihain-Tasseur for valuable advice.

Author details

[1]Bactéries Lactiques & Immunité des Muqueuses, Centre d'Infection et d'Immunité de Lille, Institut Pasteur de Lille, U1019, UMR 8204, Université Lille Nord de France, 1 rue du Pr Calmette, Lille cedex BP 245, F-59019, France. [2]DNAVision SA, avenue George Lemaitre 25, Charleroi B-6041, Belgium. [3]Laboratory of Microbiology, Faculty of Sciences, Ledeganckstraat 35, Ghent B-9000, Belgium.

References

1. Zalups RK, Ahmad S: **Molecular handling of cadmium in transporting epithelia.** *Toxicol Appl Pharmacol* 2003, **186**(3):163–188.

2. James HM, Hilburn ME, Blair JA: Effects of meals and meal times on uptake of lead from the gastrointestinal tract in humans. *Hum Toxicol* 1985, **4**(4):401–407.

3. O'Hara AM, Shanahan F: The gut flora as a forgotten organ. *EMBO* 2006, **7**(7):688–693. Rep.

4. Sekirov I, Russell SL, Antunes LC, Finlay BB: Gut microbiota in health and disease. *Physiol Rev* 2010, **90**(3):859–904.

5. Leser TD, Molbak L: Better living through microbial action: the benefits of the mammalian gastrointestinal microbiota on the host. *Environ Microbiol* 2009, **11**(9):2194–2206.

6. Nicholson JK, Holmes E, Wilson ID: Gut microorganisms, mammalian metabolism and personalized health care. *Nat Rev Microbiol* 2005, **3**(5):431–438.

7. Claus SP, Ellero SL, Berger B, Krause L, Bruttin A, Molina J, Paris A, Want EJ, de Waziers I, Cloarec O, et al: Colonization-induced host-gut microbial metabolic interaction. *MBio* 2011, **2**(2):e00271–10.

8. DuPont AW, DuPont HL: The intestinal microbiota and chronic disorders of the gut. *Nat Rev Gastroenterol Hepatol* 2011, **8**(9):523–531.

9. Clemente JC, Ursell LK, Parfrey LW, Knight R: The impact of the gut microbiota on human health: an integrative view. *Cell* 2012, **148**(6):1258–1270.

10. Lozupone CA, Stombaugh JI, Gordon JI, Jansson JK, Knight R: Diversity, stability and resilience of the human gut microbiota. *Nature* 2012, **489**(7415):220–230.

11. Breton J, Le Clère K, Daniel C, Sauty M, Nakab L, Chassat T, Dewulf J, Penet S, Carnoy C, Thomas P, et al: Chronic ingestion of cadmium and lead alters the bioavailability of essential and heavy metals, gene expression pathways and genotoxicity in mouse intestine. *Arch Toxicol* 2013, **87**(10):1787–1795.

12. Matsuda K, Tsuji H, Asahara T, Matsumoto K, Takada T, Nomoto K: Establishment of an analytical system for the human fecal microbiota, based on reverse transcription-quantitative PCR targeting of multicopy rRNA molecules. *Appl Environ Microbiol* 2009, **75**(7):1961–1969.

13. Andersson AF, Riemann L, Bertilsson S: Pyrosequencing reveals contrasting seasonal dynamics of taxa within Baltic Sea bacterioplankton communities. *ISME J* 2010, **4**(2):171–181.

14. De Filippo C, Cavalieri D, Di Paola M, Ramazzotti M, Poullet JB, Massart S, Collini S, Pieraccini G, Lionetti P: Impact of diet in shaping gut microbiota revealed by a comparative study in children from Europe and rural Africa. *Proc Natl Acad Sci U S A* 2010, **107**(33):14691–14696.

15. Yu Z, Morrison M: Comparisons of different hypervariable regions of rrs genes for use in fingerprinting of microbial communities by PCR-denaturing gradient gel electrophoresis. *Appl Environ Microbiol* 2004, **70**(8):4800–4806.

16. Temmerman R, Scheirlinck I, Huys G, Swings J: Culture-independent analysis of probiotic products by denaturing gradient gel electrophoresis. *Appl Environ Microbiol* 2003, **69**(1):220–226.

17. Vanhoutte T, Huys G, De Brandt E, Swings J: Temporal stability analysis of the microbiota in human feces by denaturing gradient gel electrophoresis using universal and group-specific 16S rRNA gene primers. *FEMS Microbiol Ecol* 2004, **48**(3):437–446.

18. Fazeli M, Hassanzadeh P, Alaei S: Cadmium chloride exhibits a profound toxic effect on bacterial microflora of the mice gastrointestinal tract. *Hum Exp Toxicol* 2011, **30**(2):152–159.

19. Lepage P, Häsler R, Spehlmann ME, Rehman A, Zvirbliene A, Begun A, Ott S, Kupcinskas L, Doré J, Raedler A, Schreiber S: Twin study indicates loss of interaction between microbiota and mucosa of patients with ulcerative colitis. *Gastroenterology* 2011, **141**(1):227–236.

20. Brinkman BM, Hildebrand F, Kubica M, Goosens D, Del Favero J, Declercq W, Raes J, Vandenabeele P: Caspase deficiency alters the murine gut microbiome. *Cell Death Dis* 2011, **2**:e220.

21. Berry D, Schwab C, Milinovich G, Reichert J, Ben Mahfoudh K, Decker T, Engel M, Hai B, Hainzl E, Heider S, et al: Phylotype-level 16S rRNA analysis reveals new bacterial indicators of health state in acute murine colitis. *ISME J* 2012, **6**(11):2091–2106.

22. Falk A, Olsson C, Ahrné S, Molin G, Adawi D, Jeppsson B: Ileal pelvic pouch microbiota from two former ulcerative colitis patients, analysed by DNA-based methods, were unstable over time and showed the presence of *Clostridium perfringens*. *Scand J Gastroenterol* 2007, **42**(8):973–985.

23. Bosshard PP, Zbinden R, Altwegg M: *Turicibacter sanguinis* gen. *nov.*, sp. *nov.*, a novel anaerobic, Gram-positive bacterium. *Int J Syst Evol Microbiol* 2002, **52**(Pt4):1263–1266.

24. Werner T, Wagner SJ, Martínez I, Walter J, Chang JS, Clavel T, Kisling S, Schuemann K, Haller D: Depletion of luminal iron alters the gut microbiota and prevents Crohn's disease-like ileitis. *Gut* 2011, **60**(3):325–333.

25. Presley LL, Wei B, Braun J, Borneman J: Bacteria associated with immunoregulatory cells in mice. *Appl Environ Microbiol* 2010, **76**(3):936–941.

26. Po C, Klaassens ES, Durkin AS, Harkins DM, Foster L, McCorrison J, Torralba M, Nelson KE, Morrison M: Draft genome sequence of *Turicibacter sanguinis* PC909, isolated from human feces. *J Bacteriol* 2011, **193**(5):1288–1289.

27. Upreti RK, Shrivastava R, Chaturvedi UC: Gut microflora & toxic metals: chromium as a model. *Indian J Med Res* 2004, **119**(2):49–59.

28. Lemon KP, Armitage GC, Relman DA, Fischbach MA: Microbiota-targeted therapies: an ecological perspective. *Sci Transl Med* 2012, **4**(137):137. rv5.

29. Quigley EM: Prebiotics and probiotics; modifying and mining the microbiota. *Pharmacol Res* 2010, **61**(3):213–218.

30. Breton J, Daniel C, Dewulf J, Pothion S, Froux N, Sauty M, Thomas P, Pot B, Foligné B: Gut microbiota limits heavy metals burden caused by chronic oral exposure. *Toxicol Lett* 2013, **222**(2):132–138.

31. Rappaport SM, Smith MT: Epidemiology environment and disease risks. *Science* 2010, **330**(6003):460–461.

Permissions

The contributors of this book come from diverse backgrounds, making this book a truly international effort. This book will bring forth new frontiers with its revolutionizing research information and detailed analysis of the nascent developments around the world.

We would like to thank all the contributing authors for lending their expertise to make the book truly unique. They have played a crucial role in the development of this book. Without their invaluable contributions this book wouldn't have been possible. They have made vital efforts to compile up to date information on the varied aspects of this subject to make this book a valuable addition to the collection of many professionals and students.

This book was conceptualized with the vision of imparting up-to-date information and advanced data in this field. To ensure the same, a matchless editorial board was set up. Every individual on the board went through rigorous rounds of assessment to prove their worth. After which they invested a large part of their time researching and compiling the most relevant data for our readers.

The editorial board has been involved in producing this book since its inception. They have spent rigorous hours researching and exploring the diverse topics which have resulted in the successful publishing of this book. They have passed on their knowledge of decades through this book. To expedite this challenging task, the publisher supported the team at every step. A small team of assistant editors was also appointed to further simplify the editing procedure and attain best results for the readers.

Apart from the editorial board, the designing team has also invested a significant amount of their time in understanding the subject and creating the most relevant covers. They scrutinized every image to scout for the most suitable representation of the subject and create an appropriate cover for the book.

The publishing team has been an ardent support to the editorial, designing and production team. Their endless efforts to recruit the best for this project, has resulted in the accomplishment of this book. They are a veteran in the field of academics and their pool of knowledge is as vast as their experience in printing. Their expertise and guidance has proved useful at every step. Their uncompromising quality standards have made this book an exceptional effort. Their encouragement from time to time has been an inspiration for everyone.

The publisher and the editorial board hope that this book will prove to be a valuable piece of knowledge for researchers, students, practitioners and scholars across the globe.

List of Contributors

Stephanie Berthet
Unité INSERM 1027, Equipe de Pharmacoépidémiologie, Université de Toulouse (Université Paul Sabatier), Toulouse, France

Pascale Olivier
Unité INSERM 1027, Equipe de Pharmacoépidémiologie, Université de Toulouse (Université Paul Sabatier), Toulouse, France
Centre Régional de Pharmacovigilance, de Pharmacoépidémiologie et d'Information sur le Médicament, Service de Pharmacologie Clinique, Hôpitaux de Toulouse, Toulouse, France

Jean-Louis Montastruc
Unité INSERM 1027, Equipe de Pharmacoépidémiologie, Université de Toulouse (Université Paul Sabatier), Toulouse, France
Centre Régional de Pharmacovigilance, de Pharmacoépidémiologie et d'Information sur le Médicament, Service de Pharmacologie Clinique, Hôpitaux de Toulouse, Toulouse, France

Maryse Lapeyre-Mestre
INSERM 1027, Equipe de Pharmacoépidémiologie, Université de Toulouse (Université Paul Sabatier), Toulouse, France
Centre Régional de Pharmacovigilance, de Pharmacoépidémiologie et d'Information sur le Médicament, Service de Pharmacologie Clinique, Hôpitaux de Toulouse, Toulouse, France

Elmira Far
Department of Clinical Pharmacology and Toxicology, University Hospital Zurich, Rämistrasse 100, 8091 Zurich, Switzerland

Ivanka Curkovic
Department of Clinical Pharmacology and Toxicology, University Hospital Zurich, Rämistrasse 100, 8091 Zurich, Switzerland

Kelly Byrne
Department of Clinical Pharmacology and Toxicology, University Hospital Zurich, Rämistrasse 100, 8091 Zurich, Switzerland

Malgorzata Roos
Division of Biostatistics, ISPM, University Zurich, Hirschengraben 8, 8001 Zurich, Switzerland

Isabelle Egloff
Department of Clinical Pharmacology and Toxicology, University Hospital Zurich, Rämistrasse 100, 8091 Zurich, Switzerland

Michael Dietrich
Department of Orthopaedic, Balgrist University Hospital, Forchstrasse 340, 8008 Zurich, Switzerland

Wilhelm Kirch
Institute of Clinical Pharmacology, Medical Faculty Technical University of Dresden, Fiedlerstrasse 27, D - 01307 Dresden, Germany

Gerd-A Kullak-Ublick
Department of Clinical Pharmacology and Toxicology, University Hospital Zurich, Rämistrasse 100, 8091 Zurich, Switzerland

Marco Egbring
Department of Clinical Pharmacology and Toxicology, University Hospital Zurich, Rämistrasse 100, 8091 Zurich, Switzerland

Clémence Perraudin
Faculté de Médecine Paris-Sud Paris XI, Le Kremlin-Bicêtre, France
Institut National de la Santé et de la Recherche Médicale (INSERM) Unité 988, Villejuif, France
Centre National de la Recherche Scientifique (CNRS) UMR 8211, Villejuif, France
Ecole des Hautes Etudes en Sciences Sociales (EHESS), Paris, France

Françoise Brion
Faculté de Pharmacie, Université Paris Descartes, France
APHP Hôpital Robert Debré, Paris, France

Olivier Bourdon
Faculté de Pharmacie, Université Paris Descartes, France
APHP Hôpital Robert Debré, Paris, France

Nathalie Pelletier-Fleury
Institut National de la Santé et de la Recherche Médicale (INSERM) Unité 988, Villejuif, France
Centre National de la Recherche Scientifique (CNRS) UMR 8211, Villejuif, France
Ecole des Hautes Etudes en Sciences Sociales (EHESS), Paris, France

Steven T Bird
Department of Health and Human Services/Food and Drug Administration/ Center for Drug Evaluation and Research (CDER)/Office of Management/ CDER Academic Collaboration Program, Bldg 22, 10903 New Hampshire Avenue, Silver Spring, MD USA 20993
University of Florida, College of Pharmacy, Pharmaceutical Outcomes & Policy, 101 S. Newell Drive (HPNP), PO Box 100496, Gainesville FL, USA 32611

Salvatore R Pepe
Department of Health and Human Services/Food and Drug Administration/ Center for Drug Evaluation and Research (CDER)/Office of Management/ CDER Academic Collaboration Program, Bldg 22, 10903 New HampshireAvenue, Silver Spring, MD USA 20993
University of Florida, College of Pharmacy, Pharmaceutical Outcomes & Policy, 101 S. Newell Drive (HPNP), PO Box 100496, Gainesville FL, USA 32611

Mahyar Etminan
University of British Columbia, Pharmaceutical Outcomes Programme, 709-828 West 10th Avenue, Vancouver, British Columbia, Canada V5Z1M9

Xinyue Liu
University of Florida, College of Pharmacy, Pharmaceutical Outcomes & Policy, 101 S. Newell Drive (HPNP), PO Box 100496, Gainesville FL, USA 32611

James M Brophy
McGill University, Royal Victoria Hospital, 687 Pine Street West, Montreal, Quebec H3A 1A1, Canada

Joseph AC Delaney
University of Florida, College of Pharmacy, Pharmaceutical Outcomes & Policy, 101 S. Newell Drive (HPNP),PO Box 100496, Gainesville FL, USA 32611

Joyce H You
School of Pharmacy, The Chinese University of Hong Kong, Shatin, N.T., Hong Kong

Fiona Y Wong
School of Public Health and Primary Care, The Chinese University of Hong Kong, Prince of Wales Hospital, Shatin, N.T., Hong Kong

Frank W Chan
School of Public Health and Primary Care, The Chinese University of Hong Kong, Prince of Wales Hospital, Shatin, N.T., Hong Kong

Eliza L Wong
School of Public Health and Primary Care, The Chinese University of Hong Kong, Prince of Wales Hospital, Shatin, N.T., Hong Kong

Eng-kiong Yeoh
School of Public Health and Primary Care, The Chinese University of Hong Kong, Prince of Wales Hospital, Shatin, N.T., Hong Kong

Roderick Clark
Department of Community Health and Epidemiology, Dalhousie University, Halifax, NS, Canada

Judith E Fisher
College of Pharmacy, Faculty of Health Professions, Dalhousie University, Halifax, NS, Canada
Pharmaceutical Services, Department of Health and Wellness, Halifax, NS, Canada

Ingrid S Sketris
College of Pharmacy, Faculty of Health Professions, Dalhousie University, Halifax, NS, Canada

Grace M Johnston
School of Health Administration, Faculty of Health Professions Dalhousie University, Halifax, NS, Canada

Santosh KC
Faculty of Pharmacy, Mahidol University, Bangkok, Thailand
Bir Hospital, Kathmandu, Nepal

Pramote Tragulpiankit
Faculty of Pharmacy, Mahidol University, Bangkok, Thailand

Sarun Gorsanan
Faculty of Pharmacy, Siam University, Bangkok, Thailand

I Ralph Edwards
Uppsala Monitoring Centre, Uppsala, Sweden

Manu Shankar-Hari
Division of Asthma, Allergy and Lung Biology, King's College London, London, UK
Critical Care and Anesthesia Research Group, King's Health Partners Academic Health Sciences Centre, London, UK
Department of Critical Care Medicine, Guy's and St Thomas' NHS Foundation Trust, London, UK

Peter S Kruger
Princess Alexandra Hospital, Wooloongabba, Brisbane, Australia
University of Queensland, Brisbane, Australia

Stefania Di Gangi
Division of Asthma, Allergy and Lung Biology, King's College London, London, UK
Department of Critical Care Medicine, Guy's and St Thomas' NHS Foundation Trust, London, UK

Damon C Scales
Interdepartmental Division of Critical Care, University of Toronto, Toronto, Canada
Department of Critical Care Medicine, Sunnybrook Health Sciences Centre, Toronto, Canada

Gavin D Perkins
Warwick Clinical Trials Unit, Warwick Medical, University of Warwick School, Warwick, UK

Danny F McAuley
Centre for Infection and Immunity, The Queen's University of Belfast, Belfast, UK

Marius Terblanche
Division of Asthma, Allergy and Lung Biology, King's College London, London, UK
Critical Care and Anesthesia Research Group, King's Health Partners Academic Health Sciences Centre, London, UK
Department of Critical Care Medicine, Guy's and St Thomas' NHS Foundation Trust, London, UK

Márcia Germana Alves de Araújo Lobo
Hospital Geral de Palmas, Av NS1, s/n Conj. 02 - Lote 01, Palmas 77.054-970, Brasil

Sandra Maria Botelho Pinheiro
Curso de Medicina, Universidade Federal do Tocantins, Av. NS 15 s/n (109 Norte), Palmas 77001-090, Brasil

José Gerley Díaz Castro
Curso de Enfermagem, Universidade Federal do Tocantins, Av. NS 15 s/n (109 Norte), Palmas 77001-090, Brasil

Valéria Gomes Momenté
Curso de Engenharia de Alimentos, Universidade Federal do Tocantins, Av. NS 15 s/n (109 Norte), Palmas 77001-090, Brasil

Maria-Cristina S Pranchevicius
Curso de Medicina, Universidade Federal do Tocantins, Av. NS 15 s/n (109 Norte), Palmas 77001-090, Brasil

Reeta Heikkilä
University of Eastern Finland, Faculty of Health Sciences, School of Pharmacy, Social Pharmacy, P.O.Box 1627, FI-70211 Kuopio, Finland

Pekka Mäntyselkä
University of Eastern Finland, Faculty of Health Sciences, School of Medicine, Department of Primary Health Care, P.O.Box 1627, FI-70211 Kuopio, Finland
Kuopio University Hospital, Unit of Primary Health Care, P.O.Box 1777, FI-70211 Kuopio, Finland

Riitta Ahonen
University of Eastern Finland, Faculty of Health Sciences, School of Pharmacy, Social Pharmacy, P.O.Box 1627, FI-70211 Kuopio, Finland

Annika Nordén-Hägg
Department of Pharmacy, Uppsala University, Box 570, Uppsala S-751 23, Sweden

Sofia Kälvemark-Sporrong
Department of Pharmacy, Uppsala University, Box 570, Uppsala S-751 23, Sweden

Åsa Kettis Lindblad
Department of Pharmacy, Uppsala University, Box 570, Uppsala S-751 23, Sweden

Vivienne J Zhu
Regenstrief Institute, Inc, IndianapolisIndiana, USA
Indiana University School of Medicine, Indianapolis, IN, USA. 3Siemens Healthcare, Malvern, PA, USA

Anne Belsito
Regenstrief Institute, Inc, IndianapolisIndiana, USA

Wanzhu Tu
Regenstrief Institute, Inc, IndianapolisIndiana, USA
Indiana University School of Medicine, Indianapolis, IN, USA

J Marc Overhage
Indiana University School of Medicine, Indianapolis, IN, USA
Siemens Healthcare, Malvern, PA, USA

Rafael Bonfante-Cabarcas
Biochemistry Research Units, Health Sciences School, Universidad Centro Occidental Lisandro Alvarado, Barquisimeto, Lara, Venezuela
Libertador Av. con Andrés Bello, Unidad de Bioquímica, Decanato de Ciencias de la Salud, Universidad Centro-Occidental "Lisandro Alvarado", Barquisimeto, Estado Lara Código Postal: 3001, Venezuela

Erlymar López Hincapié
Biochemistry Research Units, Health Sciences School, Universidad Centro Occidental Lisandro Alvarado, Barquisimeto, Lara, Venezuela
Libertador Av. con Andrés Bello, Unidad de Bioquímica, Decanato de Ciencias de la Salud, Universidad Centro-Occidental "Lisandro Alvarado", Barquisimeto, Estado Lara Código Postal: 3001, Venezuela

Eliezer Jiménez Hernández
Biochemistry Research Units, Health Sciences School, Universidad Centro Occidental Lisandro Alvarado, Barquisimeto, Lara, Venezuela
Libertador Av. con Andrés Bello, Unidad de Bioquímica, Decanato de Ciencias de la Salud, Universidad Centro-Occidental "Lisandro Alvarado", Barquisimeto, Estado Lara Código Postal: 3001, Venezuela

Ruth Fonseca Zambrano
Biochemistry Research Units, Health Sciences School, Universidad Centro Occidental Lisandro Alvarado, Barquisimeto, Lara, Venezuela
Libertador Av. con Andrés Bello, Unidad de Bioquímica, Decanato de Ciencias de la Salud, Universidad Centro-Occidental "Lisandro Alvarado", Barquisimeto, Estado Lara Código Postal: 3001, Venezuela

Lady Ferrer Mancini
Biochemistry Research Units, Health Sciences School, Universidad Centro Occidental Lisandro Alvarado, Barquisimeto, Lara, Venezuela
Libertador Av. con Andrés Bello, Unidad de Bioquímica, Decanato de Ciencias de la Salud, Universidad Centro-Occidental "Lisandro Alvarado", Barquisimeto, Estado Lara Código Postal: 3001, Venezuela

Marcos Durand Mena
Biochemistry Research Units, Health Sciences School, Universidad Centro Occidental Lisandro Alvarado, Barquisimeto, Lara, Venezuela
Libertador Av. con Andrés Bello, Unidad de Bioquímica, Decanato de Ciencias de la Salud, Universidad Centro-Occidental "Lisandro Alvarado", Barquisimeto, Estado Lara Código Postal: 3001, Venezuela

Claudina Rodríguez-Bonfante
Medical Parasitology Research Units, Health Sciences School, Universidad Centro Occidental Lisandro Alvarado, Barquisimeto, Lara, Venezuela
Libertador Av. con Andrés Bello, Unidad de Bioquímica, Decanato de Ciencias de la Salud, Universidad Centro-Occidental "Lisandro Alvarado", Barquisimeto, Estado Lara Código Postal: 3001, Venezuela

Niels Bindslev
Synagics Lab, Endocrinology Section, Department of Biomedical Sciences, The Medical Faculty, Panum Building, University of Copenhagen, Blegdamsvej 3, DK-2200, Copenhagen N, Denmark

Yoshinori Inagaki
Laboratory of Microbiology, Graduate School of Pharmaceutical Sciences, The University of Tokyo, 7-3-1 Hongo, Bunkyo-ku, Tokyo 113-0033, Japan

Yasuhiko Matsumoto
Laboratory of Microbiology, Graduate School of Pharmaceutical Sciences, The University of Tokyo, 7-3-1 Hongo, Bunkyo-ku, Tokyo 113-0033, Japan

Keiko Kataoka
Genome Pharmaceuticals Institute Co., Ltd., The University of Tokyo Entrepreneur Plaza, 7-3-1 Hongo, Bunkyo-ku, Tokyo 113-0033, Japan

Naoya Matsuhashi
Genome Pharmaceuticals Institute Co., Ltd., The University of Tokyo Entrepreneur Plaza, 7-3-1 Hongo, Bunkyo-ku, Tokyo 113-0033, Japan

Kazuhisa Sekimizu
Laboratory of Microbiology, Graduate School of Pharmaceutical Sciences, The University of Tokyo, 7-3-1 Hongo, Bunkyo-ku, Tokyo 113-0033, Japan
Genome Pharmaceuticals Institute Co., Ltd., The University of Tokyo Entrepreneur Plaza, 7-3-1 Hongo, Bunkyo-ku, Tokyo 113-0033, Japan

Lina M Hellström
eHealth Institute and School of Natural Sciences, Linnaeus University, Kalmar, Sweden

Åsa Bondesson
Department of Medicines Management and Informatics, Skåne Regional council, Malmö, Sweden

Peter Höglund
Department of Clinical Pharmacology, Lund University, Lund, Sweden

Tommy Eriksson
Department of Clinical Pharmacology, Lund University, Lund, Sweden

Carolien GM Sino
University of Applied Sciences Utrecht, Research Centre for Innovation in Healthcare, Bolognalaan 101, 3584 Utrecht, CJ, The Netherlands

Rutger Stuffken
Department of Pharmacoepidemiology and Clinical Pharmacology, Utrecht University, Faculty of Science, Utrecht, The Netherlands
Department of Clinical Pharmacy, Tergooi Hospitals, Blaricum/Hilversum, The Netherlands

Eibert R Heerdink
Department of Pharmacoepidemiology and Clinical Pharmacology, Utrecht University, Faculty of Science, Utrecht, The Netherlands

Marieke J Schuurmans
University of Applied Sciences Utrecht, Research Centre for Innovation in Healthcare, Bolognalaan 101, 3584 Utrecht, CJ, The Netherlands
Department of Rehabilitation, University Medical Centre Utrecht, Nursing Science and Sports, Utrecht, The Netherlands

Patrick C Souverein
Department of Pharmacoepidemiology and Clinical Pharmacology, Utrecht University, Faculty of Science, Utrecht, The Netherlands

Toine (A) CG Egberts
Department of Pharmacoepidemiology and Clinical Pharmacology, Utrecht University, Faculty of Science, Utrecht, The Netherlands
Department of Clinical Pharmacy, University Medical Centre Utrecht, Utrecht, The Netherlands

Adriana Isvoran
Department of Biology and Chemistry, West University of Timisoara, 16 Pestalozzi, Timisoara 300115, Romania
Advanced Environmental Researches Laboratory, 4 Oituz, Timisoara 300086, Romania

Dana Craciun
Teacher Training Department, West University of Timisoara, 4 Blvd. V. ParvanTimisoara 300223, Romania

Virginie Martiny
Université Paris Diderot, Sorbonne Paris Cité, Molécule Thérapeutiques in silico, Inserm UMR-S 973, 35 rue Helene Brion, Paris 75013, France
INSERM, U973, Paris F-75205, France

Olivier Sperandio
Université Paris Diderot, Sorbonne Paris Cité, Molécule Thérapeutiques in silico, Inserm UMR-S 973, 35 rue Helene Brion, Paris 75013, France
INSERM, U973, Paris F-75205, France

Maria A Miteva
Université Paris Diderot, Sorbonne Paris Cité, Molécule Thérapeutiques in silico, Inserm UMR-S 973, 35 rue Helene Brion, Paris 75013, France
INSERM, U973, Paris F-75205, France

Urs E Gasser
ClinResearch Ltd, Aesch, Switzerland

Anton Fischer
F. Hoffmann-La Roche Ltd, Basel, Switzerland

P Timmermans
F. Hoffmann-La Roche Ltd, Basel, Switzerland

Isabelle Arnet
Pharmaceutical Care Research Group, Department of Pharmaceutical Sciences, University of Basel, Klingelbergstr. 50, 4056, Basel, Switzerland

Mohiuddin Hussain Khan
Drug Management & Policy, Kanazawa University, Kakuma-machi, Kanazawa, Ishikawa 920-1192, Japan
Médecins Sans Frontières, 14 Sayat-Nova street, Vanadzor, Lori, Armenia

Kirara Hatanaka
Drug Management & Policy, Kanazawa University, Kakuma-machi, Kanazawa, Ishikawa 920-1192, Japan
Department of Pharmacy, Saiseikai-Nakatu Hospital, Shibata, Osaka 530-0012, Japan

Tey Sovannarith
National Health Product Quality Control Center, Ministry of Health, Phnom Penh, Cambodia

Nam Nivanna
National Health Product Quality Control Center, Ministry of Health, Phnom Penh, Cambodia

Cecilia Cadena Casas
Drug Management & Policy, Kanazawa University, Kakuma-machi, Kanazawa, Ishikawa 920-1192, Japan
Becton Dickinson de México, S.A.de C.V. Km 37.5 – Aut. México-Qro. Parque Industrial Cuamatla, Cuautitlán Izcalli., Edo. De México, CP 54730, México

Naoko Yoshida
Drug Management & Policy, Kanazawa University, Kakuma-machi, Kanazawa, Ishikawa 920-1192, Japan

Hirohito Tsuboi
Drug Management & Policy, Kanazawa University, Kakuma-machi, Kanazawa, Ishikawa 920-1192, Japan

Tsuyoshi Tanimoto
Department of Analytical Sciences, Faculty of Pharmaceutical Sciences, Doshisha Women's College, Kyoto, Japan

Kazuko Kimura
Drug Management & Policy, Kanazawa University, Kakuma-machi, Kanazawa, Ishikawa 920-1192, Japan

Yumei Fan
The Key Lab of Animal Physiology, College of Life Science, Hebei Normal University, Hebei Province, Shijiazhuang 050024, China

Caizhi Liu
The Key Lab of Animal Physiology, College of Life Science, Hebei Normal University, Hebei Province, Shijiazhuang 050024, China

Yongmao Huang
Laboratory of Medical Biotechnology, Hebei Chemical and Pharmaceutical College, Hebei Province, Shijiazhuang 050026, China

Jie Zhang
The Key Lab of Animal Physiology, College of Life Science, Hebei Normal University, Hebei Province, Shijiazhuang 050024, China

Linlin Cai
The Key Lab of Animal Physiology, College of Life Science, Hebei Normal University, Hebei Province, Shijiazhuang 050024, China

Shengnan Wang
The Key Lab of Animal Physiology, College of Life Science, Hebei Normal University, Hebei Province, Shijiazhuang 050024, China

Yongze Zhang
The Key Lab of Animal Physiology, College of Life Science, Hebei Normal University, Hebei Province, Shijiazhuang 050024, China

Xianglin Duan
The Key Lab of Animal Physiology, College of Life Science, Hebei Normal University, Hebei Province, Shijiazhuang 050024, China

Zhimin Yin
Jiangsu Province Key Laboratory of Molecular and Medical Biotechnology, College of Life Science, Nanjing Normal University, Nanjing 210046, China

Solomon Yu
Aged and Extended Care Services, Level 8B Main Building, The Queen Elizabeth Hospital, Central Adelaide Local Health Network, 21 Woodville Road, 5011 Woodville South, SA, Australia
Adelaide Geriatrics Training and Research with Aged Care (G-TRAC) Center, School of Medicine, University of Adelaide, South Australia, Australia
Discipline of Medicine, School of Medicine, Faculty of Health Science, University of Adelaide, Adelaide, SA, Australia
The Health Observatory, Discipline of Medicine, School of Medicine, Faculty of Health Science, University of Adelaide, Adelaide, South Australia, Australia

Thavarajah Visvanathan
Department of Anaesthesia, The Queen Elizabeth Hospital, Central Adelaide Local Health Network, South Australia, Australia

John Field
Discipline of Medicine, School of Medicine, Faculty of Health Science, University of Adelaide, Adelaide, SA, Australia

Leigh C Ward
School of Chemistry and Molecular Biosciences, The University of Queensland, Brisbane, QLD, Australia

Ian Chapman
Discipline of Medicine, School of Medicine, Faculty of Health Science, University of Adelaide, Adelaide, SA, Australia

Robert Adams
The Health Observatory, Discipline of Medicine, School of Medicine, Faculty of Health Science, University of Adelaide, Adelaide, South Australia, Australia

Gary Wittert
Discipline of Medicine, School of Medicine, Faculty of Health Science, University of Adelaide, Adelaide, SA, Australia

Visvanathan
Aged and Extended Care Services, Level 8B Main Building, The Queen Elizabeth Hospital, Central Adelaide Local Health Network, 21 Woodville Road, 5011 Woodville South, SA, Australia.
Adelaide Geriatrics Training and Research with Aged Care (G-TRAC) Center, School of Medicine, University of Adelaide, South Australia, Australia
Discipline of Medicine, School of Medicine, Faculty of Health Science, University of Adelaide, Adelaide, SA, Australia
The Health Observatory, Discipline of Medicine, School of Medicine, Faculty of Health Science, University of Adelaide, Adelaide, South Australia, Australia

Megan Morse
Department of Pharmacology, Pennsylvania State University College of Medicine, Hershey, PA, USA

Haiyan Sun
Biochemical Technologies, Science and Technology Division, Corning Inc., Corning, NY, USA

Elizabeth Tran
Biochemical Technologies, Science and Technology Division, Corning Inc., Corning, NY, USA

Robert Levenson
Department of Pharmacology, Pennsylvania State University College of Medicine, Hershey, PA, USA

Ye Fang
Biochemical Technologies, Science and Technology Division, Corning Inc., Corning, NY, USA

Andrew Walubo
Department of Pharmacology, University of the Free State, P. O. Box 339 (G6), Bloemfontein 9300, South Africa

Jérôme Breton
Bactéries Lactiques & Immunité des Muqueuses, Centre d'Infection et d'Immunité de Lille, Institut Pasteur de Lille, U1019, UMR 8204, Université Lille Nord de France, 1 rue du Pr Calmette, Lille cedex BP 245, F-59019, France

Sébastien Massart
DNAVision SA, avenue George Lemaitre 25, Charleroi B-6041, Belgium

Peter Vandamme
Laboratory of Microbiology, Faculty of Sciences, Ledeganckstraat 35, Ghent B-9000, Belgium

Evie De Brandt
Laboratory of Microbiology, Faculty of Sciences, Ledeganckstraat 35, Ghent B-9000, Belgium

Bruno Pot
Bactéries Lactiques & Immunité des Muqueuses, Centre d'Infection et d'Immunité de Lille, Institut Pasteur de Lille, U1019, UMR 8204, Université Lille Nord de France, 1 rue du Pr Calmette, Lille cedex BP 245, F-59019, France

Benoît Foligné
Bactéries Lactiques & Immunité des Muqueuses, Centre d'Infection et d'Immunité de Lille, Institut Pasteur de Lille, U1019, UMR 8204, Université Lille Nord de France, 1 rue du Pr Calmette, Lille cedex BP 245, F-59019, France

www.ingramcontent.com/pod-product-compliance
Lightning Source LLC
Chambersburg PA
CBHW080254230326
41458CB00097B/4448